MW00837556

EDUCATIONAL AUDIOLOGY
FOR THE
LIMITED-HEARING
INFANT AND PRESCHOOLER

Third Edition

EDUCATIONAL AUDIOLOGY FOR THE LIMITED-HEARING INFANT AND PRESCHOOLER

An Auditory-Verbal Program

By

DOREEN POLLACK, CCC SPL-A.

*Emeritus Director, Auditory Verbal International
and formerly Director, Speech and Hearing Services
Porter Memorial Hospital
Denver, Colorado*

DONALD GOLDBERG, PH.D., CCC SPL-A, Cert. AVT

*Director, Beebe Speech and Hearing Center
Easton, Pennsylvania*

NANCY CALEFFE-SCHENCK, M.ED., CCC-A, Cert. AVT

*Coordinator, Children's Comprehensive Program
Denver Ear Institute
Englewood, Colorado*

With a Foreword by

Erik Wedenberg, M.D.
Stockholm, Sweden

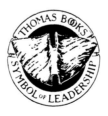

CHARLES C THOMAS · PUBLISHER, LTD.
Springfield · Illinois · U.S.A.

Published and Distributed Throughout the World by

CHARLES C THOMAS • PUBLISHER, LTD.
2600 South First Street
Springfield, Illinois 62794-9265

© *1997 by* CHARLES C THOMAS • PUBLISHER, LTD.
ISBN 0-398-06750-3 (cloth)
ISBN 0-398-06751-1 (paper)
Library of Congress Catalog Card Number: 96-49202

First Edition, 1970
Second Edition, 1985

With THOMAS BOOKS *careful attention is given to all details of manufacturing and design. It is the Publisher's desire to present books that are satisfactory as to their physical qualities and artistic possibilities and appropriate for their particular use.* THOMAS BOOKS *will be true to those laws of quality that assure a good name and good will.*

Printed in the United States of America
SC-R-3

Library of Congress Cataloging-in-Publication Data

Pollack, Doreen.
    Educational audiology for the limited-hearing infant and
preschooler : an auditory—verbal program / by Doreen Pollack, Donald
Goldberg, Nancy Caleffe-Schenck ; with a foreword by Erik Wedenberg.
—3rd ed.
        p.   cm.
    Includes bibliographical references and index.
    ISBN 0-398-06750-3 (cloth). — ISBN 0-398-06751-1 (paper)
    1. Children, Deaf—Rehabilitation.   I. Goldberg, Donald Michael.
II. Caleffe-Schenck, Nancy.   III. Title.
    [DNLM: 1. Hearing Disorders—in infancy & childhood.   2. Hearing
Disorders—rehabilitation.   WV 271 P771e 1997]
RF291.5.C45P65   1997
618.92'0978—dc21
DNLM/DLC
for Library of Congress   96-49202
                                                                                                          CIP

FOREWORD

It is a great pleasure for me to write a foreword to a book for limited hearing infants, because I have a deaf son and have made every effort to give him the best possible training and start in life. The problems for parents of deaf children are certainly the same all over the world.

At first, the news that a child is deaf comes as a stunning blow. My wife and I were dentists in 1939 when our son was diagnosed as probably totally deaf. We wondered if there was a tiny remnant of hearing left, and if it might be possible to train this remnant. I thought one might speak into the ear without giving the child any chance of lipreading, and diminish the visual impression in order that the auditory stimuli might exercise a first claim upon consciousness. I did not give the method any name. Today, it is called the *Uni-Sensory Approach.*

We began the training by crawling on the floor and saying vowels. That was fun for a two-year-old! An important principle in all training for infants is that it should be fun. It is also very important that the hearing defect is discovered as early as possible, and that the mother is given the opportunity to learn as much as she needs in order to succeed. The most important work takes place in the home, and I have found that it is the mother's efforts which will decide whether the work will succeed or not.

My wife gave up her profession and devoted all her time to our son. And it took time. It took one year to teach this very gifted three-year-old child twenty-five words. Parents should therefore not despair if progress is very slow in the beginning. I remember a friend's words to me in a dark moment: "Parents of many deaf children will gratefully see how many joys the Creator has hidden in this trial when he made it possible for man, through these trials, to get a tiny glimpse of creative work." All of the parents will feel what we experienced when we made communication with our son—a joy, which I can only describe as a ceasing of the sorrow we had felt for a long time.

Later on, I worked with other pupils who came from various countries. They are grown up now, and the oldest is thirty years old. Just as Mrs.

Pollack advocates, I worked only with auditory training and never taught lipreading. In spite of this, my pupils became the best lipreaders because they acquired through the intensive auditory training a much larger vocabulary than normal.

Fortunately, there has been a great change in the attitude of the community. As late as 1936, pupils in large schools for the deaf went around like prisoners in striped clothes. In 1951, preschools started throughout our country. In 1953, the name *deaf-mute* was changed to *deaf.* Now we say, "He has a hearing defect."

During recent years, integration in preschools has started, which is growing into real integration in all schools. This way, children with normal hearing begin at a very early age to understand that there are others who are like themselves in every way except for the hearing defect. This deep understanding between children will help the deaf become truly part of the community.

Mrs. Pollack's book is needed by students and teachers who, for the first time, have the opportunity to guide the development of very young children. Her teaching reflects the ideas of the old Greek philosophers in 400 B.C., that "the eye is the mirror of the soul but the ear is the gate of the soul."

ERIC WEDENBERG

INTRODUCTION

The history of education for the hearing-impaired child spans centuries. It is the story of many dedicated people in different parts of the world, working empirically to meet the needs of a group usually called "the deaf" within a framework of the knowledge and equipment available to them.

In all educational fields today dramatic changes are taking place, and educators are reevaluating time-honored concepts. In the field of audiology, two important new facts have emerged as a result of technological progress and audiological research in the last two decades: *first,* that less than 5 percent of so-called deaf children are totally deaf, and *second,* that even a profoundly deaf child can wear hearing aids and develop hearing perceptions.

As soon as audiologists were able to test reliably the hearing of a child within the first three years of his life, and initiate training during the period of life normally critical for speech and language development, *the need arose for a new approach to management of hearing impaired infants.* This book describes the thinking and experiences of those who have been using new techniques to keep pace with the tremendous advances made in audiological instrumentation and in psycholinguistic and communications research.

In the United States, a program was begun in 1948 at Columbia Presbyterian Medical Center, New York City, under the direction of the late Dr. E. Prince Fowler, Jr., to determine how early congenital hearing impairment could be tested, how soon hearing aids could be fitted upon infants, how hearing aids could be selected, and how infants should be trained to use them. The author was part of a small group[1] who developed an experimental approach. She found that babies could be given a screening test soon after birth and successfully fitted with

---

[1]The group in New York City consisted of Mrs. Lorraine Amos Roblee, Supervisor; Dr. Jon Eisenson, Consultant; Mrs. Doreen Pollack and Miss Sylvia Morgan, paedoaudiologists.

hearing aids, provided that the parents received adequate instruction and support.

At first it was assumed that hard-of-hearing children who wore aids from an early age would develop hearing perceptions normally, while those who were profoundly deaf would still learn through lipreading. Both assumptions proved to be erroneous.

When formal lipreading training was given, even the hard-of-hearing children continued to recognize speech primarily by lipreading. No usable recognition of words by auditory cues was learned spontaneously. The selection of a hearing aid then posed a problem. In order to measure the benefit derived from the use of a specific aid, children had to be able to respond to sounds without visual clues. Subsequently all formal training was structured to teach attention to sound and response to sound. The results were far beyond those predicted, and showed us that the profoundly deaf child did not have to be dependent upon lipreading at all times.

In 1949 to 1950, the program aroused the interest of Dr. Huizing, who had come to New York to engage in research. He returned to Holland and directed an experimental program in his own country. The author moved to Denver and started a preschool program sponsored by Dr. Richard Winchester of the University of Denver, and The Denver Hearing Society. In 1954, Mrs. Marion Downs became the University Hearing Services Director and later suggested the use of Dr. Huizing's new term, *acoupedics.* [2]

In London, during the same period of time, Dr. Whetnall was developing her "auditory approach," which was advocated by Dr. Ciwa Griffiths in California under the name "H.E.A.R. Foundation." At the same time, Dr. Froeschels and Mrs. Beebe in New York, and Dr. Wedenberg in Sweden were using a "uni-sensory approach."

Subsequently, Dr. Guy Perdoncini in France and Dr. Tsunoda in Japan described uni-sensory auditory training programs, and similar methods were being used in other parts of the world.

It was again much like the story of the Salk vaccine, as Dr. Jonas Salk described it: a ball bouncing around from group to group, and he was fortunate enough to be in the right place at the right time to catch it.

---

[2]In Denver, Mrs. Kathleen Bryant, Mrs. Marion Downs, Mrs. Marion Ernst, Miss Elaine Freeland, Mrs. Alice Melville, Mrs. Pollack, Mrs. Bunny Rubin, and Dr. Joseph Stewart (who directed a five-year research grant at the University of Denver) used an acoupedic approach.

"The past is prologue"—many people's ideas have been absorbed into educational audiology in order to help the hearing-impaired child succeed in a hearing world. Some readers may respond enthusiastically to these ideas, while others may reject them completely. It has been said that the greatest tyrants over men's minds are their own unexamined ideas. This book will have been worthwhile only if a large number of audiologists and teachers look at the training of hearing-impaired youngsters from a different viewpoint, and seek a better way of teaching communication.

DOREEN POLLACK

NOTES AND ACKNOWLEDGEMENTS
FOR THE THIRD EDITION

When the publisher asked me to update the Second Edition of *Educational Audiology*, I hoped to report on major advances in the field of education for limited-hearing infants and preschoolers. There have been changes, but primarily in audiology, as, for example, acceptance of universal newborn screening, new instrumentation for assessment, and improved amplification technology. Most exciting was the development of the 22-channel cochlear implant which brought more auditory information to the profoundly-deaf child. Another development was the formation of Auditory Verbal International (which now has more than one thousand members worldwide) and the initiation of a certification examination for auditory-verbal therapists.

In the educational field, there is little change to report. Educators continued to focus on "Total Communication," that is, sign language and interpreters. Many members of the Deaf community said TC did not work and they advocated returning to American Sign Language and special schools.

Therefore, I have retained the historical references which led me to develop Acoupedics. The therapy has not changed because it was successful in producing children who could speak for themselves.

I am deeply grateful to the graduates who shared their lives with the readers. I wish to thank Donald Goldberg and Nancy Caleffe-Schenck for their substantive contributions to this edition, and Pat Greene of LISTEN, Inc., who gave permission to publish her beautiful poetry. And last, but not least, thanks to my typists, Bonnie Barlow and Cindy Rusch.

Two explanatory notes in response to readers of the second edition: the term "educational audiology" was coined from the term "audiological education" used by Dr. Huizing. Some years later, this term was adopted by educators who had introduced audiology services into the schools.

Secondly, it was my call to refer to clinicians as "she" and the child as "he" in order to make the narrative read more smoothly, instead of so many his/her's, he/she's and so on. In many instances, however, I have changed "mother" to "parent" in deference to the number of dads who now participate actively in the therapy program.

D. P.

ACKNOWLEDGMENTS FOR
THE SECOND EDITION

I wish to express my appreciation to the administration of Porter Hospital and the LISTEN Foundation for giving me the opportunity to develop these ideas, and to my professional colleagues whose commitment resulted in an inspiring program. Since the publication of the First Edition, more than two hundred families have been enrolled in the Acoupedic Program.

The unexpected rewards of publishing have been the letters from readers, describing the impact upon their children's lives, and the response of other professionals in the field. Requests for workshops and lectures have been received from all over the United States, Canada and Mexico. All of these shared experiences helped to reaffirm and expand the basic principles of Acoupedics.

For this new edition, my heartfelt thanks go to Cherie Neerhof, my typist, who deciphered the manuscript, and to my husband, who was responsible for the charts and for building a "writing room."

D.P.

ACKNOWLEDGMENTS FOR
THE FIRST EDITION

This is a wonderful opportunity to thank all the people who have made this book possible, beginning with our nephew, Jan, whose hearing loss started my involvement with hearing-impaired infants, and ending with my typist, Trudy Vander Veen, and illustrators, Mr. William Sanderson of the University of Denver, and Mr. Ray Nelson of Porter Hospital. To single out each individual would be impossible, for the list includes all my teachers and professional colleagues; all the parents who brought their delightful infants to me; and, most surely, my own three children who taught me a mother's role and shared me "with all my other children," as they used to describe them.

D.P.

The Gift of Language

Language.
a gift
received,
expressed.
the gift of spoken language
often
taken for granted,
unless
it is absent
then
the gift must emerge
through
the efforts of people
working together
cooperatively
with great skill,
nurturing,
repeating,
waiting,
accepting
small efforts to speak,
until
the gift in measured growth
bursts forth
and another child
speaks for herself, himself,
in gift.

PAT GREENE

CONTENTS

EDUCATIONAL AUDIOLOGY
FOR THE
LIMITED–HEARING
INFANT AND PRESCHOOLER

Chapter 1

HISTORICAL REVIEW OF THE CONCEPT OF AUDITORY TRAINING

Since "All Past Is Prologue" and most ideas evolve from previous concepts, it is important to review briefly the contributions of deaf education and audiology to an auditory approach for young children.[1]

Realization of the importance of utilizing residual hearing has a very long history, dating back to the first century when Archigenes used a hearing trumpet and intensified sound. Alexander did the same in the sixth century. Ernaud, in 1761, used analytic exercises, and Pereire said that total deafness did not exist. In 1802, Itard claimed that the deaf could be trained to hear words, and in 1860, Toynbee wrote that the great advantage of calling forth the auditory power of so-called deaf mutes is that they can be enabled to hear their own voices and to modulate them.

In the United States, the leading proponent of "acoustic exercises" was Dr. Max Goldstein who was inspired by Urbantschitsch of Vienna (translated by Silverman, 1982). He defined his Acoustic Method (1939) as the stimulation of the hearing mechanism and its associated sense organs by sound education. He said that the teacher must not allow the child's body to touch her, must not place her own hand on the child, and must either hold a piece of stiff paper between her mouth and the child's ear, or speak through a simple megaphone or a simplex hearing tube.

However, few children actually received auditory training and Dr. Goldstein's ideas were far ahead of his time, for the following reason: The term *deafness* was used to denote hearing losses ranging from moderate to total, and the condition which came to be associated with the word "deaf" was that one either heard or one did not hear. As late as 1962, Bernero wrote as follows: "A popular misconception is that students in a school for the deaf have no useful hearing."

The literature of deaf education is permeated with statements which emphasize that the severity of a hearing handicap is irreversible and a

---

[1]For a detailed history of deaf education, the student is advised to read Markides (1986).

hearing-impaired child must be trained to depend upon visual and kinesthetic cues because he can learn very little, if anything, through his hearing. The title of a widely known book epitomizes this philosophy: *They Grow in Silence* (Mindel and Vernon, 1971).

AN AUDIOMETRIC DEFINITION OF DEAFNESS

It was not until after 1940 that the use of audiometers, together with conditioning techniques, such as the peep show (Dix and Hallpike, 1947) and the psychogalvanometer (Hardy, 1966), gave specific information about the type and degree of a hearing loss. Audiograms demonstrated what the young child was unable to hear with his own ears, and made it possible to describe what was really meant by deafness. Dr. Clarence O'Connor (1954) defined it in the following manner:

> The Deaf, who make up about 4 percent of the hearing impaired children, are those who are unable to hear spoken language either with or without amplification, or who hear spoken language only imperfectly with amplification. They are the children whose impairment is greater than 60 db (A.S.A. standard).

For example, the child whose audiogram is given in Figure 1.1 would be described as having an average 82 decibel loss for the speech frequencies in the right ear with a more severe loss for the high frequencies than for the lower frequencies.

Since average conversation varies from a whisper at approximately 20 decibels to a loud sound at 80 decibels (A.S.A. standard) and the most comfortable listening level is 55 decibels to 65 decibels, this child is certainly deaf to conversation, although she is not totally deaf.

It was indeed logical to assume on the basis of such a severe loss that the child should be taught through the unimpaired sensory pathways, that is, visual and kinesthetic, which were assumed to be unimpaired.

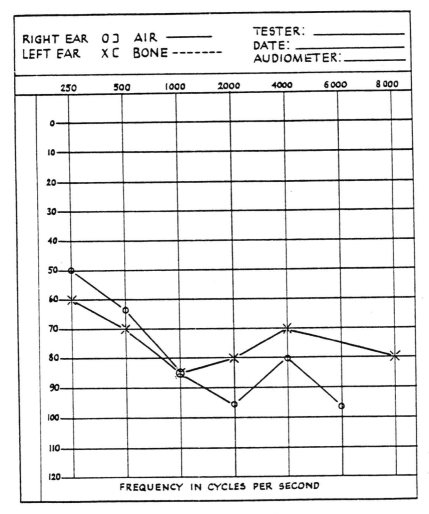

Figure 1.1. Audiogram of Valerie, tested by Mrs. Ewing in October, 1945, and found to be profoundly deaf. The parents were told that Valerie would have to learn to lipread, and they were informed about the education of deaf children. Courtesy of Ewing, I., and Ewing, A.: *New Opportunities for Deaf Children*. London, U. of London, 1961.

The Use of Audiometric Classification

In time these audiological data were used not only to describe the communication difficulties related to the hearing loss (see Table 1-I) but also for classification of education needs and methods to be used (see Table 1-II).

Although such a classification system gives useful descriptions of the untrained, unaided child, it may do serious injustice to many acoustically handicapped children because audiometric information can be misinterpreted. This is discussed fully in Chapter 2.

TABLE 1-I
RELATION OF AMOUNT OF HEARING LOSS
TO COMMUNICATIVE EFFICIENCY*

Amount of Hearing Loss (dB)	Effect
1. Less than 30	May have difficulty in hearing faint or distant speech; is likely to "get along" in school, and at work requiring listening.
2. 30 to 45 [41 to 55 I.S.O.]	Understands conversational speech at 3 to 5 feet without too much difficulty; may have difficulty if talker's voice is faint or if face is not visible.
3. 45 to 60 [56 to 70 I.S.O.]	Conversational speech must be loud to be understood; considerable difficulty in group and classroom discussion and perhaps in telephone conversation.
4. 60 to 80 [71 to 90 I.S.O.]	May hear voice about a foot away; may identify environmental noises and may distinguish vowels, but consonants are difficult to perceive.
5. More than 80 [90 I.S.O.]	May hear only loud sounds.

*From Silverman, S. R.: The education of children with hearing impairments, *J. Pediat.*, *62:*254–260, 1963.

TABLE 1-II
EDUCATIONAL NEEDS OF CHILDREN
WHO ARE HARD OF HEARING*

1. *Hearing loss less than 30 dB*
   Lip reading and favorable seating.

2. *30 to 45 dB loss* [41 to 55 I.S.O.]
   Lip reading, hearing aid (if suitable) and auditory training, speech correction and conservation, favorable seating.

3. *45 to 60 dB loss* [56 to 70 I.S.O.]
   Lip reading, hearing aid, and auditory training, special language work, favorable seating or special class.

4. *60 to 80 dB loss* [71 to 90 I.S.O.]
   Probably special educational procedures for deaf children with emphasis on speech, auditory training, and language with the possibility that the child may enter regular school.

5. *More than 80 dB loss* [90 I.S.O.]
   Special class or school for the deaf. Some of these children eventually enter regular high schools.

*From Silverman, S. R.: The education of children with hearing impairments, *J. Pediat.*, *62:*254–260, 1963.

THE DEVELOPMENT OF
A MULTISENSORY APPROACH

The second important technological development in the middle forties (1940s) was a small monopac hearing aid which could be worn by very young children. Subsequently, more time was allotted to auditory training in the special schools. Such an approach came to be known as the multi-sensory approach, or "look and listen." Kinesthetic stimuli were also given by placing the child's hand upon the teacher's face and neck. Reading was taught at an early age, utilizing the Fitzgerald Key (Pugh, 1955), a system of teaching which emphasizes the syntactical structure of language.

A case history representative of this approach has been given by the Ewings (1961):

> At two, Valerie could lipread 160 words. She went to a special school at three years, three months. Her mother used her aid constantly and had five requirements when presenting new words:
>
> 1. Listen to it and lipread it.
> 2. Understand it.
> 3. Read it.
> 4. Say it.
> 5. Incorporate it in conversation, and look for it being used by the child.

This approach is widely used today, and many children taught multisensorily have acquired excellent language skills. Some have been able to integrate with the normal-hearing in regular high schools, to attend college, and to enter professions such as geology, orthodontics, and so on (Star, 1980).

But, despite these years of work in special schools, the *majority* of these children do not approach the flow of conversation acquired by their normal-hearing peers, and a large number are scarcely intelligible to people outside their families. Their attitude toward themselves remains as follows: "I am a deaf person," and they associate mainly with other deaf people. During this time they do not use voice or much speech, but communicate by signs and finger spelling. This is equally as true of children educated in oral day schools as of those educated in the residential schools.

Levine (1956) related the story of Anna as representative of this group:

> To the hearing world Anna is different. She may even seem odd, backward, peculiar. Her voice and speech grate upon hearing ears. Her language has mechanical rigidity. She is uninformed or misinformed about many things of

common knowledge. She is unbelievably naive for her age. The hearing world stares at her with puzzled eyes. She shrinks back to the comfort of her own deaf society. She is at ease in hearing company only when it consists of her family group.

In reality, the *multisensory* approach has continued to emphasize visual skills, as pointed out by Oyer and O'Neill (1961):

> The combined use of visual and auditory modalities in aural rehabilitation seems to be an established, if not necessary approach.... A great deal of verbal emphasis is placed upon a combined approach, but in actual practice, major attention is directed toward the use of only one of the sensory modalities. *Auditory training is neglected, with the result that lipreading becomes the major therapeutic technique.* The existence of residual hearing is accepted but very little auditory training is provided. Such an approach is especially prominent in the majority of the public school programs. Auditory training, when it does occur, is confined to the audiology clinic. Even in this instance, it receives only moderate attention.... Aural rehabilitation work should be directed toward the use of this residual hearing and not toward the determination of how well the individual can do without it.

THE DEVELOPMENT OF AN AUDITORY APPROACH

The third important development in the 1940s was the emergence of a new professional group, the audiologists, who became responsible for diagnosis and habilitation of deaf preschoolers.

In 1947, Dr. Louis Di Carlo (1947), speaking in the United States, stated the following:

> The tendency to compensate through other sense avenues minimized the early importance of rehabilitation through hearing. Moreover, since the emphasis favored visual and tactical stimulation, language habits and abilities which develop most adequately through the ear, proceeded rather slowly. Research is beginning to reveal that hearing aids intelligently used offer a most promising outlook for speeding education and social growth of little children with impaired hearing.

European literature of the 1950s began to include increasing references to *hearing* rather than to *deafness*. In 1954, in England, Fry and Whetnall (1954) used the term "auditory training" and defined it as the means by which the cortical areas are given additional practice in the discrimination of sounds, both the background sounds of everyday life, and speech patterns.

> As far as possible we should try to reproduce the conditions in which the normal child learns to listen during the first years of life. There is no short cut

which will eliminate the need for repetition of sounds if the auditory areas in the cortex are to learn.

Doctors and clinicians revived Dr. Goldstein's idea that all other cues should be excluded during training sessions, so that the child's attention would be primarily upon sound.

Helen Beebe (1953), an American working with Dr. Emil Froeschels, wrote the following:

> Both in home training and in work done by the therapist, lip-reading should be avoided as much as possible. Otherwise the child may easily become dependent upon lip-reading and will not use his hearing. After it is assured that he will use his hearing to understand and to engage in conversation, he can be taught to lip-read, which he will need in school for example, where the speaker is too far away.

In Sweden, Wedenberg (1961) advocated beginning auditory training as early as possible, and described his listening exercises. They were given *ad concham*. One of his colleagues, Bengt Barr (1954), stressed that hearing is the "port of entry" for speech, and speech development is important to general development. He advocated a method built primarily upon the auditory sense, with the visual sense used as a complement. He reported great possibilities for correct interpretation of a speech message since less than one-half of what is spoken can be lipread, which gives no redundancy of information-bearing elements. He concluded that by *commencing* with the auditory senses as the first basis of learning, we can recreate the natural synergy between hearing and vision.

In 1958, a progressive international conference took place in England which indicated that audiologists and educators were beginning to communicate and share similar philosophies.

Among the papers given was one by a principal of a New York City School for the Deaf, Harriet McLaughlin (1960). She reported changing her program after visiting Dr. Whetnall in London. She began to work at Bellevue Medical Center, where no attempt was made to have the child watch the face of the teacher. Because they knew that these children were fixed visualizers, they tried to stress the auditory approach and to underplay the use of the other senses. They also limited the use of headphones as they believed that they adversely affect wearing and listening with an individual hearing aid.

At the same conference, the Reverend Father Van Uden of Holland (1960) described the object of their *Sound-Perceptive Method* to be to educate deaf children to live as far as possible in a world of sound, so that sound becomes their companion in life. They establish an integration of sound perception and bodily movement.

Beckman and Schilling of Germany (1959) advocated the avoidance of speech-reading development until after auditory orientation has been established. They emphasized the importance of retraining normal rhythmic patterns and inflections and the development of interpolative skills in listening and contextual speech.

Ethel Goldsack demonstrated to many members of the National College of Teachers of the Deaf that she had succeeded in developing speech perception and the capacity to talk well in a class of six-year-old children, all of them profoundly deaf, *by using hearing as a main factor.* Her methods included not less than one period of individual speech-hearing training of ten minutes duration for every pupil, every day. Rather rapid reading aloud of whole sentences with normal continuity of phrase pattern, normal intonation, and rhythm is an essential feature of this method.

The changes which had taken place between 1940 and 1960 were summed up by another British teacher of the deaf who wrote the following:

> We can admire the work of early oralists while being aware that in the learning of speech and language there is no substitute for hearing, and we must try to develop even the smallest remnants. *For many children today, lipreading is taking second place as a complement to an imperfect acoustic impression* (Richardson, 1962).

There was now a large body of literature in foreign journals on auditory training—too large to quote—and all indications were that this was considered to be the keystone in modern educational treatment of deaf children in other countries. Quigley (1966) gave many references.

Early in 1964, an eleven-member advisory committee was appointed by the government to study the educational opportunities for the deaf in the United States. In the summarization and recommendations made by the committee are the following statements:

> The American people have no reason to be satisfied with their limited success in educating deaf children and preparing them for full participation in our society.
>
> Less than half of the deaf children needing specialized preschool instruction are receiving it.
>
> The average graduate of a public residential school for the deaf—the closest we have to generally available "high school" for the deaf—has an eighth grade education.

Five-sixths of our deaf adults work in manual jobs, as contrasted to only one-half of our hearing population.

The infant should have a better chance of being identified in the early months of life and to be put in touch with better and more generally available clinical facilities. . . . Parents of deaf children need more readily available counsel, guidance and instruction. Programs designed to facilitate language and speech preparation for very young children, as well as *programs to make maximum use of residual hearing, should also be more generally available.* [2]

The results of such a critical report were as follows:

1. The United States Office of Education began to fund a large number of parent-infant and preschool programs. Most school boards elected to provide programs for the three to six year olds, with private agencies and/or the State Department of Public Health under the Handicapped Children's Fund, taking financial responsibility for the zero to three population. However, the state of Minnesota, whose special consultant was Dr. Winifred Northcott, legislated that every school district or unorganized territory could provide special instruction and services *from birth,* or as soon as the diagnosis of hearing loss had been established (Educational Guidelines, Minnesota Department of Education Amendment to M120.17, Subdivision 1, 1965).

    On the other hand, as late as 1975–1976, the state of Colorado reported that only forty-two preschoolers were being serviced, thirty-one of them in self-contained or residential units, with an estimated 562 preschoolers not being serviced by the public schools. The National Advisory Commission on the Handicapped estimated that 80 percent of 49,000 deaf children and 80 percent of 328,000 hard-of-hearing children were not being serviced nationally in 1976.

2. In 1975, the United States Congress passed the Education for All Handicapped Children Act of 1975 (Public Law 94-142). This law implies a tremendous change in the attitude toward handicapped persons. A free and appropriate public education was considered to be the right of children, ages three to eighteen, by September, 1980. When a state accepted federal funds, a full educational goal had to be set for ages zero to twenty-one. Local educational authorities were given the responsibility to develop an

---

[2]This study was sponsored by the U. S. Dept. of Health, Education and Welfare, and is frequently referred to as the Babbidge report (1964).

individualized educational program, the I.E.P., for each handicapped child served, which must involve the consent of the parents.

The law also required, to the maximum extent appropriate, that handicapped children be educated with children who are not handicapped, and they could receive supplementary aids and services.

Due Process procedures were built into the law, thus giving parents important rights such as independent educational evaluation (Nix, 1977).

These legislative enactments impacted positively the placement of handicapped children who traditionally had been educated in segregated environments throughout the nation. In order to ensure success and acceptance of the hearing-impaired child in the regular classroom and in the community at large, the law appeared to give support to oral education, since learning, socializing, and communicating with the normal-hearing is best accomplished through the use of residual hearing and speech (Froelinger, 1981).

Among subsequent laws which were written to cover all disabilities were the following:

1. ADA, Americans with Disabilities Act (1990). This prohibited discrimination on the basis of disability.
2. IDEA, the Individuals with Disabilities Education Act, Part B. This ensures a free, appropriate public education in the least restrictive environment, for children with disabilities, ages three to twenty-one years of age (1990).
3. IDEA, Part H. This assures services for infants and toddlers with disabilities ages 0 to three.

THE DEVELOPMENT OF TOTAL COMMUNICATION

The actual result of these laws has been a total swing of the pendulum back to manual communication in the public schools. Several factors combined in the United States to produce this result:

1. Oral education had not been generally successful in the majority of public school settings. Few university programs of special education prepared young teachers to teach speech effectively or to appreciate and use the potential of modern amplification or cochlear implants.
2. There were many audiologists who could measure residual hearing but did not know how to teach young children to use it, and

classroom teachers who knew very little about amplification or cochlear implants.

3. There was a significant dichotomy between the clinician, who could evaluate hearing, developmental and learning problems, and the teacher who was educated to teach subject matter to "deaf children."

4. The sociological climate of the country emphasized minority rights and among the rights demanded by the leaders of the deaf community were the use of manual communication and interpreters. The needs of deaf adults had indeed been neglected.

5. School districts rarely had either the financial resources or the trained personnel to implement an individualized program for every kind of problem. Financial assistance to schools was usually given on the basis of a grouping of six to eight handicapped students. Because deafness is a low incidence handicap, schools offered only one educational option or formed noncategorical classes.

At this critical time, spokesmen for the deaf community introduced the concept of Total Communication for all hearing-impaired children. This was defined as a combination of all forms of communication which had been used in deaf education: the language of signs and fingerspelling, lip or speech reading, speech, the use of residual hearing, reading and writing, and an arsenal of hardware and software were to be used simultaneously (Dicker, 1970). The emphasis was to be on the development of *language,* not speech.

The United States government began to give large grants to the universities and schools for Total Communication. Immediately, there was controversy about the type of manual communication to be used and many new systems were proposed because American Sign Language (ASL) could not be used simultaneously to represent spoken or written English. ASL is a language system with a different structure; that is, meaning is indicated by the place, movement, and direction of the sign rather than by the grammatical structure of spoken English.

Rather than preparing children for integration into the normal-hearing population, the concept of "reverse mainstreaming" was introduced. Normal-hearing children were to learn manual communication and all hearing-impaired were to learn manually and be accompanied by interpreters. Classes to teach sign language to the lay public were offered and every television station included a manual adult in its shows.

The option of manual communication was indeed needed in the cascade of services envisioned by P.L. 94-142, but most schools simplified their problems by offering the same program to all hearing-impaired children. Enormous pressure was, and is being placed upon parents to conform to one system.

Unfortunately, these major changes were made on the basis of the failure of traditional oral, that is, lipreading, programs and on the basis of very sparse and incomplete research on manual, rather than total communication, in spite of historical evidence that reliance upon interpreters and manual communication segregates the deaf and limits their full participation in a community (Nix, 1972).

The concept that a small child who knows nothing of speech and language can learn simultaneously through many different systems was inferred from the progress of older children who had begun their education in traditional oral schools and had added manual communication later. It was also assumed that *all* hearing-impaired children were excellent candidates for manual communication without any tests for visual perception, visual acuity, learning disabilities, motor disabilities, and so on (Dinner, 1981).

Also overlooked was the fact that 90 percent of the children with a hearing loss have two normal-hearing parents who will have to learn manual communication before they can stimulate their own child, and they live in a neighborhood where few, if any, of their neighbors understand or use manual communication. This ultimately limits the opportunity to learn language.

The oralness of the environment has long been considered essential in teaching spoken language to a child. Even Quigley (1969), who attempted to study two groups of children, one being trained orally and the other through the Rochester method, carried out his studies in state residential schools, "where the communication of children out of class is through the language of signs and fingerspelling with very little oral communication, at least on the part of the student."

When schools offer only one option—Total Communication—they overlook the fact that the majority of children who are labeled deaf are not profoundly deaf (see Demographics in Chapter 2, Table 2-IV), and many of them have multiple problems (see Chapter 14). This again points out the danger of classifying children on the basis of their "deafness."

The long-term results of mandatory Total Communication are not in, but personal observation of programs defined as Total Communication has shown both a lack of emphasis on speech teaching and on the effective use of residual hearing in the majority of programs. Some of the statements made by Total Communication proponents have undoubtedly contributed to this attitude. For example, Mindel and Vernon (1971) wrote that "one can generally say that the child with a profound loss does not have the equipment to learn language and speech through hearing. Continuous efforts to expose the child to sound are an exercise in futility." These authors also state that children who were thought to have significant hearing losses but who eventually develop greater vocabulary and language ability than anticipated are usually children who were originally misdiagnosed!

Bilingualism-Biculturism

The 1990s brought a movement on the part of the Deaf community away from Total Communication and inclusion which, they claimed, did not work. Deafness was not a pathology which needed treatment, but a social condition. American Sign Language was the natural language of the Deaf and should be used for communication for all children with a hearing loss. English should be taught as a second language for reading and writing. Residential schools were important because Deaf culture is emphasized there. (At present, approximately one-quarter of the deaf are educated in private or public residential schools.)

Two normal-hearing authors endorsed this concept: Oliver Sachs, a neuropsychiatrist who had been innovative in his own field, wrote a book, *Seeing Voices,* in which hearing aids were barely acknowledged; and Harlan Lane wrote *The Mask of Benevolence—Disabling the Deaf Community* (1992). Dr. Lane inveighs against cochlear implants and hearing aids, mainstreaming, Oral and Total Communication, and all the audiologists or professionals of the "Hearing Establishment." After fifty years in this field, the author feels that we have come full circle. The Deaf wish to return to segregated education using their own language, ASL. There are no new ideas in deaf education, only new names for the old ones. It is technology which moves forward, not backwards.

Alexander Graham Bell was indeed prophetic when he said in 1894: "These discussions and controversies may continue to the end of time until some new elements can be introduced into the problem."

THE DEVELOPMENT OF AN ACOUPEDIC APPROACH

None of the references quoted thus far use the term *acoupedics,* although they place emphasis upon utilization of residual hearing at an early age. Instead they use the term *auditory training.* What, then, is the difference?

The best definition of the goals of an *auditory training approach* is given by T.J. Watson (1961):

> (a) Better understanding of the spoken language of others, (b) More rapid development of the use of language by the child and its extension in the direction of normality, (c) Better speech by the child in terms of voice quality, articulation, and rhythm, (d) Higher attainment in school subjects, especially in the basic skills, and (e) Better social and emotional adjustment through the provision of a direct link, however tenuous, with hearing people.

He feels that these goals are well-known to an oral education and that auditory training is merely an extension and an improvement rather than a different type of method. He feels that one of the newer accomplishments in auditory training has been improvement in amplifying equipment combined with much earlier diagnosis of deafness, with the earlier use of hearing aids and the development of language through the natural method at a much earlier age. He concludes with a discussion of the clinic as a place in which parents are educated so they can carry on a program within the home, since the child will be with them much more than with a trained teacher of the deaf.

In comparison, Henk Huizing (1959) defined *acoupedics* in the following manner:

> This new philosophy is principally based on the education or re-education of the function of hearing. *Our ultimate goal is the successful biosocial integration of the deaf child in a normal environment.* The child must now build up a new source of information and understanding by the development of an adequate auditory memory. This will tie him much closer to his surrounding world than was formerly the case. He must learn to penetrate the space around him by the formation of a foreground background relation between various auditory clues and by grasping the sound patterns which are concomitant with motion. He must learn to understand what kind of information is relevant in a given situation, and which is not. He must learn to use these stimuli for improving his language skill and for better understanding of life situations and human relations. *This is a process of integrating hearing in the deaf child's personality.*

Integrating hearing into the child's personality goes far beyond auditory training, and for this reason alone the new term *acoupedics* is necessary. But there are reasons for defining and differentiating the type of training given today. The term *auditory training* had been used for many years before the wearing of a powerful hearing aid was possible for the limited-hearing infant. It has acquired several connotations. It is the term used in many schools where auditory training is a short lesson in the daily curriculum, and may only mean the use of headphones. It is used to describe training with hearing aids for adults who have had normal hearing before the acquisition of a hearing loss. In almost all cases it refers to a specific type of training given in conjunction with, *or supplementary to,* other types of training, as for example, lipreading.

The term *Acoupedics* refers to a comprehensive habilitation program for all hearing-impaired infants and their families which includes an emphasis upon learning through hearing aids, without formal instruction in lipreading or any form of manual communication. Its ultimate goal is preparation for independent participation in the normal hearing community to the fullest extent possible, considering the abilities of each child (Pollack, 1974).

Chapter 2

THE ACOUPEDIC APPROACH AND ITS CHANGE TO AUDITORY–VERBAL

THE deprivation caused by a severe hearing loss traditionally has been described in terms of communication. However, this does not reach the heart of the problem, because we live in a veritable ocean of sound. Abnormal hearing means much more to a limited-hearing child than defective speech, language, or communication.

THE IMPORTANCE OF HEARING

The Ewings (1961) describe other ways in which hearing is important to living. The reasons are as follows:

1. It is a continual source of information about things and happenings within our immediate physical environment.
2. It provides warning signals that are important to physical safety.
3. It gives help to the individual in acquiring and maintaining physical skills.
4. It forms a link with the rest of the world and instinctively becomes an emotional link that contributes to mental health and social ease.

The Ewings discuss the full consequences of deafness and its influence on mental growth, mental health, and social security. They list some of the effects of deafness in relation to every aspect of living today as "a narrowing of social experience, a limitation of information and social contacts, a feeling of helplessness in the dark." They believe that a child actually learns to mistrust and disregard hearing and rely wholly upon vision because of the difficulty in localization.

Myklebust (1960) also believed deafness has been described too narrowly in terms of communication without describing the effect upon the total organism. Hearing is the main distance sense. It has important repercussions on homeostatic equilibrium; for example, there may be a lack of shifting figure-ground.

18

He described many tests of intellectual development, memorization abilities, motor capacities, social maturity, and concreteness-abstractness, which demonstrated the effect of hearing impairment. The more behavior is limited and restricted to the stimulus, the more concrete it appears.

Myklebust concluded that difficulty in exploring and knowing the environment as a result of sensory deprivation causes the individual to *behave* differently. He perceives differently and his personality adjustment is different. *It is a total basic organismic deprivation.* Myklebust mentioned difficulties in realism and the need for an internal fantasy world; also a difficulty in understanding and forming a close contact with the environment.

Bowlby (1958) expounds upon the essential role played by hearing and speech in the development of attachment to, or oneness with, the mother. The nurturing effect of sound in growth and in the generation of an emotional response may be seen in a baby at a few weeks of age, when he is quieted by his mother's voice and when he responds to her vocalization. Later on, when the baby is moving from oneness to separateness (Kaplan, 1978), separation can be tolerated if a baby is reassured by the sound of his mother in the next room.

In simple terms, hearing is a sense which functions before birth and which gives us important information about ourselves and our environment which no other sense can give. It is the one sense which is never "turned off": we can hear when we are awake or asleep or in a coma; we can hear in the dark, around corners, and behind our backs. Eventually we respond to many environmental sounds without being consciously aware of them.

One may conclude that hearing is a prerequisite for normal personality development and that there is no substitute for hearing, yet we have been trying to educate deaf children without this all important information. Without hearing, it is true the deaf can make an adjustment to the world, but it is not the *same* world.

Therefore, one of the major goals of an Acoupedic Approach is to integrate hearing into the personality of a young deaf child. How can this be accomplished?

THE BASIC PRINCIPLES OF ACOUPEDICS

The Hearing Impairment Is Detected at an Early Age

A congenital hearing loss can and should be detected shortly after birth because both volunteers and nursery nurses can be trained to do screening tests. Unfortunately, it is still quite common for parents who express anxiety about their baby's hearing to be reassured by their doctors that the baby is just slow, or that it is too early to test hearing. Hearing should always be tested when the infant is a "high-risk" baby, when parents express anxiety, when any change is observed in a child's responses to sound, or when speech and language development is delayed or defective.

Audiologic assessment must be ongoing. Thresholds of young children may appear to be more severe at an early age because of the prevalence of conductive overlay. It has been reported that up to 60 percent of the infant population has one or more incidents of otitis media (Brooks, in Mencher, 1981).

On the other hand, hearing loss can be progressive. In the case of KK, in Figure 2.1, the left ear improved and the right ear deteriorated over time.

Two Hearing Aids or a Cochlear Implant Are Fitted to Provide the Maximum Amount of Potential Hearing

Aids are fitted as soon as the diagnosis of hearing loss has been made by an otologist and medical treatment has been completed. A binaural fitting, that is, a separate aid for each ear, should be made if there is residual hearing in both ears. At this time, research is continuing with binaural fitting when one ear is functionally deaf (Markides, in Libby (Ed.), 1980). The hearing aid should be worn throughout the child's waking hours and can be worn at night, too.

In an Acoupedic Program, a child is not classified and labeled on the basis of his unaided audiogram (as in Tables 1-I and 1-II in Ch. 1), but upon *his ability to use his potential hearing obtained by wearing aids throughout his waking hours.* This permits our expectation level to be raised.

It is worth comparing the problem of the visually handicapped person who wears corrective glasses throughout his waking hours. He is not classified and limited on the basis of his *unaided* vision when he applies

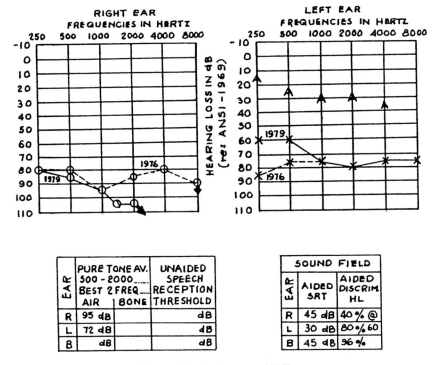

Figure 2.1. Audiogram of K.K.

EAR	PURE TONE AV. 500 - 2000 BEST 2 FREQ AIR	BONE	UNAIDED SPEECH RECEPTION THRESHOLD
R	95 dB		dB
L	72 dB		dB
B	dB		dB

SOUND FIELD		
EAR	AIDED SRT	AIDED DISCRIM HL
R	45 dB	40 % @
L	30 dB	80 % 60
B	45 dB	96 %

for a driving license. If he were, few myopic adults would be permitted to drive.

There are a number of reasons why a classification system based on the child's audiogram should not be used:

1. Audiometric standards are subject to change. The following chart illustrates that children now appear to be deafer than they used to because of the change from ASA (American Standard) to ISO (International Standard), or ANSI 1969 which is similar to ISO.

Case SH, in Figures 2.2 and 2.3, when tested at two years of age, was said to have an average loss of 85–90 dB for the speech frequencies. At ten years of age, when the audiometric standards had changed, her loss appeared to be greater; an average of 103 dB.

2. An audiogram does not tell us the degree of residual hearing possessed by a child. The majority of American audiometers in use amplify pure tones only to an intensity of 110 decibels (ANSI 1969). The human ear is able to hear some frequencies at approximately 120 to 130 dB without pain. Thus, the child who does not respond to a pure tone at

TABLE 2-I
SCALE OF HEARING IMPAIRMENT

Hearing Level in dB 1951 ASA Reference	Descriptive Term	Hearing Level in dB* 1964 ISO Reference
-10 to 15 dB	Normal Limits	-10 to 26 dB
16 to 29	Mild	27 to 40
30 to 44	Moderate	41 to 55
45 to 59	Moderately Severe	56 to 70
60 to 79	Severe	71 to 90
80 plus	Profound	91 plus

*Average of Hearing Levels in Speech Range (500--2000 cps.)

110 dB may respond to an audiometer which can produce tones at 115 dB or even 125 dB. This hearing is used with the hearing aid.

It is frequently stated that a child with a left corner audiogram has no high frequency hearing. In Figure 2.4 it will be seen that RA did respond to higher frequencies in both ears when tested by intensities beyond the limits of the standard audiometer, a threshold which is reflected in his aided responses. He can now use a telephone. A cochlear implant may give even more auditory information in the high frequencies.

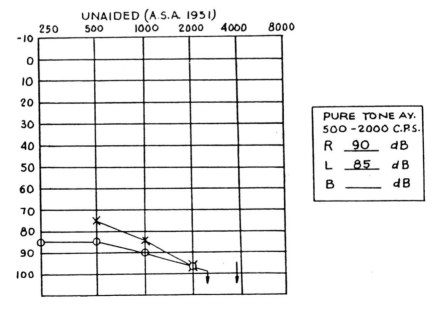

Figure 2.2. First audiogram of Cindy (A.S.A. Standard).

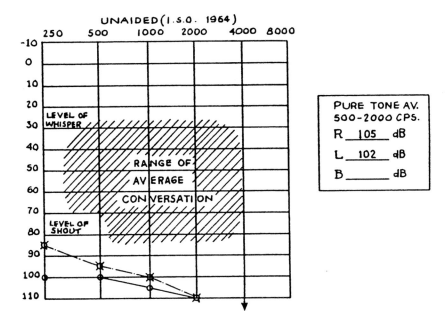

Figure 2-3. Audiogram of Cindy (I.S.O. Standard).

Berlin (1982) has shown that some children (usually those with losses in the moderate to severe range) respond to suprahigh frequencies which are never tested routinely.

3. An audiogram does not tell us what the potential hearing will be when appropriate hearing aids are worn binaurally.

The emphasis upon audiograms has been misleading to those who are not audiologists. For example, the range of normal hearing is defined as -10 dB to 25 dB in Table 2-I (although many audiologists feel that losses greater than 15 dB are handicapping to a child). However, we do not have to listen at those intensities. Normal conversation ranges from a quiet voice of 40 dB to a voice heard in close proximity at 60 to 70 dB (ANSI), a range which is easily obtainable with present day amplifiers. Thus, the child who does not respond to the human voice with his own ears is able to discriminate words *without visual clues,* at the level of a quiet conversational voice when aided. The aided audiogram in Figure 2.4 shows that when RA is wearing hearing aids, he is no longer *deaf*—he is only hard-of-hearing.

The child who has a *severe* hearing loss and does not respond to the human voice unaided until it is 70 decibels loud receives even more benefit from current hearing aids; he may almost respond within normal limits when aided (see case history C.M. in Ch. 15).

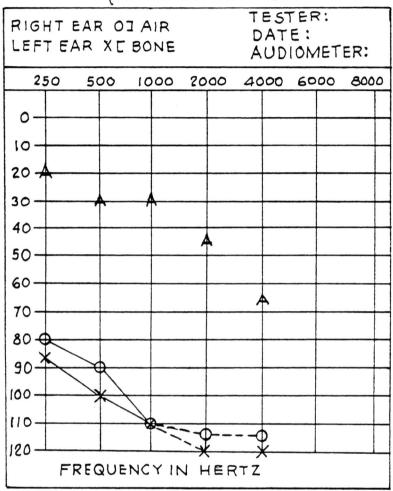

Figure 2.4. Audiogram of RA.

4. An audiogram does not tell us what each child will do with his residual hearing. It is well known to teachers that a child with a mild loss is not always less handicapped than one with a severe loss. The presence of learning disabilities and other factors such as intelligence, age of onset and etiology of the hearing loss, age of audiological and educational intervention, and quality of home training are all virtually important factors.

5. An audiogram does not tell us how speech sounds when it reaches

the brain, nor how the brain will process those sounds. Above all, it does not tell us what we can educate the brain to do with amplified sound. We are not educating the peripheral mechanism, but a *mind.*

If Cindy, in Figures 2.2 and 2.3, was judged by the classification system reprinted in Chapter 1, and if her teachers approached her with the attitude that she is deaf because of the severity of her hearing loss, all kinds of limitations would be placed upon her—orally, educationally, and vocationally. In actual fact, she has worn hearing aids since she was eighteen months of age, has attended schools for normal-hearing children since kindergarten, and she has learned a foreign language (French) which she speaks fluently. She graduated from law school and won a prize as one of three best speakers in a national competition for law students (Pollack, 1982; Harris, 1983).

The use of the term *deafness,* with its semantic connotations, is outdated for such a child and sets up barriers to communication. The term *limited-hearing,* coined by Lorraine Amos Roblee, is more descriptive of the majority of those we call *deaf.* If we refer to them as "children with a hearing loss," then we recognize that there are many different kinds of children who have a hearing impairment, and they do not fit neatly into two groups: the *deaf* and the *hard-of-hearing.*

The Limited-Hearing Child Is Given the Fullest Opportunity to use His Residual Hearing

Norbert Wiener (1954) has said that there are many possibilities built into man, but all must be made good by learning. The two basic techniques for learning in an auditory approach are as follows:

1. Uni-sensory training to develop hearing perception.
2. Use of the auditory feedback mechanism to develop speech.

Uni-sensory Training: For too long, teachers have fitted children with amplification and then diverted their attention away from listening by teaching them to look and *depend* upon looking at the speaker's face or hands. The emphasis upon *visual* skillfulness, which was essential before early fitting of modern hearing aids, is no longer necessary. The essential goal now is to educate the child to use his aided hearing to its full potential, and this has to be accomplished by training the aided hearing maximally and intensively at an early age.

In an Acoupedic Approach, one neither trains awareness of, nor attention to, visual cues through lipreading, cued speech, early training of reading, or finger spelling. All of the training is concerned with awareness and interpretation of sounds heard through a cochlear implant or hearing aids which are worn throughout the child's waking hours.

There can be no compromise because, once emphasis is placed upon "looking," there will be divided attention, and vision, the unimpaired modality, will be victorious. This fact cannot be denied since schools for the deaf provide many examples: the child who has only a moderate hearing loss but speaks as if he is deaf because of his training, the older child who is unable to adjust to wearing hearing aids although he is only "hard-of-hearing," and children who gradually discard their aids and depend upon lipreading or signing. (In a similar way, the unimpaired eye will "take over" and the impaired eye will become "blind"; or the use of a stronger set of muscles after polio will result in the atrophy of weaker muscles.)

This approach involves a complete change of attitude for the "teacher of the deaf." She is no longer teaching a child who is *deaf* but a child who hears something. Thus, she must go to the heart of the problem and constantly direct attention to listening and response to sound, until hearing is part of everything the child experiences. He will begin to depend on his aids and develop confidence in his listening skills. Although good eye contact is important, the teacher never diverts the attention of a young child to staring at her hands or face in an Acoupedic Approach. On the other hand, this does not mean that she has to blindfold him or make him sit on his hands!

A *uni-sensory* approach to developing perception is not, of course, a new idea. Alcorn's "Tadoma" method (Gruver, 1955) for the deaf-blind is an example. Miss Sullivan (1961) observed that Helen Keller learned quickly because she learned through one sense (i.e., pressure upon the hand) without distraction from other cues. Montessori (1914) also noted that children naturally isolate a sense when they are learning something new: they close their eyes in "touch" activities.

The application of uni-sensory methods to oral education (i.e., auditory training without emphasis upon visual or kinesthetic cues) was advocated by Goldstein (1939) in his *Acoustic Method,* and he recommended it for *all degrees of hearing loss.*

In a larger group residual hearing remains latent because of insufficient stimulation. *In all cases* it should be given a reasonably long try-out, for these auditory remnants are peculiarly sensitive to stimulation and re-education, and in a large percentage of cases the perseverance and resourcefulness of the teacher will be rewarded by surprisingly good results.

Goldstein used both analytical and synthetic listening exercises. But his book included chapters by teachers who added tactile and visual training. He later wrote that his method had failed because it had not been applied with sufficient care, detail, and persistence, without sufficient regard for the fundamental principles on which the method depended for success.

It is now clear to us that it failed because Dr. Goldstein's students remained deaf through most of their waking hours. They were not able to wear hearing aids and develop normal, consistent hearing perceptions. Sessions of acoustic exercises are not the answer to the child's needs. *Listening must be a continuous activity.*

Once a listening function has become an integral part of all his experiences, the child can use visual cues to a greater or lesser degree, depending upon several factors such as degree of loss, amount of environmental noise, position of speaker, type of activity, and so on. He *becomes* multisensory and *integrates* all the sensory stimuli in a natural way. Nevertheless, auditory skills training should be continued into the teen years. As one teenager reported: "I hear more, or am aware of more, all the time." One of the problems during the school years is the emphasis placed upon visual learning in a group situation.

Uni-sensory training is based upon the psychological laws and the physiological mechanism governing the development of perception, and is discussed fully in the next chapter.

The Use of the Auditory Feedback Mechanism

Development of speech is accomplished through the child's auditory feedback mechanism and innate echo-reaction. Speech is normally learned because a baby enjoys sounds and identifies with the sounds of his mother. He hears his own voice, he hears his mother's voice, and tries to imitate her—a process of unconscious identification. Then he hears himself matching her sounds.

When appropriate hearing aids are worn continuously, speech, for the most part, can be learned in the normal way. Again, it must be stressed that it is not beneficial to draw attention to visual cues at this stage. In an Acoupedic Program, a child is stimulated constantly by sound, his attention is directed toward sounds, and he is rewarded for imitating sounds. Thus, an acoupedically trained infant uses his voice naturally and *constantly,* and he controls it by hearing. Most traditionally trained teachers find this difficult to believe until they have visited an acoupedic or auditory program and witnessed a demonstration with children who have a profound hearing loss.

The dilemma of a *visual approach* in fostering oralism was laid bare by Mowrer (in Morkovin, 1960) in the foreword to *Through the Barriers of Deafness and Isolation.* He wrote thus:

> Expensive experience has shown that speech reading is the most promising key for unlocking a child's mind from the prison of deafness and social deprivation. But . . . *it is far more difficult to develop this skill and subsequent speech in children who have been deaf or seriously hard of hearing from birth.* . . . Now, we have a clear understanding of *why* this should be the case. Normal infants are said to learn to talk through imitation—they first hear the speech of others, *in a meaningful context,* and then begin trying to reproduce it themselves. But what is equally important—and commonly overlooked—is that, in the process, they are also able to hear themselves. . . . By means of the immediate auditory "feedback" from their own vocal behaviour, they can tell, quite precisely, when they are "tracking," that is, matching the model, and when they are not.
>
> However, in the child deaf from birth or early infancy, all this is changed. Since he cannot hear others, he has no auditory "model" for his own speech responses, regardless of whether he can to some degree hear himself or not. If the mouth movements which accompany speech in others are brought to his attention the child can, of course, *see* them, but he does not ordinarily see his *own* mouth movements. Thus, although he has ever so clear a memory or image of the mouth movements of others, he lacks the necessary visual feedback[1] for comparing and guiding his would-be "imitative" reproduction thereof. . . .
>
> However, it should be realized that visual feedback is by no means a perfect substitute for normal hearing. It is generally known among educators of the Deaf that lip movements are often ambiguous and that *not more than* 40 percent of them can be precisely identified.

This is our dilemma when we use a visual approach—the problem is to unlock the child from a "prison of deafness." The question is from deafness to what? From deafness to sound. What kinds of sounds? Noises, music, and so on, in the environment. Obviously the utmost skill in "speech reading" will fail to detect these. Not only are these

---

[1] Visual feedback is given during therapy by the use of mirrors. The teacher and child sit side by side, looking at each other and themselves in the mirror, but this can occur for only limited periods of time and is not an adequate substitute for the continuous auditory feedback which is part of a normal hearing child's daily life.

visually ambiguous, but the pitch, inflection, and volume of the voice are not visible at all.

Lipreading involves a cross modality transfer. If a child watches the lip movements for the word *shoe*, imitates them, and checks for results in a mirror, he is reproducing visual patterns, not the speech sounds *shoe*. If he then supplements the visual with tactile clues, he is still not imitating the sounds *shoe*. If he wears a hearing aid but his teacher directs his attention to visual clues at the same time, again the child will not repeat the sounds *shoe* normally.

This may well explain the number of oral failures and the strong influence of manualism in the United States. Acquisition of oral speech through a visual approach has been too difficult. Yet speech has been called "the greatest interest and the most distinctive achievement of man" (Wiener, 1954), and Helen Keller wrote: "If you knew the joy I feel in being able to speak to you today, I think you would have some idea of the value of speech to the deaf. One can never consent to creep when one feels an impulse to soar!"

Normal Sequential Patterns of Language Development are Followed

The phonetic aspect of language (i.e., the sound itself) is learned through the development of a listening function. The *semantic* aspect (the meaning) and the *behavioral* aspect (the translation of sound and meaning into action) are acquired through experiences which are highly motivating to an infant, and after a tremendous amount of verbal input. Ideas and activities are verbalized and the words accompany the experience *simultaneously*. Consider, in contrast, a visual approach in which a child experiences something and then has to interrupt what he is doing to look up at the speaker's face, hands, blackboard, or chart.

"A semantic receiving apparatus neither receives nor translates the language word by word, but idea by idea" (Wiener, 1954).

Although the auditory approach means a largely nonanalytical approach, careful planning is involved to expose the infant to all the patterns of his language in a normative way. The child learns to interpret and imitate the language patterns he hears through his hearing aids because they accompany his most meaningful experiences. Vocabulary learning can proceed much more rapidly. In particular, *abstract* concepts are understood because they are acquired primarily through hearing in the preschool years. Where's the *pet?* He ran *away.* The boy came *too late.* He was *very* sad. Which one is your *favorite?*

A study by Templin (1966), "Vocabulary Problems of the Deaf Child," reemphasizes the need for helping deaf children develop greater sensitivity to the flow and function of language, and states that the inferiority of deaf children in vocabulary development has been generally accepted. Templin studied knowledge and use of vocabulary—definition, synonym recall, synonym recognition, words with more than one meaning, sentence construction, similarities, and analogies. The deaf were tested at eleven, twelve, and fourteen years of age, and the hearing subjects at six, eight, nine, eleven, twelve, and fourteen years of age. The deaf responded by writing their answers; the hearing spoke or wrote. They did not differ substantially in intellectual ability, but the inferiority of the fourteen-year-old deaf varied from two or three years to more than eight years among the several tests. The greatest inferiority was apparent in the analogies, words with more than one meaning, and the synonyms recognition tests. Templin found no major differences between the performances of residential and oral day school subjects except that the day school subjects scored consistently higher on the analogies test.

It has been suggested that manual teaching would correct this situation, but a study by Quigley (1982) which examines reading, written language, and educational achievements focuses on the rather dismal performance within those areas by the majority of deaf children, and explores the question whether development of reading can take place without a preestablished internal *auditory*-based language. Dinner (1981) found that even her groups of intact children, many of whom had been exposed to sign language since birth, seemed to plateau after the fourth grade. This is in direct contrast with the achievements of the acoupedic group (see case histories in Chapter 15 and outcome studies in Chapter 4).

A Normal Living and Learning Environment: An Acoupedic Attitude and Atmosphere Are Created

In order to develop an auditory function for a child with a severe to profound hearing loss, it becomes of the utmost importance to create the right learning environment. It has to be one in which the child is bathed in sound, and surrounded by people who have normal hearing, speech, and behavior . . . people who believe he can hear, who expect him to listen and respond, and who show him how to communicate normally. It is a learning situation in which all his education can be given in the relevant and meaningful context of his daily experiences, not in sessions of auditory training.

Although the auditory approach is rooted in the oral tradition, the change is not only one of methodology. Richard Silverman has said that oralism is as much an ATTITUDE and an ATMOSPHERE as it is a METHOD OF TEACHING. The traditional attitude, which permeates all the literature of "deaf education," is that (1) a deaf child has an irreversible loss; (2) he cannot acquire much speech and language through the auditory pathway and must be taught compensatory techniques; and (3) he must be placed as soon as possible in a special group.

The attitude inherent to educational audiology is that (1) a child today needs to spend very little time in a silent world if his hearing impairment is diagnosed at an early age, and if he is wearing hearing aids or a cochlear implant continuously; (2) hearing can be integrated into the personality of a deaf child and a fundamental part of speech and language can be learned through hearing *if the emphasis is placed upon training audition;* and (3) he should be in an atmosphere which provides the fullest opportunity to use his residual hearing.

One-to-One Teaching

Individualized one-on-one teaching is essential when a developmental approach is used. The program must be designed specifically to meet each child's needs, with intervention beginning at a point slightly below the developmental stage reached so that failure is obviated and progress flows easily to the next milestone.

Mainstreaming

If young children are learning to listen, they must listen to normal voices, normal speech, and normal language. The environment required for this type of learning means that special grouping with other deaf children should be postponed until it becomes necessary within the public school system, *if ever.*

The child can be placed, almost without exception, in a normal hearing nursery program if the object is socialization. This is just as beneficial to the normal-hearing children, for they develop understanding and friendship with a handicapped child at an early age. There is a need, however, for specially trained nursery teachers for children whose parents are unable or unwilling to devote the time required in home training.

Although integration within normal-hearing classrooms has to be considered cautiously with regard to many factors, there are many disadvantages to being in a special group which may well outweigh the possibility of failure in a normal-hearing school, when we consider that we are preparing a child for life in a hearing world. Wiener (1954) has said, "Those who would organize us according to permanent individual functions and permanent individual restrictions condemn the human race to move at much less than half-steam."

Parents Are the First Models for Communication

Speech and language are first learned in a deeply emotional, one-to-one relationship, not in a teacher-class relationship. In educational audiology, the mother is given back her natural role. As she goes about the daily routine, she draws her child's attention to all the environmental sounds, and supplies the words he needs to talk about his experiences and feelings. Parents and siblings are still the best models for communication and only they can give frequent repetition and reinforcement in small doses as an infant needs them. The role of parents as partners in the education of a hearing-impaired child is so crucial that it is discussed in Chapters 12 and 13 and throughout the book.

THE EXPECTED RESULTS
OF AN ACOUPEDIC APPROACH

1. Hearing is integrated into the total personality development of a child with a hearing loss so that he is in continuous contact with, and fully responsive to the total environment.
2. Auditory information upon which the normal-hearing depend is now available to the hearing-impaired so that he is able to follow normal developmental sequences.
3. Voice quality is improved: it has melody, inflection, a range of tones, and other normal parameters.
4. Speech and language development are accelerated: it becomes easier to learn to speak because normal mechanisms can be used instead of visual-proprioceptive mechanisms; there is a simultaneous association between activity and verbalization so that meaning is acquired in the normal way and by contact with everyone in the community.

5. Lip or speech reading is easier when residual hearing is used.
6. Abstract words, jokes, riddles are understood. Psychologists report that ability to give similarities and analogies is improved.
7. A temporal or sequencing sense is restored: many hearing-impaired persons report that "time seems to stop" when they remove their hearing aids.
8. Educational and vocational expectations can be raised.
9. There are more opportunities to stay in the mainstream and to be independent; that is, without reliance upon an interpreter.
10. Improved self-concept: the ability to perceive oneself as a normal person who happens to have a hearing loss, rather than as a handicapped person who is outside the "in group," is one of the most outstanding characteristics of a graduate of an Acoupedic Program.

THE ACOUPEDIC APPROACH AND THE CHANGE TO AUDITORY–VERBAL

In 1977, at the instigation of George Fellendorf, the Executive Director of the Alexander Graham Bell Association for the Deaf, a meeting was held at the Helen Beebe Speech and Hearing Clinic in Easton, Pennsylvania, to discuss the formation of a group of clinicians who advocated an auditory approach. The following year, Pollack chaired a meeting in Washington in which it was decided to form a special committee subsequently called the International Committee on Auditory-Verbal Communication (ICAVC) based on the principles of Acoupedics. Daniel Ling suggested the term "Auditory-Verbal."

During its early years, ICAVC was a chapter of the A.G. Bell Association, but it became evident that the group would be able to advocate its approach more effectively if it became a separate organization. In 1987, ICAVC changed to Auditory-Verbal International, Inc.[2]

AVI now has a worldwide membership and has published a Code of Ethics, a Scope of Practice document, and has defined the required knowledge, skills and abilities, and developed an examination for certification as "CERT.AVT" (auditory-verbal therapist).

---

[2] AVI, Inc.'s offices are located at 2121 Eisenhower Avenue, Suite 402, Alexandria, Virginia 22314.

THE SETTING FOR A PROGRAM
OF EDUCATIONAL AUDIOLOGY

As this is a program designed primarily to meet the needs of young children, it has to be organized in a flexible manner. Ideally, because its success depends upon continuity and teamwork, it should take place within one setting. Some parents consult general practitioners, specialists, a speech clinic, an audiology clinic, an allergist, and educators, from whom they receive widely different diagnoses and advice. It is terribly unfortunate when parents are caught in the center of professional controversy.

The best environment would seem to be a center where medical, audiological, psychological, and other professional personnel work as a team. A university, associated with, or in close proximity to, a medical center, can train students, provide opportunities for research, and even set up a nursery school or home demonstration center in addition to offering low-cost education to the children. In this case, an experienced clinician, or parent facilitators, not students, must be responsible for the parent-infant program.

For example, the author opened a Speech and Hearing Service at Porter Memorial Hospital, Denver, in 1965. The Acoupedic Program was part of this service. The staff included clinical audiologists, educational audiologists, speech and language pathologists, and teachers of the deaf. The services of the hospital occupational and physical therapists and social worker were also available.

In 1970, some of the parents formed the LISTEN Foundation as a fund-raising and public relations organization. They raised funds for scholarships, equipment, teacher training, workshops, publications, and movies. In time, they purchased a house near the hospital where out-of-state families could stay and where all the families could receive "home therapy." A part-time family counselor was then hired (Pollack, in Ling and Pollack, Volta, 1983).

Another alternative, which has been used in a number of United States programs such as Ski-Hi in Utah, and CHIP in Colorado (Itano, 1994) is for professional workers to visit the homes. This may be an expensive and time-consuming solution unless the home visitors live in the same area, and it does not always provide opportunities for the parents to meet other families and successful "graduates." Also these professionals may not have the education or expertise for developing spoken language through listening.

In all countries there are some communities which are far from a center. It has long been a custom for schools, universities, or other agencies to arrange an intensive course where parents can "live-in" and meet other families. Unfortunately, this does not usually offer the long-term support needed by the family of an exceptional child.

A speech and hearing clinician with well-rounded experience can undertake an Auditory-Verbal Program alone if she can refer her patient to other professional services. In such an arrangement there is a danger that the specialists who see the child for only a short time may make independent recommendations which conflict with those given by the clinician, thus causing unnecessary trauma to the family. It is strongly advised that the clinician accompany the family or meet with the consultants for a staffing.

However, attachment to one individual has been criticized by a number of writers for several reasons. One person cannot provide the necessary array of services, audiologic, medical, counseling, and so on, or the skills which are of a multidisciplinary nature. Any habilitationist needs the opportunity to have assistance and supervision by more experienced colleagues (Mencher, 1981). Luterman (1979) points out that it is all too easy for the professional to assume responsibility for the parent and become "the savior," whereas the goal of a good clinical program is not to foster dependency upon one person but to support growth and confidence in the parents. Luterman calls this the "Annie Sullivan Syndrome" and cites as an example how ineffectual the parents are portrayed in "The Miracle Worker." However, when parents form a close attachment to a clinician, it does assure a continuity of programming which has been lacking in a number of school and university programs.

The Personnel

This approach requires a background of audiology and normal child growth and development, including normal speech and language development, in addition to a knowledge of multiple handicaps and special techniques (Ling and Ling, 1978). The clinician needs to possess diagnostic as well as remedial skill so that she can plan an individualized program based upon each child's needs, and refer to other specialists when it is appropriate.

The clinician must also be able to function on a "feeling" level which places a responsibility to work with, and maintain, his/her own personal congruence (Luterman, 1979). Unfortunately, professional training programs rarely provide experiences in counseling parents.

The person undertaking an Auditory-Verbal Program needs to have clinical insight, infinite patience, imagination, and a love of children. But she must not be too permissive; rather she must know when to direct and when to suggest.

An Auditory-Verbal Program does not end with school entry, but continues until each child no longer requires services. Therefore, it is important for the team to include an educational audiologist who knows the demands of the schoolroom and can coordinate clinic and school programs.

Who Are the Candidates for an Auditory-Verbal Approach?

Auditory-Verbal is a program of educational audiology which is designed to meet the needs of children whose hearing losses are detected at a very early age—as newborns, as infants, or preschoolers.

There is no need to "select" the candidates on the basis of hearing loss because total deafness in a young child is very rare, and all young children with residual hearing can learn to use it optimally. A cochlear implant may be an option for the totally deaf. Table IV compares the degrees of hearing loss in students enrolled in special educational programs in the United States with the students enrolled in an Acoupedic Program. This graph remains remarkably consistent from year to year.

TABLE 2-II
DEGREE OF HEARING LOSS OF CHILDREN
IN THE ACOUPEDIC PROGRAM

	Acoupedic Program *Percent*	*National* *Percent*
Total known information	100.0	100.0
Normal (under 27 dB)	0.0	2.4
Mild (from 27 to 40 dB)	3.8	4.0
Moderate (from 41 to 55 dB)	5.7	8.2
Moderately Severe (56–70 dB)	17.0	13.3
Severe (from 71 to 90 dB)	24.5	26.3
Profound (91 dB and above)	49.1	45.8

Who are the most successful candidates? Those children whose families share the same goals and participate as fully as possible in the program and those children who receive the remedial services which are appropriate to their special needs. Many of the young children will be found to have other problems, some more handicapping than the hearing loss, which does not exclude them from an Auditory-Verbal Program but may require modification of the teaching strategies.

It is interesting to note that the most successful candidates for "total communication" are also described in the same way by Meadow (1980) as being children with varying degrees of residual hearing, adequate medical attention, and parents who are very much involved in their development and committed to working closely with them and with the helping professionals. However, Meadow warns that it is an open question whether this same kind of language approach is optimum for children with additional handicapping problems and busy or noninvolved parents.

When intervention occurs after the preschool years, some of the principles of the Acoupedic Approach can still be applied, and the developmental sequence adapted and made relevant to the needs of an older child, but it is very difficult to obtain the same results, and especially if the child has become visually-oriented and dependent upon visual or manual cues.

Problems in Acceptance in this Approach

Why, one may ask, has there been so much reluctance on the part of the deaf educator to abandon traditional methods? Most teachers have seen few successful auditory-verbal children because hearing loss has not been detected routinely at an early age when it is easier for the child to acquire certain types of learning. This seems to apply to auditory and verbal communication more than to any other skill. In addition, the successful auditory-verbal child does not attend special education classes but merges into the mainstream.

A second problem stems from the dichotomy between the audiologist and the teacher, and from the unreliability or misinterpretation of early audiograms, which leads to underestimation of residual hearing.

The third problem involves the use of amplification. Not only does the idea still exist that you can hang a hearing aid upon a child and he will automatically use his residual hearing even if you divert his attention to the mouth or hands, but all recent studies show that few personal amplification systems in the schools are in good working order (Gaeth, 1966; Northern et al., 1972, and Zink, 1972), nor are they worn consistently.

The fourth problem involves the learning environment. Not only are educators trying to develop oral communication during a minimum number of hours spent in classrooms in contrast to the thousands of hours available to the normal-hearing child outside the classroom, but they have created a learning environment in which there is little oral communication among the children nor the motivation to use it. In general, it is true to say that expectations for children with hearing impairments are still very low indeed in many countries.

The last major problem seems to be the tendency to place blame on the communication methods used or on the lack of support from parents when a child does not develop good communication skills, rather than studying each individual child's needs and abilities. Diagnostic services have become more readily available, especially since the advent of P.L. 94-142, and hopefully it is now recognized that children with a hearing loss are as subject to learning disabilities and other problems as are their normal hearing peers. There is no panacea for *all* children.

SUMMARY

A program of educational audiology includes the following:

1. **Early Detection:** A complete and ongoing audiological evaluation begun at the earliest possible age.
2. **Early Fitting of Hearing Aids or Cochlear Implants:** This is to be accomplished as soon as a diagnosis has been made by an otologist and medical evaluations completed. (These first two aspects are discussed in Chapters 5 and 6.)
3. **An Auditory Approach to Training:** Intensive, individualized uni-sensory training is designed to develop perception and to use the amplification technology maximally. The child is taught to listen, not to lip read or sign. (The procedures to be used for development of a listening function are described in Chapter 8.)
4. **Development of Language Following Normal Sequential Patterns:** A largely nonanalytical approach is used in the early years with all acoustic, speech, and language stimulation given in

a rich, meaningful context of the child's play and daily experiences. (This is described in Chapters 9 and 10.)

5. **Parents as Partners and the First Models of Communication:** Parental guidance is accomplished in several ways: by participation in the child's therapy sessions, by individual counseling, by home visits, by group meetings, and by contact with experienced parents and their children, or graduates of the program. (This is discussed in Chapters 12 and 13.)

6. **Retention of a Normal Learning and Living Environment:** The young child is not placed in a special group situation with other handicapped children, and educational placement is not made on the basis of the *unaided* audiogram.

The Goals of an Auditory-Verbal Approach

The Auditory-Verbal Approach has two different goals from traditional deaf education:

1. Hearing is to be integrated into the total personality development of a young child with a hearing loss regardless of the severity of that loss.
2. The child is being prepared for full participation and independence within his community, not for special education.

In no way is the Auditory-Verbal Approach a denial of the problems associated with deafness nor is it offered as a panacea for *all* deaf children. It is never easy to be a hearing-impaired person in a normal-hearing world. The child with a hearing loss does not have to feel that he has to be the *same* as a normal-hearing child. He cannot be. But neither does his whole life have to be circumscribed and restricted by his hearing loss. An Auditory-Verbal Approach represents a viewpoint that a handicap *can* be overcome because it is only part of a person. For too many years, the child with a significant hearing loss has been restricted to a subculture. An Auditory-Verbal Approach raises the expectation level and gives him a choice.

Chapter 3

DISCUSSION ABOUT THE
BASIC AUDITORY–VERBAL PRINCIPLES

Since the 1960s, there have been many changes in the detection and intervention of children with hearing impairments:

1. The age of identification has decreased.
2. The etiology has changed—for example, no rubella epidemics in the United States.
3. Technology has improved dramatically, resulting in the development of FM units, cochlear implants, frequency transposition aids, and improved hearing aid fitting.
4. The incidence of multiply-handicapping conditions has increased, due to medical progress in saving infants from illness, prematurity, and trauma.
5. The number of parent-infant programs has increased in both the public and private sectors.

Research on all the different approaches to intervention remains sparse, but there are many studies and surveys which support the Auditory-Verbal Approach as a first option. They will be discussed in this chapter and throughout the book.

EARLY DETECTION

The success of educational audiology depends first and foremost upon early identification of the hearing impairment, and ideally, this should take place soon after birth. Strong and Clark (1994) reported that, unfortunately, one year may elapse before an intervention program begins. In the case of less severe losses, such as those caused by otitis media, diagnosis and treatment may not take place until the child is two-and-a-half years old when the normal-hearing preschooler has between three and six thousand words.

NEONATAL SCREENING

Early attempts to screen neonates relied upon observation of reflexive responses to loud tones. The responses include:

1. Acoustical palpebral reflex (APR) or blink
2. Acoustic muscle reflex (AMR), a tensing movement of a limb or the whole body, as for example, a Moro's reflex
3. Acoustic ocular-gyric reflex (AOR) usually seen at four months or older
4. Orientation reflex response (ORR). An early orientation response can often be seen when a neonate is propped up against the mother's body in a sitting position and facing the tester who makes a loud sound about twelve inches from the baby's ear but slightly behind its head. The eyes will be seen to move rapidly and briefly in the direction of the sound.

Other responses may be cardiac acceleration, arousal from light sleep, cessation of ongoing activity, facial grimaces, raising of eyebrows, and so on (Froeschels and Beebe, 1946).

In addition to these observations was added the completion of a High Risk Register. Such programs were described in the earlier edition of this book and by Downs and Sterritt (1967).

Marlowe (1993) describes in detail the preparation and organization of a neonatal screening program in a community hospital, using automated ABR equipment and trained volunteers. More than 1700 infants are admitted annually. Volunteers are required in three to four shifts, seven days a week, 365 days a year. Because of the current rapid discharges, some babies are inevitably missed, so the supervising audiologist contacts the family by telephone or letter. The results of the test are released only to the infant's physician.

Restrictions on insurance benefits pose a challenge to neonatal screenings. At this hospital, a one-time charge is included in the nursery charges for the test, and a fee for supplies under the supply code. No family is denied the test because of inability to pay, but most costs are covered by third party payors. The screening is a standing order for every infant.

THE 1994 NATIONAL CONSENSUS STATEMENT

In 1994, the Joint Committee on Infant Screening endorsed the goal of universal screening before the age of three months and intervention by six months. The Consensus Statement recommended a two-stage protocol consisting of evoked oto-acoustic emissions testing (EOAE) for all infants, followed by auditory brain stem responses (ABR) for those infants who failed EOAE.

CONTROVERSY AROUND SCREENING

There remains some opposition to neonatal screening expressed in an article by Paradise and Bess (1994). Objections include the following:

1. The large numbers to be tested (4 million babies born in the U.S. annually) compared to the small number of infants with a hearing loss (said to be 4000).
2. Cost of this protocol.
3. The reliability and validity of the test if volunteers are used may result in overreferral for retest.
4. Many babies are born at home.
5. Some babies who respond normally after birth suffer from a progressive loss.
6. A neonatal screening program may arouse unnecessary anxiety in the mothers.
7. Mass screening is useless unless treatment programs are immediately accessible.

Northern and Hayes (1994) responded to these charges, pointing out that babies are screened for other problems, and the numbers of those with all types of hearing loss are closer to six per thousand rather than one per thousand which was quoted for profound loss. The three-month period gives audiologists the opportunity to organize a program for babies who were born in rural areas or at home.

REAL COSTS OF BABIES WHO ARE NOT SCREENED

Downs (1994) writes that the initial cost does not take into consideration the economic, educational, and vocational costs of a deaf population which is not identified at an early age. The current cost of educating deaf children in a U.S. state school is 35,780 dollars annually, and for self-contained classes 9,689 dollars, compared with 3,383 dollars in regular classes.

Educationally, all children with a hearing loss are subject to delay in language development and academic skills. A significant study by Levitt (1987) reports on longitudinal data for 120 children. Speech was related to the severity of the hearing loss, but the only variant for language and educational achievement was the age of identification and intervention.

Vocationally, the yearly income of 350,000 manually-communicating deaf adults in the U.S. was reported as 30 percent less than that of the general public, and an IRS report stated that 24 percent of deaf college graduates did not have any income.

OTHER ADVANTAGES OF SCREENING

Mass screening contributes to our knowledge of hearing loss. It has been said that 40 percent of hearing impairments are of unknown etiology, and in the past it was not known if the loss was present at birth. Certainly it contributes to the awareness of physicians and the general public of the importance of testing hearing. With regard to the fear of causing anxiety and interfering with bonding on the part of mothers, the author's experience over many years was that mothers were interested in the concern which was shown and asked if they could bring in their older children for testing. In this way, we sometimes found a two-year-old with a loss which had never been detected before.

Lexington School for the Deaf described their study of infants who had entered their program by sixteen months of age and those admitted at later ages. In all measures of parent-infant communication, the younger group was statistically superior.

THE COLORADO NEONATAL SCREENING PROGRAM

Universal hearing screening has become the standard of care in Colorado since 1991, when it was ascertained by many reports that the High-Risk Registry method missed at least 50 percent of newborns. The Health Care Program for Children with Special Needs in the Colorado Department of Public Health and Environment is responsible for management and implementation of the program.

Due to the distribution of the hospitals in the major metropolitan districts, 30 out of 80 hospitals account for 80 percent of the deliveries. A three-year goal was established that 30 hospitals would be enrolled, thus ensuring that at least 80 percent of neonates would be screened. Since neonatal screening programs had been conducted in some Colorado hospitals for many years, as, for example, the ones described by Downs (1994) and by this author (1985), this should have been feasible. In fact, it has taken five years.

Other goals of this project include the following:

1. Support of the physicians, which is critical.
2. Parent education, through childbirth classes, pamphlets given to parents, etc. This included information about rehabilitation programs available to them.
3. The organization of a data system which could be shared with other states which planned to set up a screening program.

CHALLENGES IN MANAGING A NEONATAL SCREENING PROGRAM

1. Reimbursement: At present, Medicaid does not cover the cost of testing, but since hospitals are usually well-paid by third party payors, there can be some cost-shifting. It helps if the physician writes a standing order for every baby.
2. Choice of instrumentation and personnel responsible for the testing. This must be a decision made by each hospital. Volunteers have been effective with training and a supervising audiologist, but they must be covered by the malpractice insurance of the hospital. In small hospitals with fewer than 300 births annually, the nursing staff enjoys doing the screening; in larger hospitals, the audiology staff may be responsible.
3. Instrumentation: Currently, Colorado is using conventional ABR, automated ABR (using the Algol Plus) and some audiologists are trying EOAE with very good results. A 35dB click stimulus has been used.
4. Purchase of Equipment: This has been accomplished in various ways: Hospital foundations, hospital auxiliary fund-raisers, private donations, and gifts from community service organizations.
5. Time to fill out the High-Risk Register.
6. Turnover of personnel: Volunteers are asked to commit for a six-month tenure.

7. The overreferral rate: This has ranged from 3 percent to 8 percent, apparently depending upon the experience of the tester or the equipment used.
8. The follow-up system, especially in migrant populations.

The project holds monthly meetings and distributes a quarterly newsletter to audiologists, which includes a report on the risk factors found and the degrees of loss detected.

The project has received strong support from the group known as the Hearing-Impaired Family Support Network, which is composed primarily of parents, many of whom had not had the opportunity for early intervention.

THE IMPORTANCE OF
EARLY AUDITORY STIMULATION
SENSORY DEPRIVATION

Morphological Changes

The literature of psychology and physiology contains many references to sensory deprivation. Although most of the writers are concerned with animal studies, there is such general agreement across species that Riesen (1974) does not doubt applicability to human infancy. He states that disuse during early sensory periods leads to permanent alterations in the functions and structures of the relevant brain areas.

Webster quotes older studies of brains of congenitally sensorineural deaf persons that indicate poor development of the central auditory pathway. In their studies of mice, Webster and Webster (1977) found quantitative differences in the brain stem auditory nuclei and other morphological changes. All their data shows that both conductive losses and auditory deprivation during a postnatal period cause behavioral, physical and anatomical deficiencies in the central auditory system.

Ruben and Rupin (1980) stated that the infant's auditory system is plastic and can be modified by anatomical alterations that result from variations of acoustic stimuli. The input of the peripheral auditory system is critical to the maturation of portions of the cerebral auditory system. P.E.T. scans are now being used to show activity in various parts of the brain.

Relation Between Audition and Vision in the Newborn

Although some studies have taken the position that the perceptual systems are unrelated at birth, others have stressed the reflexive relation between audition and vision, in that certain combinations of auditory intensity, frequency, and rise time cause eye opening or closing (Kearsley, 1973).

Other studies have shown nonreflexive relations between audition and vision in the infant, because sound can affect visual attention in various ways as, for example, in attempts at localization; and the orientation reaction can affect processing in all modalities (Lyons-Ruth, 1974–75). *Lack* of sound can also alert visual attention. Mendelson and Haith (1976) studied the relationship between vision and audition in infants one to four days old. The importance of their studies lies in the use of darkness and a blank field to show that newborn activity is not merely reflexive and responding to visual stimulation. The sound used was a recording of a male talking in a highly modulated voice, and the conclusion reached was that sound influences visual epistemic behavior even at birth.

EMOTIONAL DEPRIVATION

Much has been written in recent years about the bonding which is said to take place between parent and infant in the early postnatal period, and specifically the importance of the reciprocal vocal play which takes place. This is felt to contribute to the feeling of "oneness" which is appropriate during the first year of life, and to the development (because of distance hearing) of "separateness" which should take place after the first birthday (Kaplan, 1978). Many emotional problems are said to be caused when a child does not separate but remains dependent upon the parent.

Bowlby (1958) says that speech and hearing play an essential role in the development of the child's attachment to his mother. Without the contact afforded by the voice, this bond is distorted or attenuated. As a consequence, an emotional separation exists. The nurturing effect of sound in growth and in the generation of emotional response can already be seen at a few weeks of age when a baby is quieted by the sound of his mother's voice. Later, when vacillation between growth and attachment is at its peak, separation can be tolerated if he is reassured by the sound of an unseen mother in the next room. Apparently, sound is a necessary part of those cognitive stimuli through which the child defines his own boundaries and his relationship to the world (Bruner, 1961). According to Spitz (1959), the normal appearance of speech is one of the first organizers of the psyche. He calls it a prerequisite for the development of object relationships in the human pattern which stimulates interchange between child and parent. In adaptation terms, it may be said that without speech, the development of such welfare emotions as mutuality, empathic feelings and tender regard is hindered.

Rainer et al. (1969), in describing personality traits in the deaf, stated that he feels sensory isolation created by deafness has far-reaching effects.

An infant, however, is highly adaptable, and some of this deprivation may well be ameliorated for the child of deaf parents who develop their own system of bonding (Schlesinger and Meadow, 1972), but the majority of deaf infants have *normal-hearing* parents. In any case, the use of sign language does not preclude mental health problems in the deaf (Rainer et al., 1969).

Communication Deprivation

There are a number of studies of hearing infants which attempt to differentiate the factors that affect development of social communication in the prelinguistic period. These studies illustrate how communication precedes language and stress the importance of the home setting because that is where most of the infant's social interaction occurs.

Brazelton et al. (1974) found that the type and amount of interaction between parent and child vary as a function of the situation and the environment. For example, in studying the vocalizations in different environments, Lewis and Freedler (1973) observed that a twelve-week-old vocalizes most often in playpens, but less frequently on the floor, in infant seats, and so on.

Differential response to sound occurs very early. Condon and Sander (1974) describe how infant movements become coordinated with adult speech within twelve to fourteen days after birth, and Spring and Dale (1977) describe the neonate's sensitivity to rhythm, intensity, and so on. Prosodic patterns also appear to communicate affect.

Eilers and Gavin (1977, 1980) demonstrated how infants discriminate some phonetic elements of their own language at a very early age, and actively improve their own skills during the first months after birth.

Trehub (1981) showed that young infants develop the ability to detect speech embedded in noise.

Other studies strongly suggest that there is a relationship between the type and amount of early linguistic input and the quality of the child's language later in life. Ringler (in Waterson and Snow, 1978) and Piaget (1952) show hearing and verbal language to constitute one of the foundations of intelligence.

Critical Periods

It is now widely accepted that there are *critical periods* for developing perception.

A critical period has been defined as a fairly well-delineated period in which a specific stimulus must be applied to produce a particular action. A "sensitive" period is the optimal time for application of such a stimulus. After this, it becomes increasingly difficult to learn. Apparently a certain degree of maturation has to be achieved before the applied stimulus permits a certain milestone of development to occur (Illingsworth and Lister, 1964; Ebbin, 1974).

The neuropsychological development of any child is directly dependent upon his participation in appropriate experiences at all stages of his growth. Particularly at the early ages, development of any skill is necessarily related to both the state of readiness and the opportunities available for developing the skill.

It would seem that the first years of life are critical for learning to listen. Fry and Whetnall (1954) say that the cortical centers can learn to discriminate between auditory stimuli readily during the first three years of life, whereas after this period learning becomes increasingly difficult. This also applies to learning a foreign language. The first year, which has been called by Whetnall (1965) the "Readiness to Listen" year, is the most important. Wedenberg (1961) also stressed that it is necessary to begin auditory training as early as possible after birth. It is in these early months that infants learn that sound has meaning. They are not just aware of environmental sounds—they learn that these sounds *mean* something. They are associated with something, and they become symbolic of something or someone. This is basic to learning that *spoken* sounds mean something and are symbolic.

Another important fact which is applicable to early training is that an infant can receive auditory impressions in close proximity, at a high level of intensity, and with little distraction; acquisition of more complex abilities, perceptions, and skills, together with interest in exploring the environment, renders the child less willing to restrict his attention.

The early years also constitute a critical period for the acquisition of *language*, not only for biological reasons, but because they are socially critical. The child can devote a large amount of time in the development of linguistic skills and he is not ridiculed for his errors. His maximal dependence on others makes him easily susceptible to influence—he *needs* to communicate (Halle, 1964). Ritchie Russell (1939) stated that it is clear that the early months of life are the most important for the planning of brain mechanism. The neuronal patterns used to learn a word in childhood will probably be the same as those used in old age.

Since a neonate moves from maturational stage to maturational stage, including the maturation of the speech coordinating mechanisms, loss of the first nine months may be crucial.

EARLY FITTING OF HEARING AIDS

All deaf children should be given the opportunity to use amplification, even when no overt responses are seen initially, unless tomography shows cochlear agenesis or postmeningitic invasion by bone, in which case evaluation for an implant can be recommended. The following case histories illustrate this principle.

Case Histories

Jay came to the acoupedic program five months after he had meningitis. He had become silent, and was reported to be unresponsive to all sounds, even to a home organ. He was just two when he became deaf. His mother said he had been an active youngster who had used less than six words (e.g., "no," "Coke," and so on). He was tested by electroencephalogram audiometry, which showed a possible "island" of hearing at 500 Hz. of 90 decibels (ASA). However, the audiologist was not optimistic, since he had seen a cochlea ossified after meningitis. He felt this could be a tactile sensation.

Jay had many other problems when he began therapy—for example, he had poor balance, was extremely distractible and "wild" in behavior, and much given to throwing things and hitting. His parents were deeply unhappy because Jay was their first child after twenty years of marriage.

Vocalization was reestablished by placing Jay's hand on the clinician's neck when she said *bye-bye.* Then his hand was placed upon his own neck. As soon as he felt his voice again, he began to use it spontaneously, *without tactile cues.* His responsiveness to sounds increased slowly until the second year of therapy, when he was able to echo (in a very quiet voice) all words spoken. He loved music, he always indicated that he heard noises outside, and he also indicated that he recognized what made the sounds. Within a few months, Jay was imitating consonants *k*, *t*, *p*, and others *without lipreading*, and using them at the ends of words, but a recheck of his hearing by EEG when he was 3.6, gave the following results:

Air Conduction	250	500	2000
Right Ear	No Response	80–90 dB	No Response
Left Ear	No Response	75–80 dB	No Response
(A.S.A.Standard)			

Jay was very resistant to wearing headphones, and the author felt this did not show all of his residual hearing.

The lesson to be learned from this case is that nothing is lost by assuming that hearing exists — *there is everything to gain*. The author believed that Jay's auditory memory should be preserved if it was at all possible. He progressed like other children with profound congenital hearing loss at first, but in a short time he showed a mature understanding of concepts and interests appropriate to an older child; he was accurate in counting, matched alphabet letters, made rapid associations between immediate and past experiences, and pronounced many words normally. At four years of age, he was participating in a Montessori preschool.

Jay's most recent audiogram shows the following configuration (ANSI 1969 Standard):

Air Conduction	125	250	500	1000	2000	4000	80000	P/T Ave.
Right Ear	65	90	95	110	120	125	NR	108+
Left Ear	60	75	90	105	115	125	NR	103

Jay's binaural aided speech detection threshold was 35 dB.

He attended a residential oral school because of his mother's illness and subsequent death, but returned home for his high school years in a private school for normal-hearing boys. He is now a student at N.T.I.D.

Infants who have profound congenital losses may also fail to respond during their first testing session because sound has been too quiet and meaningless to them.

R.T. is a very good example of this (see Figure 3.1). He was tested at fifteen months of age and gave no overt response to any frequency with the exception of a questionable response to 125 dB. The author noticed that he had an unusually pleasant voice quality and surmised that he had suffered a progressive loss from birth. He was fitted with two body aids and soon began to show awareness of sound. He was conditioned to play audiometry very easily and the next audiogram was as follows:

Air Conduction	250	500	1K	2K	4K	P/T Average	Aided SAT
Right Ear	75	90	105	NR	NR	105+	55 dB
Left Ear	65	80	105	110	105	98+	40 dB

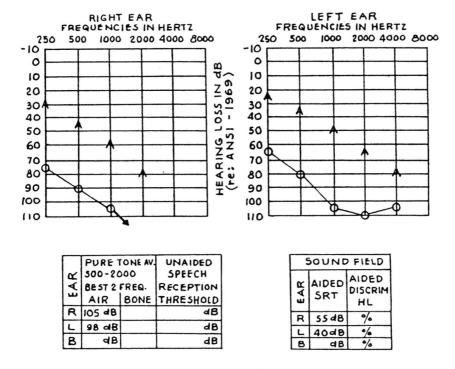

Figure 3.1. Audiogram of RT after training.

After the first year of listening, he made rapid progress and was eventually mainstreamed in public school. Subsequent audiograms showed fluctuations, especially in the right ear, and a shunt was inserted in the hope of stabilizing his residual hearing.

With the progress made in electrophysiologic testing, this type of case would now be tested with brain stem audiometry emissions. Even so, there are still audiologists using ABR who make diagnostic errors such as the following case (as reported by the mother):

Mrs. T., your daughter has a very profound loss. There are no actual sounds that she hears; she responds only to vibrations. Her loss is permanent and there is nothing medically that can be done. Hearing aids will do her very little good; don't waste your money on them. Start immediately to teach her sign language so that she will have some way to communicate with you.

Fortunately, this mother could not accept "the hopelessness of his verdict," and sought help from the Acoupedic Program. Her daughter proved to have a severe to profound loss and was an excellent candidate for both hearing aids and an auditory-verbal method of communication.

Hanners also describes the "state of the art" and the misfitting that occurs when clinical audiologists test infants without a program of habilitation and accompanying feedback from a teacher (in Nix, 1976).

THE USE OF BINAURAL HEARING AIDS

Nature provides us with two ears apparently for localization, spatial awareness, and intelligibility in noise. The benefits of binaural amplification have been investigated and summarized by Markides (in Libby, 1980).

1. Binaural fitting gives the ability to "squelch" reverberation and background noise.
2. It gives the power to select one stimulus from a number of stimuli, as in the "cocktail party" effect, thus improving the understanding of speech under extremely unfavorable conditions.
3. It gives enhanced location.
4. It gives the benefit of summation of energy at threshold and supra-threshold levels. For example, the same loudness sensation will occur binaurally with 6 dB less sound pressure than monaurally, thus decreasing the possibility of trauma.
5. It gives summation of information content, especially when the two ears are dissimilar in frequency distribution.
6. It avoids the "head shadow effect."
7. It gives a better quality of sound.
8. It gives ease of listening.
9. It gives better discrimination of speech.

It is easy to demonstrate the improvement binaural amplification gives to children with symmetrical losses. For example:

Case 1: Molly, Congenital, Etiology: Maternal Rubella. Fitted at 12 months.

Right Ear	75	90	85	80	75	65	85	45	60% at 60 dB
Left Ear	90	90	95	90	80	70	92	45	56% at 60 dB
Binaural								40	80% at 60 dB

Case 2: Congenital, Etiology Unknown. Fitted at 2 years.

Right Ear	80	100	110	115	110	NR	108	45	36% at 70 dB
Left Ear	80	95	105	125	125	NR	108	45	48% at 70 dB
Binaural								40	68% at 70 dB

But sometimes a child will discard the hearing aid in the worst ear as she grows older. This has been most frequent in the Rubella children who seem to suffer from a progressive loss in one ear while the better ear remains the same (see cases K.K. and Ryan T.). This happened to the author's nephew when he was a teenager. He complained that although he could hear in the worse ear, it was an unpleasant and distracting noise. At age 54, his better ear remains as it did in childhood.

In the following congenital case, the etiology was unknown:

Case 3: Etiology Unknown. Fitted binaurally at 2 years of age but Rejected Aid on Left Ear at 10 years.

Right Ear	50	70	80	70	60	70	75	30	76% at 60 dB
Left Ear	90	100	105	110	NR	NR	105	NR	CNT
Binaural	20	30	35	40	35			30	76% at 60 dB

Nothing is lost by stimulating both ears until it can be verified that a particular infant does not benefit from binaural amplification. A cochlear implant is, of course, fitted monaurally.

THE POWER CONTROVERSY: DO HEARING AIDS DAMAGE RESIDUAL HEARING?

The reluctance of many audiologists to fit power aids stems from two fears:

1. That the results of exposure to the maximum power output of current hearing aids may cause the same kind of threshold shift experienced by normal listeners after exposure to continuous, high-intensity sound.
2. That some subjects suffer additional hearing loss after using amplification so one ear should be "saved."

A review of the literature shows a few instances in which hearing improved after temporary removal of the aid. Early studies in the 1950s and 1960s were often contradictory, some asserting that aided ears deteriorated and nonaided ears remained the same, while others asserted that deterioration occurred in nonaided ears also, and powerful aids had little or no effect on the residual hearing of deaf children. Some concluded that progressive loss was probably due to the pathology of deafness.

Whetnall (1964) pointed out that acoustic trauma results from long exposure to a continuous noise at a high level of intensity or from a sudden explosion. Aided speech sounds are not continuous, however, and children do not wear aids at intolerable levels—they adjust the volume controls.

Markides (in Libby, 1980) gives an excellent description and comparison of all the studies related to hearing aid usage and its relationship to progressive hearing loss, and concludes that there does not yet appear to be any conclusive *scientific* evidence that powerful aids do or do not have a deleterious effect on residual hearing, and therefore, if power aids are needed, it is better to use them rather than deny auditory experiences to a child.

Ott studied twenty-two patients from the Acoupedic Program and reported her findings (Balkany, Ott, and Pollack, 1980). There were eleven females and eleven males who had been wearing aids with MPOs greater than 125 dB for periods averaging fifteen years. All had been fitted binaurally with the exception of two cases, one of whom had been monaural until age fourteen, and the other had changed from binaural to monaural at ten years of age.

The etiology of these patients was as follows:

Unknown:	10
Rubella:	7
Rh Factor	2
Familial	2
Meningitis:	1

Ott used a battery of tests which included air and bone conduction, speech tests using the WIPI for the younger children, and PBK lists for the older cases. The Tullio phenomenon was explored and also the patient's subjective uncomfortable loudness threshold. ABR was used in some of the patients. Hearing aids were analyzed with Phonic Ear equipment. The patients clustered into three groups:

1. Those now wearing aids with MPOs of 119–124 dB: minimal changes were noted over the years.
2. Those now using MPOs of 125–130 dB: 41 percent showed changes but only minor changes in the speech tests.
3. Those now using MPOs of 130–139 dB: 55 percent had significant changes in residual hearing at two frequencies; 39 percent had losses in the pure tone averages; 50 percent showed changes in their SRT. One of these cases is shown in Figures 2.2 and 2.3 in Chapter 2. She has been using aids with an MPO of 136 dB for twenty-four years and all her audiograms are remarkably consistent.

There was no *statistical* difference in the progression between groups two and three, and the conclusion was that power hearing aids could not be blamed for the progression. We need long-range studies which duplicate exactly the data collected and the tests used.

In conclusion, it must be stated that if audiologists make the statement that hearing aids damage hearing, they must also be prepared to explain why these aids do not cause any change in at least 50 percent of the cases, and why progressive loss occurs in patients who are *not* wearing power aids. They must also be asked why they are "saving" hearing which cannot be used without appropriate amplification, and why they recommend aids which will put children "off the air" when they are learning to talk.

The author recommends approaching every child as an individual. Consistent, ongoing audiologic management will monitor threshold changes and then appropriate modifications of the hearing aid fitting can be made.

THE UNI–SENSORY APPROACH

Normal Development of Perception

A uni-sensory method for development of hearing perception is based on the psychological laws and physiological mechanisms governing the normal development of perception. These are as follows:

1. Awareness of the stimulus
2. Attention to the stimulus
3. Motivation
4. Learning

Awareness

Awareness is a complex phenomenon, and what little is known of its anatomical and physiological substrata suggests that it is dependent upon the reticular formation, which is a diffuse system of cells and fibres in the brain stem concerned with maintaining consciousness and the perception of the external world.

Luria (1973) describes the reticular formation as having the structure of a "nerve net" with ascending and descending systems. It is a powerful mechanism for maintaining cortical tone and regulating the functional state of the brain.

Attention

Krech and Crutchfield (1959) describe *attention,* or the *perceptual set,* as a selective focus for awareness. The human organism functions, not with a multisensory response, but with constant shifting of attention.[1] With divided attention perception discrimination is poorer. The main target for focus is generally the clearest and most differentiated in the field.

Studies of sensory interaction have a long history. Urbantschitsch, in 1888, pointed out that if one stimulus is strong enough to become the figure in the figure-ground relationship (as in normal vision and abnormal hearing), it *inhibits.* If both stimuli occupy the ground (as with normal hearing and normal vision), it facilitates.

Negus (1963) also states that there is interference of sense perception on one part of the cortex by excessive stimulation of another area. It appears impossible to receive more than one stimulus to the full at one and the same time, and it is possible to reject one sense in favor of another of more immediate importance. He gives as examples, lovers of music who shut their eyes when listening, loud music used as anaesthetic during dentistry, and so on.

Razran (1955) described this as a theory of dominance. When competing or conflicting attention tendencies are aroused, the rule is not compromise, but victory of one and defeat of the other.

Audiologists have found that children do not respond to auditory stimuli during an EEG hearing test when they are deeply engrossed visually (Gordon and Taylor, 1964), and similar "behavioral curtains" have been observed during hearing tests with the psychogalvanometer. The blanket or bottle held by the child seemed to inhibit the CNS so that poor responses were obtained (Hardy, 1966).

In simple words, if we want a child to attend to sound we must emphasize listening, not looking.

The psychological findings quoted above have been well supported *physiologically* by human and animal research. Only a few examples will be given.

Negus (1963) describes the physiological basis for inattention as follows:

> Extending throughout the length of the brain in all vertebrate animals, including man, there is a long column of interconnected cells known as the

---

[1] A child also has a more restricted span of what can be taken in at one time. His simultaneous perception of parts and whole is limited.

reticular system. The cells of this system receive afferent connections from all the sensory tracts ascending into the brain from the spinal cord, and from the sensory roots of the cranial nerves.

It has been established that incoming sense impulses from sense receptors can be selectively facilitated or inhibited at their point of entry in the neuraxis. This perceptual selection is *attention*. *If attention is directed to a visual stimulus, then simultaneously evoked acoustic potentials are blocked by discharge of inhibitory impulses from the reticular system.*

The existence of peripheral inhibition, presumably from fibres traversing the basilar mechanism, was directly observed by Galambos (1958) and inferred from some experimental results by Lowry in Harris (1950) who concluded that the nervous system overcomes its diffuse nature by setting up inhibitory processes which sharpen discrimination.

Hubel et al. (1959) demonstrated that the auditory cortex of the cat can be activated only when the cat attends, that is, orients himself toward the source of the auditory stimulus. Other studies show that if an animal deploys his available free energy in attending to a given stimulus, there is less energization of other physiological mechanisms responsible for other forms of stimulation. In general, these men feel that contribution of attention is undoubtedly great, particularly in the area of sensory preconditioning (Hernandez-Peon, 1956).

Motivation

Motivation has been described as the main factor for voluntary attention. It can arouse or alert the cortex before normal perception can take place. Having aroused the cortex to perceive one set of signals, another set, arriving at the same time, may be inhibited.

Elonen and Zwarensteyn (1964) describe how a blind child can very selectively deafen himself to all sound, and do it so effectively that he is labeled deaf. This is also true in cases of brain damage or receptive aphasia. These are the children who have failed to discover that the sounds with which they are bombarded could be used as a means of communication with those around them. They are not *motivated* to hear.

Learning

Psychologists have come to realize the immense importance of learning in perception. The human being is constantly bombarded with physical stimuli, but out of this chaos order is achieved — perceptions are organized into meaningful objects and relations.

Senden and Hebb discovered that *visual* perception has to be learned. Patients whose congenital cataracts had been newly removed and were undergoing, like a baby, their first experiences of visual pattern, could not master the discrimination of form for several weeks. For example, they could not distinguish a triangle from a circle. The ability to perceive stimuli was present; the ability to organize them had not been developed—*learning was lacking* (see Newsom, 1962).

The integration of *auditory* information belongs to the brain, not to the peripheral mechanism.

Krech and Crutchfield (1959) show that the properties of a whole cannot be considered simply as an adding up of the separate properties of its parts. It is the *pattern* of the parts which contributes the essential perceptual qualities of the whole. Once a pattern has been learned, the organism shows a readiness to make a particular response to it. In another context, the more familiar a word, the greater the set toward its perception. For example:

> Understanding, which is a psychological skill, is more significant for language development than the ability to make sounds. We cannot remember and repeat the sixty or so phonemes which a sentence may contain, but we can understand the sentence because the sequence of phonemes within words, and the sequence of words within sentences, fall into familiar patterns that help to organize the stimuli and enable us to program the response.

By grouping, the span of comprehension is thus extended. Organization has the function of enabling the perceiver to cope with more material.

The perceptual act has been diagrammed by Solley and Murphy (1960).

INFORMATION PROCESSING

Recent publications on "information processing" substantiate the Auditory-Verbal Approach. Shatz (1977) points out that we have limits on the amount of information we can process at any one time, and we allocate our skills depending on the complexity of the task. To accomplish complex, cognitive tasks, we can operate only within our limits. Studies have shown that we learn best by the method by which we are taught because we are given a "set" in that direction (Bendet, 1977). Thus we select information according to that set which, in turn, is reinforced by the new information acquired. For example, if a child is

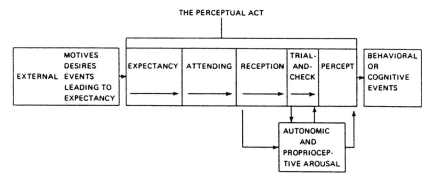

THE PERCEPTUAL ACT

Figure 3.2. Diagrammatic Schematization of the Perceptual Act. Courtesy of Solley, C.M., and Murphy, G.: *Development of the Perceptual World.* New York, Basic, 1960.

constantly required to look at the speaker's hands or face, he selects visual information and his visual orientation is reinforced when that information becomes meaningful. Similarly, when directed to *listen*, the child is "programmed" to process auditory information.

Although sensations from one modality can enhance perception in another modality, they can also interfere, *especially in the learning phase,* and especially if the reticular formation is not adept at inhibiting the imposing stimuli (Ayres, 1972).

Luria (1973) gives an illustration of modality interference:

> The simple arousing (or "impulsive") action of a verbal instruction can be observed in a normal-hearing child by the end of the first or beginning of the second year of life in response to the mother's simple question, "Where is the doll?" or "Where is the cup?" The infant directs his fixation toward the object named and reaches out for it. However, this takes place only in the most simple conditions, *namely when there are no distracting objects in the field of vision.* As soon as the test is repeated under different conditions, and the child is instructed to "give the doll," while at the same time another distracting or unfamiliar toy, such as a fish or a bird, is placed alongside it, a different result will be obtained. In this case the child's fixation wanders between all these objects, and it frequently rests not on the doll ... but on the brightly distracting object which happens to be near and gives it instead. At this stage of development a spoken instruction cannot yet overcome factors of involuntary attention competing with it, and victory in the struggle goes to the factors of the direct field of vision. The direct orienting response to a new, informative or distracting stimulus, formed in the early stages of development, easily suppresses the higher, social form of attention which has only just begun to appear. Not until four and a half to five years of age is this ability to obey a spoken instruction strong enough to evoke a dominant connection.

The application of this to an Auditory-Verbal Approach is as follows: The infant is motivated to listen and other cues are de-emphasized. He attends to sounds and receives them with the least possible distraction, thus achieving better discrimination. He does not perceive speech in terms of single sounds, but in patterns, and he understands the meaning of these patterns because of the context in which he hears them.

Uni-Sensory Versus Multi-Sensory

The term uni-sensory has often been misinterpreted by the advocates of the multi-sensory approach to mean *deprivation* of other clues. Of course, the child is not deprived of the use of his unimpaired senses during auditory training; rather, through intensive training of the impaired modality, he is enabled to respond *multi-sensorily*, whereas a multi-sensory approach, which in fact emphasizes visual-motor skills, leads to "overcompensation" by the unimpaired modalities. (For the brain-injured child, multi-sensory stimuli have been observed to be more confusing than therapeutic.)

Facilitation

A great deal of the criticism stems from research into "facilitation" which proves that a combined method (i.e., audiovisual) gives higher scores for understanding spoken material than either visual or auditory. This is not disputed by the advocates of uni-sensory training; *the integration of all cues for effective communication is the end toward which they strive.* Interaction is the rule in psychological processes, and the stimulation by one sensory modality can facilitate perception in another sense modality because it sets off ascending reticular formation.

The disagreement then lies wholly in the means by which this goal is to be reached. Most facilitation experiments have been conducted with a population of normal-hearing adults, or of hearing-impaired adults whose training has been visually-oriented (lipreading, and so forth). But Gaeth (1963) showed that his training of very young children gave evidence that auditory orientation could be improved by *emphasis upon audition.* In other experiments, the performance on the combined method of presentation was not superior to that on the auditory or the visual method in *learning.* Gaeth, like Urbantschitsch, felt that the effect of bisensory presentation is likely to be different when one sense modality is deficient.

Ling, Leckie, Pollack, Simser, and Smith (1982) studied syllable reception by twenty-four profoundly hearing-impaired children trained from infancy in auditory programs. Stimuli were presented under three conditions: through audition, lipreading, and a combination of the two. Syllable identification was chosen because syllables are the most difficult verbal stimuli to perceive accurately. Although most of the children showed relatively limited ability to identify syllables through audition alone, their use of residual hearing clearly led to a 20 percent overall gain when used as a supplement to lipreading. An increase of such magnitude had not previously been reported. A further striking difference (relative to previous studies) is the finding that scores for the AL condition were, except in three cases, larger than the sum of each subject's scores in the A and L conditions.

Stone (1983) repeated these tests within self-contained classrooms to twenty-one profoundly deaf children who had received uni-sensory instruction for a minimum of three years. His results were similar to those obtained by Ling, et al.

One must also question the assumption that the child's vision and visual perception are unimpaired. Myklebust and Brutten (1953) found that visual defects occurred in their sample more frequently than in a normal-hearing control group. Even when vision was normal, visual perception was not, and they concluded the following:

> A *deficiency in abstraction* seems to explain the distinct perceptual inferiority of deaf children and underlies the disturbed perceptual functioning of the deaf. The perceptual stimuli used posed unmanageable perplexities to the mental equipment of the deaf child. The deaf were characterized by a perceptual approach which was largely concrete. The deaf child's visual perception was more adequate in the structuring of stimuli which were tractable to concretization or association with things of experience.

Steritt et al. (1966) also compared a group of normal-hearing and a group of hearing-impaired children in an oral day school and found that the hearing-impaired group was inferior in visual as well as auditory temporal pattern reproduction.

Joseph Stewart demonstrated, using tests by Elkind, Koegler, and Elsie (1964) that facilitation of a higher order may result from an auditory approach (see Table 3-I). This was not a rigorously controlled research experiment but a pilot investigation to determine the future usefulness of these items on a larger scale. The tests were used for a thesis by Carl Binnie, entitled *A Comparative Investigation of the Visual Perceptual Ability of Acoustically Impaired and Hearing Children* (unpublished, University of Denver, 1963), in which subjects from a residential school and an oral day school were compared. The non-acoupedic group scored lower than the acoupedic group of six-year-olds in a test of visual perception.

TABLE 3-I
VISUAL PERCEPTION DATA, SIX–YEAR–OLDS

Sex	*Nonacoupedic Group*		*Pure Tone Average (better ear)*
	Picture Integration	*Picture Association*	
F	1	3	65
F	11	6	80
M	7	5	80
F	9	3½	90
F	11	8	90
Mean	7.8	5.1	79
Acoupedic Group			
M	15	6½	75
F	11	6	80
M	10	5½	87
M	9	7	80
M	13	10	90
Mean	11.6	7	87

Courtesy of Stewart, Joseph: *The Effectiveness of Educational Audiology on the Language Development of Hearing Handicapped Children*, U. of Denver, 1965.

These results, for these groups, indicate highly superior visual perception on the part of a group deprived of lipreading training! This shows that a uni-sensory approach does not inhibit the development of visual perception but it does emphasize the development of auditory perception, and appears to improve facilitation. One can surmise that the question of facilitation involves more than just the integration of auditory and visual clues.

THE DEVELOPMENT OF SPEECH THROUGH THE AUDITORY FEEDBACK MECHANISM

It now seems *imperative* to fit the hearing aids and begin training when the child is developing an auditory feedback mechanism. He hears not only the voices in his environment, but also his own voice, and this should be hearing controlled. Early vocalizations are acoustically very different from speech sounds, but apparently this vocal play constitutes an important part in the development of syntax, of motor skills, inflection patterns, and so on.

Lenneberg (1964) reported that babies from different countries sound similar until about nine months, when their babbling and vocalization begin to resemble the mother tongue. That is, a Dutch baby starts to sound "Dutch" and an English baby sounds "English." His study in Boston revealed that neither deafness nor deaf parents reduce the sound activity of the first six months to any appreciable extent. *The sounds of the first three months are virtually identical.* (This correlates with Irwin's study.) After the sixth month, the total range of babbling sounds appears to be more restricted. The results of absence of auditory feedback and control were also noted. One particular aspect of the vocalizations of older deaf children was surprising. It was an unassailable fact that these children would laugh and even emit certain babbling sounds in connection with emotional states displaying a perfectly normal voice with good pitch and loudness control. Yet, in the course of their efforts to speak, the quality of their voice changed entirely, frequently in some abnormal low-pitched or high-pitched tone, completely devoid of pleasing intonation patterns, and obviously uncontrolled by appropriate feedback. In other words, proprioception cannot take the place of auditory control.

An auditory approach, however, has been most rewarding in achieving normal inflection patterns and a pleasing voice in contrast to the "deaf" voice quality usually associated with severe hearing impairments.

Somatosensory and auditory feedback provide the only reliable cues an individual has regarding the accuracy of the sounds he has given forth. Visual cues and verbal explanations are relatively inadequate. The author has sometimes demonstrated this to parent groups by asking them to tell her "how to produce a *b* sound." She follows their directions with very amusing results—but cannot produce the exact sound. Then she shows how easy it is to listen to a sound and imitate it in the normal way. Even for children with a profound loss, "matching" phonemes through listening is quite easy, once they have developed a listening function with their aids, but some phonemes, such as [s] or [d3] may involve other techniques, such as listening with a transonic aid.

Luria (1973) also discusses the importance of a child's internal speech, which may have developed to such an extent by school age that it changes not only the course of movement and action but also the organization of sensory processes. He gives the example of a child being asked to make a certain movement in response to a pale pink color, but to make no movement in response to the darker shade. With an increase in the speech of presentation, the child's performance fell off sharply and many errors occurred; but when the test was carried out with the child instructed to say "pale or dark" to herself at the same time as the response was made, the accuracy was considerably increased. In a similar way, it is very difficult to add up a long column of numbers if we cannot say them to ourselves. We also use internal speech to remember telephone numbers, names, directions, and so on.

RETENTION OF A NORMAL ENVIRONMENT

There have long been two conflicting philosophical forces in deaf education: one that supports "acceptance" of a handicap as permanent and develops an educational and social system based on that handicap; and the other which believes teachers should prepare children for greater independence and for the fullest possible participation in the normal-hearing community.

Until thirty or forty years ago, the majority of children with hearing impairment did not receive special education until they were of school age. By that time, six or seven critical developmental years had been lost and teachers did not attempt to "catch up." A sheltered environment was created in residential schools, for the most part, where a different language system could be used. After school, the graduates of these programs moved into the Deaf community. This was reinforced by the fact that few of their family members used fluent sign language.

In the 1990s, the pendulum has swung back with the Deaf community demanding a bilingual-bicultural system, in which children will use ASL (American Sign Language) for communication and English for reading and writing. These children, of course, will require interpreters. (One group even advocates placing Deaf children with hearing parents in Deaf homes.)

At the same time, there have always been outstanding Deaf individuals who have not identified with the Deaf community. Almost certainly the educational and economic levels of their parents were important factors, but not all the deaf or deafened are accepted by the Deaf community which expects a commitment to being "deaf" and to using sign language.

The limitations placed upon all individuals who are grouped in a "subculture" or minority culture, and the effects upon their social-emotional life and their vocational achievements have long been recognized.

There are many studies which show the effects of an educational setting upon the performance of the hearing-impaired and among these are the National Demographic Surveys (Jenesma and Trybus, 1978). Hearing-impaired children in regular schools are found to speak more intelligibly and perform better on language and academic tests, although it is also true that they differ on a number of variables from the children in special schools, with superiority of performance generally, but not always, associated with less severity of loss. However, Reich et al. (1977) found that the longer the children were in a regular program, the more their relative performance improved, whereas those in special classes fell further behind the longer they remained in those classes.

The problem seems to be a reduction in expectation in the special schools. Much of the traditional pattern stems from a negative attitude that neither oralism nor mainstreaming can be achieved, but early intervention and technologic progress have opened up the opportunity to raise expectations.

The author discarded the idea of special preschool groups after realizing that they were self-defeating if oralism and mainstreaming were to be her goals. When you are teaching a child to *listen,* you need a quiet environment, and when you want a child to learn to talk, it does not motivate him to be in a group of nonverbal peers. If one's goal is mainstreaming, the models for both behavior and communication have to be normal hearing.

Social interaction is also a two-way process, and the concept of mainstreaming must involve changing some of the perceptions of the normal-hearing towards physical differences. Discrimination against the socially deprived is a fact, and when a child has the dual handicap of hearing loss *and* lower social class, he may indeed find the normal-hearing world a difficult environment.

The goal of retaining the most normal learning and living environment does not, however, negate the desire for socialization among persons with similar physical handicaps because of their mutual interests and understanding, but the author believes this should be a personal choice, not a foregone conclusion, recognizing that narrowing social experiences limits the source of information and gives rise to a distorted or incorrect picture of the normal-hearing world in which we all live.

Chapter 4

RESEARCH STUDIES AND OUTCOME SURVEYS

Statistical studies for all methods of teaching deaf children remain sparse, although there are many testimonial or anecdotal publications. As pointed out in Chapter 1, most studies are post-facto. It is often difficult to compare results when there are so many variables.

Available findings at this time tend to support an auditory approach in the areas of auditory functioning, speech intelligibility, language acquisition, success in independent mainstreaming and in vocations not heretofore accessible to the deaf.

Auditory Functioning

Studies in print using tests of speech reception and discrimination are limited to comparing speech reception through auditory, visual, and auditory-visual channels. Erber (1974) found the mean advantage of auditory-visual over lipreading alone to range from 19 to 28 percent.

Leckie, in 1979, showed that children with losses greater than 95 dB in the better ear have a 23 percent improvement for syllables, a 36 percent improvement for predicting the final word in a low predictable sentence, and a 36 percent one in a high predictable sentence. Similar studies have been quoted in the section on facilitation.

Improvement in speech reception and discrimination is given in case histories throughout this book. It is interesting that Moog and Geers (1994) found that no piece of equipment is a panacea for all deaf children. The most important factor is the excellence of the therapy.

Speech Intelligibility

The speech and voice quality of children with hearing impairments tend to be more deviant and less intelligible when the loss is more severe. Suprasegmental deficiencies include abnormal rate and rhythm, lack of inflection, restricted pitch range and a "deaf voice quality," that is, those aspects of spoken language which are normally acquired through hearing, auditory feedback and self-monitoring. Segmental defects include vowel distortions such as prolongation or nasalization, omission or intrusion of consonants, voiced/voiceless confusion, blurring or distortion of consonant blends, and so on. The most difficult consonants are, in fact, those which are the most difficult for normal-hearing preschooler: j, ch, sh, z, s, v, th, and r (Ling, 1992, Ross 1982, and Boothroyd 1982).

Ling (1981) studied the speech production of seven children with average hearing levels of 90 dB in the better ear and no additional handicaps. Following early parent-infant programming, the children were placed in normal-hearing schools and their conversation and that of a normal-hearing control group were recorded and analyzed. Statistical tests indicated that the hearing-impaired were no less intelligible than their normal-hearing peers, and when the study was completed three years later, all the children were judged to be 100 percent intelligible.

Bentzen (1981) reported that the speech of 3,462 children born in 1969 in nine European countries was studied in the eighth year of life (half of them had a hearing loss greater than 90 dB). The ability to speak intelligibly to strangers was judged to differ from two-thirds in some countries to only one-third in others, and the conclusion drawn was that the earliest possible provision of hearing aids and the degree of integration with normal-hearing and speaking children are critical.

Griffiths and Ebbin (1978) reported on a three-year clinical investigation of thirty-four subjects with moderate to severe hearing loss who had been enrolled in an aural/oral program before their second birthday. Some of the children had multiple handicaps. No child was older than five years of age when the study was completed, and a battery of speech, language, perceptual and cognitive tests was administered. Although the rate of accumulation of speech sounds lagged behind that of the normal-hearing group, all sounds were learned in time. There was a significant difference between the children whose hearing aids were fitted before eight months of age and those who were fitted between eight and twenty-four months.

In the reports from the Office of Demographic Studies of Gallaudet College (1975–1978), Jenesma and Trybus show clear trends that early use of hearing aids is correlated with heavier speech emphasis (and less use of signs), with higher speech intelligibility generally related to speech usage or the oralness of the environment, and that *reading scores equate speech intelligibility.*

LANGUAGE ACQUISITION

Although there is a wide range of performance, most studies have shown that there is a two- or three-year delay in the hard-of-hearing, and a four to five year gap for the deaf. For example, Davis (1974), using the Boehm's Test of Basic Concepts, found that 50 percent of the six-year-olds fell at or below the 10th percentile. However, Hannon and Owrid (1974) found that children from higher socioeconomic backgrounds did better than children from lower backgrounds although nonverbal scores were the same for both groups.

Most of the studies emphasize that hearing loss is a depressant to the development of syntax because of insufficient and improper input at the appropriate stage of development. That the basic structures are deviant becomes more apparent when one studies written language samples. Indeed, Quigley (1976) has said repeatedly that few children with a severe or profound loss have adequate reading and writing skills.

Hanners (1973) studied thirty-four children between six and nine years of age in three public school programs which spanned three thousand miles geographically. The first group, AO_1, was exclusively aural/oral; the second group, TC, was exclusively total communication; and the third group, AO_2 and TC_2, had both aural/oral and total communication classes. Only the AO_1 group had systematic audiologic management. All the children had congenital or prelingual hearing impairments of 75 dB or greater in the better ear, were free of other handicaps and had been identified or enrolled in a program no later than thirty-six months of age.

Maternal rubella was given as the etiology in twenty-two of the subjects. The primary measure studied was sentence length, using both written and developmental sentence scoring techniques. The mean sentence scores for the AO_1 group (both individually and as a group) were markedly higher than for the other groups, leading Hanners to suggest that systematic audiologic management and maximal use of residual hearing had made important differences in language acquisition. Hanners noted that programs publicizing their natural language and parent training programs vary considerably in their application of the aural/oral approach, especially with regard to maximal use of residual hearing through wearable amplification.

Luterman (1976) studied forty-nine of his students at Emerson College nursery program: twenty-two from an auditory-oral group and twenty-seven from a visual-oral group, with losses ranging from 75–115 dB in both groups. Each child was administered the five subtests of the ITPA of visual reception, visual association, auditory reception and grammatical closure, as well as the receptive and expressive subtests of the Northwestern Syntax Screening Test. The auditorially trained children were found to be superior in language skills to the visually trained in spite of a two year age advantage in the visual group.

In the most recent study conducted by the Central Institute for the Deaf (Moog and Geers, 1994), 327 children aged five to eight were tested in twelve total communication and thirteen oral programs. Each child had greater than 90 dB hearing level in the better ear and had been educated consistently since age three. Significant differences in the use of correct grammatical structures were apparent with the oral children showing a clear advantage. After the age of seven, the oral children continued to improve whereas the scores of the T.C. group declined for spoken language.

Educational Achievement and Mainstreaming

Ernst (1974) described the educational and communication achievement of twenty-three children (born in 1964 and 1965) from the Acoupedic Program, sixteen of whom were of maternal rubella etiology. McClure (1977) also studied fourteen rubella children who were mainstreamed, and found that they were working at grade level in reading and spelling as measured on the *Wide Range Achievement Test.*

Northcott described a longitudinal study of eleven auditory children who graduated from the Minnesota Infant Preschool public school program. In grades three to five, they were within the normal range as a group in achievement test scores and sociometric range of behavior. McConnell (1975) reported similar results for his graduates. For examples of mainstreaming success, see the outcome surveys of Auditory-Verbal graduates.

Balow and Brill (1975) did an extensive study of the achievement in reading and arithmetic of 590 children. They found that deaf children who had attended an early oral program scored significantly higher than those who had not. This is surprising after the students had spent several years in a nonoral school, and it contradicts studies which report that deaf children of deaf parents score higher than deaf children of hearing parents (which is usually interpreted to mean that early oral education is ineffective).

Bloom (1975) followed up the school placement of children described by Luterman and reported under the section on language tests in this chapter. She found that so many of the auditory children achieved fully integrated status (or day school placement as opposed to schools for the deaf) that the data suggests the auditory approach develops sufficient communication skills necessary to succeed in a fully integrated setting, especially since the hearing levels, when training was begun, were comparable in both groups. In addition, the results on the visual subtests of the ITPA were essentially the same for both groups which implies that normal hearing-impaired children will develop visual awareness without formal instructions, and therefore it might be wiser to use therapy time to develop better auditory skills.

Several other educators have studied educational mainstreaming of deaf infants. Tell et al. (1981) followed sixty-five children of whom twenty-nine (twelve profoundly deaf and seventeen severely deaf children) continued their education in regular schools. Tell felt that normal or above normal intelligence, good progress in language acquisition, and complete dedication of the parents were important factors.

Psycho-Social Development

Problems about social adjustment and self-confidence are not inevitable as was shown in the Kennedy et al. (1976) longitudinal sociometric and cross-sectional data on mainstreaming hearing-impaired children. However, the children did show a greater dependency on adult help.

Langston, a school psychologist, studied the results of aural-oral programming in Arkansas (Kirkman, 1975) and in the Colorado Acoupedic Program (1976, but unpublished). Langston was impressed by the fact that profoundly impaired youngsters, aged eight to thirteen, were able to perform well on the verbal portion of the Wechsler Intelligence Scale for Children (Revised) rather than with special nonverbal (or manual) testing standardly used with hearing-impaired populations. She also noted their success in mainstreaming into regular education, and their good acceptance of their hearing aids, possibly due to proper functioning and good parent education.

Langston further stressed that their ability to respond to normal conversational speech, that is, to relate in a testing situation to a stranger who used a normal tone of voice, was one of the largest differences between the children in the auditory program and other hearing-impaired children. There was a noticeable lack of internalization that they were "deaf"—that is, most self-concepts were free of seeing themselves as primarily hearing-impaired.

OUTCOME SURVEYS

The first problem facing parents with children diagnosed as deaf is the choice of habilitation program. Educators are concerned with the problem of predicting the best program for an individual. Studies have been either retrospective or they have been longitudinal.

Auditory-Verbal Surveys

1. One of the first projects to study auditory-verbal preschoolers was undertaken at the University of Denver (Stewart, 1965). He compared the vocabulary usage of A–V children with an oral (lipreading) group after five years. In spite of mostly monaural hearing aids, the A–V children scored significantly higher.

2. A retrospective study was conducted of children in the Acoupedic Program at Porter Hospital in Denver (Yoshinaga-Itano and Pollack, 1983) by studying data in hospital charts and by sending a questionnaire to parents who were listed in the metropolitan telephone directory. Out of more than 200 children who had attended the program between 1965 and 1981, 120 were contacted and 81 responded. They were felt to be representative of the total number.

    Most of the children had been referred by physicians or other parents. However, parents were encouraged to visit different programs before making a commitment to Acoupedics because parent participation was a requisite for the program.

    Itano reported on many factors:

    1. Unaided hearing loss, speech reception and discrimination.
    2. Aided audiogram, speech reception, and discrimination.
    3. Etiology of hearing loss, if known.
    4. Age of hearing aids fitting.

    5. Performance and verbal intelligence, if tested.
    6. Parents' educational and vocational levels.
    7. Children's present means of communication (speech or sign).
    8. Children's educational placement (mainstreamed without interpreter, or special education).
    9. Children's type of vocation (if school graduate).
   10. Financial cost.

Finally, Itano studied the longitudinal scores for the Peabody Picture Vocabulary Test, which was given routinely as part of the children's annual evaluations, beginning at 3 or 4 years of age and continuing until nine. Other studies have found that the PPVT is the best predictor of reading achievement (Davis et al., 1981).

Itano found that the children fell into two groups, the quicker and the slower learners. Group 1 either caught up to their normal-hearing peers or were within one year of their chronological age. Group 2 remained within two or two-and-a-half years of their peers. Although comparable in most factors, group 2 contained more children with multiple handicaps.

Degree of hearing loss and performance intelligence quotient were found to be poor predictors of language success, although the configuration of the loss was a factor to be considered. Etiology raised questions for future research. In this group of children, those with genetic losses seemed to have more language learning difficulty. Those children with rubella etiology, but no other handicaps, excelled in spoken language, probably because they had more remaining hair cells which resulted in better discrimination.

Early intervention was obviously important: 16 of the children were aided by 12 months of age, and 48 by two years. The majority had profound losses in both ears, or severe losses in one ear and profound in the other ear. But with appropriate audiological management and an auditory program, the mean aided speech reception was 41.3 dB, and discrimination was a mean of 71.6 percent without visual cues.

Parents reported that 63 used only speech for communication and 17 used speech with hearing people and sign with deaf people. One child used only sign because he was severely multicapped.

Educationally, the majority, 62, were mainstreamed without an interpreter, although they might have received some supportive services. Only 19 were in special education classes. This is surprising because 15 had severe physical or developmental problems and 18 others had received therapy for sensorimotor integration.

Ten of the group were then between 26 and 34 years of age, and were in vocations not usually open to deaf adults: lawyer, vocational counselor, bank teller, preschool teacher, accountant, cartographer, and so on.

The author feels that the most important factor was parent commitment. Although ranging from high school dropout to graduate student, mothers were homemakers, and there were few divorces. However, in the later years of the program, there were more single working mothers, a trend which may affect the quality and quantity of language stimulation for all deaf children.[1]

3. Goldberg and Flexer (1994) also conducted a survey of graduates of Auditory-Verbal programs in Canada and the United States. This survey looked only at the social validity of A–V principles. Three hundred sixty-six questionnaires were sent with a response rate of 42.9 percent. One hundred fifty-seven usable forms were returned. Ages ranged from 18 to 47 years, with the majority in their twenties.

The survey revealed the following:

Severe to Profound or Profound	93%
Hearing Loss in the Better Ear:	93%
Prelingual Loss:	95%
Etiology Unknown:	54%
Rubella Etiology (among the older graduates)	28.9%
Average Age of Hearing Aid Fitting:	27 MOS.

Educational History of Complete Mainstreaming:	
Elementary School:	78.5%
Middle School:	86.7%

One hundred twenty-four graduates attended or were enrolled in normal-hearing colleges or universities, and only 15 were in colleges dedicated to the education of the deaf.

Approximately one-third of the respondents reported having additional problems.

The jobs reported included a wide range from blue-collar to professional, including attorneys and doctors.

When queried about their families' involvement in their ther-

---

[1]A detailed copy of this report is available from the LISTEN Foundation, 3535 So. Sherman St., Englewood, Colorado 80110.

apy and education, all but one stated that their mothers were actively involved, with 76 percent staying at home during their children's preschool years. Fathers were said to have given encouragement and help, mainly with homework.

The graduates were questioned as to their perceptions of their current participation in the "hearing," "deaf," or both worlds. 72.7 percent replied that they were part of the hearing world.

The results of this survey are remarkably similar to the one conducted by Itano and Pollack.

4. Robertson and Flexer (1993) conducted a parent survey of reading levels of children who had learned speech and language through Auditory-Verbal methods. The hypothesis that guided this study was that children with hearing impairments who learn standard spoken language through using amplified hearing will learn to read in the same normal and predictable ways as normal-hearing children. Three hundred surveys were given to parents, with 76 being returned from parents in the United States and Canada, and 29 from Germany and Switzerland. (The latter were not used in the results.)

The children ranged in age from 6 to 19 at the time of the survey, with approximately 81 percent reporting severe to profound hearing loss. Approximately half were male and half female. Fifty-four children were of school age and all but one were placed in regular classrooms. Parents supplied standardized reading scores for 37 children. Seven children read below the fiftieth percentile, 14 at the fiftieth, and 16 above.

Among the interesting details in this report, 94 percent were read to daily during early childhood and liked to read. All but one participated in extracurricular activities with normal-hearing peers.

That 86 percent of the children read at or above their grade level is in stark contrast to the reports of reading achievement in the general population of persons with hearing impairment (Geers and Moog, 1989) and current reports from special education administrators that deaf children are still being graduated with third or fourth grade reading levels.

A University of Colorado Study

Although this is not an Auditory-Verbal study per se, it does include Auditory-Verbal children.

Since little is known about prelinguistic precursors of early language in very young hearing-impaired infants, an important longitudinal study is taking place in Colorado, where 55 percent of newborns are currently screened at birth. The majority of the infants are referred by the Department of Public Health and few of the parents come from middle or upper economic groups. Many of the children have multiple handicaps.

Families are enrolled in an intervention program named CHIP—Colorado Home Intervention Program. Parent facilitators visit the homes and guide and observe parent-child interactions. Parents are said to be informed by unbiased information about method options and are free to make their own choice. Surprisingly, more parents chose signing or total communication than auditory-oral. One wonders if they were informed about the long-term implications and especially their need to become fluent signers themselves.

Assessment occurs every six months by using parent questionnaires and videotapes of typical parent-child communicative interactions.

Reports[2] to date include the following:

1. From Phone to Phoneme (Itano and Stredler-Brown, 1992), using a Phonetic/Phonologic Assessment of hearing-impaired infants and toddlers. The researchers count the number of vowels and consonants, the number of speech utterances, and the mean number of speech elements per utterance. (Since 1985, when 149 infants have been tested, more sophisticated assessment procedures have been reported in the literature.)

   This paper concludes that appropriate early intervention may prevent the characteristics which have inhibited the development of intelligible speech in the past. The authors also declare that signing has not had a deleterious effect upon speech because the transition into meaningful language appears to support the development of speech production. This contradicts the findings of Moog and Geers (1994) that the more children signed, the less they spoke.

2. Learning to Communicate: Babies With Hearing Impairments Make their Needs Known (Yoshinaga-Itano and Stredler-Brown, 1992).

   This study is based on pragmatic use of indexical gestures which are critical to the development of language in hearing-impaired children. 096The Communicative Intention Inventory

---

[2]Obtainable from the Department of Communication Disorders, The University of Colorado, Campus Box 409, Boulder, CO 80209.

(Coggins and Carpenter, 1981) was used. The infant has to adopt different strategies at different stages of development.

3. Early Identification and Intervention: The Effect on Infants with Hearing Impairment (Itano and Apuzzo, 1993 and 1994).

The original study separated the infants into two groups: those identified from birth to six months, and those identified after 18 months. As the numbers grew, subjects were divided into four groups based upon age of identification: birth to two months; 3 to 12 months; 13 to 24 months; and subjects identified after 25 months. Each group contained subjects with varying degrees of hearing loss. Each category had a mean age of 40 months at the time of testing. Subjects were tested for their Development quotients on the Minnesota Child Developmental Inventories (MCDI). Subtests on the MCDI included general development, gross motor, fine motor, expressive language, comprehension-conceptual, situation comprehension, self-help and personal-social. Subjects in the earliest identification group scored significantly higher than the other groups in general development and expressive language.

4. A later report (Itano, Apuzzo, Coulter and Stredler-Brown, 1995) stated that children identified between birth and six months have significantly higher developmental functioning at 40 months of age compared with those identified after six months. Children with mild-to-severe sensorineural losses perform similarly at 40 months of age on their language functioning and general development when they are identified at birth. Only those with profound losses have significantly lower developmental functioning, but even they were only 12 to 15 months below their chronological age at 40 months.

When amplification was fit within two to three months of identification and intervention begun immediately, the advantages were found at all levels between 18 months and 36 months in the following areas: expressive language, expressive and receptive vocabulary, and number of vowels and consonants.

5. The Language Development of Young Hearing-Impaired Children, Using the MacArthur Communicative Developmental Inventories (Carey, 1986).

This study compared the CHIP infants with the norms for normal-hearing infants (Bates, Bretherton and Snyder, 1988, and Fenson, Dale, Reznick, Bates, Thal, and Pethick, 1994).

Carey looked at the many variables involved: age of identifi-

naires used, such as the MCDI, the Calhoun Play Assessment, and the Westby Symbolic Playscale.

The most interesting finding was the relationship between cognition and age of identification. Those who were identified early and had normal cognition (such as 80 and above on the MCDI) consistently performed the best on all sections of the MacArthur CDI inventories.

When analyzing age of identification only, infants identified before six months consistently out-performed those identified after six months.

The language development rate of hearing-impaired children does seem to replicate that of hearing children, although a delay is seen in each of the four sections of the MacArthur study.

The degree of hearing loss did not have an effect in gestures used or phrases understood. The only difference seen was in the Words Produced and Words Understood sections of the Inventories. For children with profound losses, their developmental trend on these sections appeared characteristically different. However, it is important to realize that even a mild loss will result in a delay in vocabulary production, thus underscoring the importance of early intervention. The amount of delay is highly dependent on cognitive status.

The two groups must be compared on the development of *spoken* language, that is, without signs, because this is the communication system used in the U.S. and the "hearing world." For a discussion of the issues related to sign language and Deaf culture, the reader is referred to *A Child Sacrificed* (Bertling, 1995).

Chapter 5

AUDIOLOGICAL ASSESSMENT

DONALD GOLDBERG

INTRODUCTION

A critical need exists for the early detection, identification, and management of infants, toddlers, and children with hearing impairments. The comprehensive audiologic management of these youngsters is a most essential component in the successful implementation of the Auditory-Verbal Approach.

The purpose of this chapter is to review the audiologic assessment of neonates, infants, and children, including objective and physiological, as well as subjective and behavioral measures. In addition, the Auditory-Verbal International Suggested Protocol for Audiological and Hearing Aid Evaluation (AVI, 1991a) will be described as the model for comprehensive audiologic diagnostics and management of these children. In this and the following chapter, it is noted that the comprehensive audiologic management of children with hearing impairment attempts to address Principles 1 and 2 from the Auditory-Verbal International, Inc. Position Statement (1991b), specifically:

(1) Supporting and promoting programs for the early detection and identification of hearing impairment and the auditory management of infants, toddlers, and children so identified.

(2) Providing the earliest and most appropriate use of medical and amplification technology to achieve the maximum benefits available.

Principles of auditory-verbal practice have been adapted from Pollack (1970; 1985).

It is the authors' hope that with a solid foundation of audiology in an auditory-verbal approach, more children will be afforded the opportunity to learn to listen and to learn spoken language.

VARIABLES OF HEARING IMPAIRMENT

Children with hearing impairment are considered to be an extremely heterogeneous population. A number of variables make comparisons among these children difficult and inherently inappropriate. A listing of several variables of hearing impairments is presented in Table 5-I. No one variable is categorically more important than another, but instead, it is the unique combination of several of these factors which result in a wide variety of outcomes.

TABLE 5-I.
VARIABLES OF HEARING IMPAIRMENTS

---

age of onset
etiology
type of hearing disorder (conductive, sensorineural, mixed or central)
degree of hearing loss (mild through profound)
configuration of hearing loss (symmetry, degree of slope, unilateral versus bilateral)
hearing age*
consistency of amplification
speech perception abilities
presence of other disabilities
learning environment
type of intervention services

Hearing (or Listening) age refers to the time that a child with a hearing impairment has consistently worn appropriate amplification.

It is not uncommon for parents to try to compare children with the same degree of hearing loss. Difficulty exists, however, in categorizing hearing impairments into discrete levels due to the fact that the degree of hearing loss exists on a continuum. Two children, even with the same audiogram, will most likely have different communication abilities due to the variety of factors noted above. Although patterns do exist, for example, children with prelingual, severe to profound hearing impairments will not learn spoken language unless intervention occurs (Ling, 1989); predictions of how children with hearing impairments *will be* when they grow up is not advisable. Generalizations from an audiogram alone are inappropriate due to the myriad of factors influencing the behavior of children with hearing impairments.

DIAGNOSIS OF HEARING IMPAIRMENT—NEONATES

High-Risk Registers

According to the National Institutes of Health (1993), there is a clear need in the United States for improved methods and models for the early identification of hearing impairment in infants and young children. The average age of identification of hearing loss in children is presently 2.5 years with some loss unidentified until six years of age. There is an inverse relationship between the average age of identification and the degree of hearing loss, with more severe hearing impairments being diagnosed earlier in life (Pappas & McDowell, 1983). The earlier a hearing impairment is identified, the sooner medical, audiological, and amplification intervention can be initiated.

The Joint Committee on Infant Hearing, formed to address this issue, recommended in 1982 that infants at high risk of hearing loss be screened, and developed the High Risk Registry. The Registry was an initial list of indicators or risk factors. In 1990 and in 1993, the Joint Committee modified the original list to improve detection (COR, 1993). Several factors have been specified by the Joint Committee on Infant Hearing Screening as placing neonates and infants at risk for hearing impairment (ASHA, 1991). Should a child present with any of the factors outlined in Table 5-II, careful audiologic follow-up is recommended.

Universal Newborn Hearing Screening

Research findings have indicated, however, that risk factors identify only 50 percent of infants with significant hearing loss (Pappas, 1983; Eissmann, Matkin, & Sabo, 1987; Mawk, White, Mortensen, & Behrens, 1991). In an effort to identify the remaining children, the National Institute on Deafness and Other Communication Disorders (NIDCD) issued a report in the spring of 1993 on early identification of hearing impairment in infants who are deaf or hard-of-hearing. With the availability of modern technology affording us with methods for the accurate and reliable assessment of newborns' hearing, it was concluded in the NIH Consensus Statement that newborn hearing screening should be universal.

According to the NIH Consensus Statement (1993), the preferred model for universal screening should begin with an evoked otoacoustic

TABLE 5-II
JOINT COMMITTEE ON INFANT HEARING RISK FACTORS (ASHA, 1991)

Neonates (Birth to 28 Days)

- Family history of childhood hearing impairment;
- Congenital infection known or suspected to be associated with sensorineural hearing impairment such as toxoplasmosis, syphilis, rubella (German measles), cytomegalovirus (CMV), and herpes;
- Unusual ear, eye, head, or neck development including cleft lip or palate, low hairline, extra skin or pits near the pinna; and so forth;
- Birth weight less than 1500 grams (3 lbs., 5 oz.);
- Severe jaundice (hyperbilirubinemia) at levels that required an exchange of blood transfusion;
- Use of certain ototoxic medications known to damage hearing, for more than 5 days and loop diuretics in combination with these;
- Bacterial meningitis;
- Birth Apgar scores of 0 to 3 at 5 minutes, or a history of failing to initiate spontaneous respiration by 10 minutes after birth, or a history of hypotonia persisting to 2 hours of age;
- Prolonged mechanical ventilation (to assist breathing) for a duration equal to or greater than 10 days;
- Indicators associated with a syndrome known to include hearing impairment (e.g., Waardenburg or Usher's syndrome).

Infants (29 Days to 2 Years)

- Presence of any of the criteria listed above for neonates at risk;
- Parents or caregivers have concerns regarding hearing, speech, language, and/or developmental delay;
- Presence of neonatal risk factors associated with progressive sensorineural hearing impairment;
- History of head trauma;
- Presence of neurodegenerative disorders (diseases that cause degeneration of the nervous system);
- History of childhood infectious diseases known to be associated with sensorineural hearing impairment (e.g., measles).

emissions test and should be followed by an auditory brainstem response test for all infants who fail the evoked otoacoustic emissions test.

Because not all hearing impairments are present at birth, the significant number of infants and children who develop hearing impairments during the first years of life, must be detected via hearing screening programs through daycare and Head Start programs; education programs of parents, primary caretakers, medical and nursing personnel; and all other professionals who have opportunity to observe the child and recognize factors that place the child at high risk for hearing impairment. School entry will also provide an additional opportunity for universal identification of children with significant hearing impairment (NIH, 1993).

Few would argue that via universal screenings, use of high-risk registers, and/or professional responsiveness to parental concerns regarding infants, toddlers, and children with hearing impairments, intervention can be initiated as soon as possible. Identification and intervention for children with hearing impairments will ideally transpire at earlier ages in our future.

Objective Measurements

The objective measurements of neonates is strongly advocated. The most frequently utilized electrophysiological measurements in the objective assessment of newborn hearing are auditory evoked potentials, specifically Brainstem Auditory Evoked Response potentials [BAER or Auditory Brainstem Response (ABR) testing] and Otoacoustic Emissions (OAEs).

Auditory Evoked Potentials (AEPs)

As noted by Martin (1991), the electrical responses to a signal propagated along the auditory pathway are typically defined based on the latency or time period that elapses between the introduction of a stimulus and the occurrence of the response. Responses in the first 10 milliseconds after the introduction of a signal are believed to originate in the brainstem and are referred to as auditory brainstem responses (ABRs) (see Figure 5.1). AEPs occurring from 10 to 50 milliseconds in latency are called auditory middle latency responses (AMLRs), and are believed to originate in the auditory cortex. Late evoked responses (LERs) occur beyond 50 milliseconds and arise in the cortex (Martin, 1991).

Auditory Brainstem Response (ABR) testing involves the attachment of electrodes to various landmarks on the head. The electrodes measure the electrical signal caused by nerves firing in response to sound stimuli presented through earphones or a bone oscillator (Flexer, 1994). Martin (1991) states that if the ABR is elicited by click stimuli, hearing sensitivity is believed to be assessed from 1000 to 4000 Hz. Threshold data is inferred based on the auditory threshold observed in the ABR tracings. Should tone pip stimuli be utilized, more specific threshold data will be obtained across a wider frequency range.

It must be noted that the ABR response will be compromised should middle ear pathology exist and is dependent on the child being relatively motionless. Sedation may be necessary depending on the state of

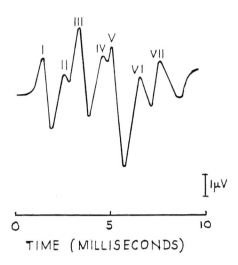

Figure 5.1. Brainstem audiometry: waves I through VII.

the child. In any case, the ABR has developed into an important test in diagnostic audiology, one which has proven sensitivity, specificity, and efficiency (Martin, 1991).

Otoacoustic Emissions (OAEs)–Kemp (1978) first reported that signals are emitted from the inner ear into the external auditory meatus in response to auditory stimulation with clicks. The two general classes of OAEs include spontaneous and evoked (Kenworthy, 1993). Spontaneous emissions (SOAEs), which occur without any external stimuli, appear in about 40 percent of subjects with normal hearing (e.g., Probst, Coats, Martin, & Lounsbury-Martin, 1986). Kenworthy (1993) stated that SOAEs appear useful in explicating cochlear mechanics but are impractical as a screening response. Nearly universal in ears with normal hearing, however, are evoked otoacoustic emissions (EOAEs) (e.g., Johnson, Bagi, Parbo, & Eberling, 1988) and not observed in the presence of peripheral hearing loss greater than 30 to 40 dB HL (Kemp, Ryan, & Bray, 1990). Today, EOAEs have been routinely utilized in many hearing screening programs. Measurement time is brief (approximately 1 to 3 minutes) and essentially noninvasive (see Figure 5.2).

Subjective or Behavioral Measurements

Subjective or behavioral measurements can play a role in the measurement of the hearing of newborns, however, clinical impressions should

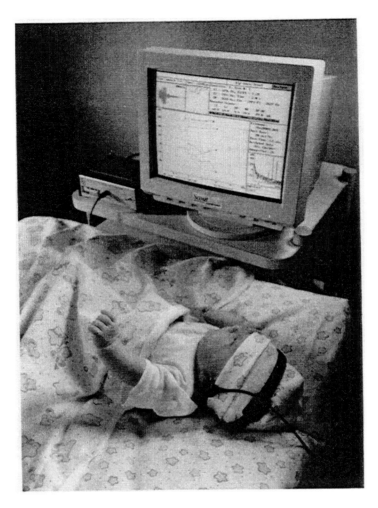

Figure 5.2. Distortion Product Otoacoustic Emission (DPOAE) screening of an infant (Photo courtesy of Bio-Logic Systems Corporation).

routinely be verified with objective measurements. Even the most experienced pediatric audiologist runs the risk of testing a newborn and making judgments which are inaccurate interpretations of the hearing status of the neonate, when relying exclusively on subjective/behavioral measures.

DIAGNOSIS OF HEARING IMPAIRMENTS—INFANTS

Infants are both a joy and a challenge to test. It is fair to state that experienced pediatric audiologists are needed to establish an optimal test situation. In the author's work site, two certified and licensed audiologists work together as a team for all pediatric assessments of children three years old and younger. One audiologist serves as the test assistant in the booth with the child and his/her parent. This audiologist has the important role of keeping the child on task, often including much direction of the child to the midline, in order that both audiologists might observe a localization response to one or both sides. The second audiologist is positioned in the examiner's area. The two audiologists are in communication with each other either via a monitor set, the bone oscillator, or headphone system, along with microphones set up to pick up all verbal communications (see Figure 5.3). It is most important for the audiologist in the booth to be made aware of the timing of presentations being delivered to the child. Therefore, if there are false positive responses, the child can be prompted that "there was no sound" and be encouraged to respond only when he/she hears the sound. The agreement between the audiologists regarding the reliability of the response behaviors observed is critical in the determination of threshold data.

Physiological Measurements

Again, the use of ABR and OAE testing would be an appropriate recommendation, especially if behavioral measurements are equivocal or if the infant is hard to test. In addition, due to the likelihood that infant testing will be accomplished in the sound field, it will not be known in which ear the tones are heard, that is, a lack of ear specificity arises. Should an ear difference exist, the child will potentially be responding with the better ear and the configuration and severity of the hearing loss in the nonsymmetrical ear will not be accurately assessed.

Behavioral Measurements

Behavioral Observational Audiometry

Typically in Behavioral Observational Audiometry (BOA), the infant is positioned upon one of the parent's lap, or is seated in a high chair. The parent is instructed to avoid making any overt responses to the

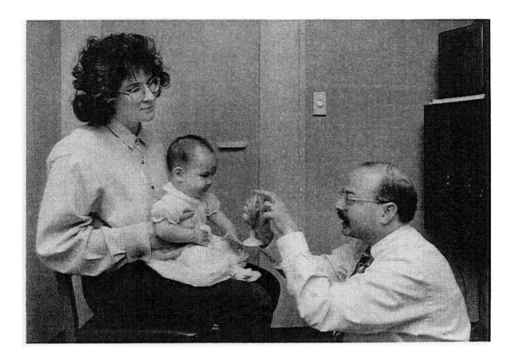

Figure 5-3. Use of a test assistant during infant audiologic testing.

sound stimuli to be presented, as the parent's response behaviors may transfer to the child and thereby confound the observation. If it is anticipated that the intensity of the testing stimuli will be loud, the parent should be provided ear plugs and/or ear muffs (the audiologist serving as the test assistant in the booth should be similarly protected).

BOA evaluates the infant's unconditioned response behaviors. The test stimuli are presented in the sound-treated room via loudspeakers and it is the audiologists' responsibility to evaluate the presence and consistency of the responses (see Figure 5.4). Various auditory milestones have been established to assist the interpretation of response behaviors of infants at varying age ranges (see McConnell & Ward, 1967; Northern & Downs, 1984). It should be noted that the response behaviors observed are often considered Minimal Response Levels (MRLs) and are not typically a "true" threshold, but instead indicative of identifiable behavioral changes which are most likely above or louder than the actual threshold. Flexer (1994) cautioned that BOA testing can be significantly influenced by the infant's state, methodology of stimulus presentation, variables of the infant's response behaviors, and observer bias.

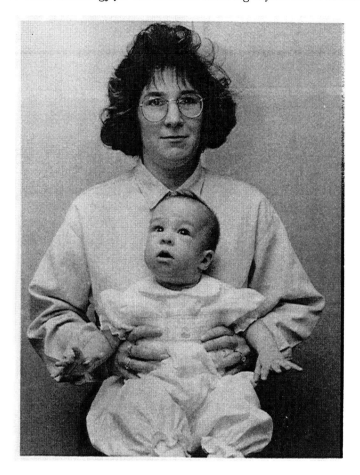

Figure 5-4. Behavioral Observation Audiometry.

Visual Reinforcement Audiometry/Conditioned Orientation (Operant) Reflex (Response) Audiometry

In Visual Reinforcement Audiometry (VRA) (Liden & Kankkunen, 1969) or Conditioned Orientation (or Operant) Reflex (or Response) (COR) (Suzuki & Ogiba, 1961) testing, sound stimuli are initially paired with the lighting and animation of characters (for examples, a panda bear, clown, or "Barney") often positioned on speakers in the sound-treated room. The child ideally makes head turn movements to each side. After the child is under stimulus:response control, the sound stimuli are presented alone. Should the child localize to a speaker, he/she is rewarded with the illumination and animation of the character (see

Figures 5.5 and 5.6). Threshold data or MRLs are subsequently determined in evaluating the hearing status of the infant.

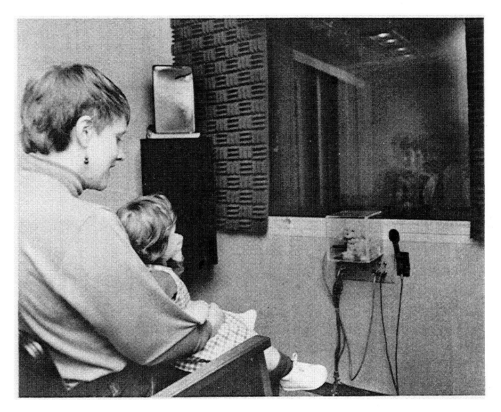

Figure 5-5. Visual Reinforcement Audiometry.

It has been this examiner's practice that should the child localize to the opposite speaker from which the sound stimuli was delivered, he/she will be reinforced by the character on the side turned to. However, a notation is made regarding the child's localization response behavior.

DIAGNOSIS OF HEARING IMPAIRMENTS—CHILDREN

Physiological Measurements

Typically, children can be tested using behavioral measurements. In the rare instance that behavioral testing does not result in the complete audiometric picture for both the right and left ears via air and bone

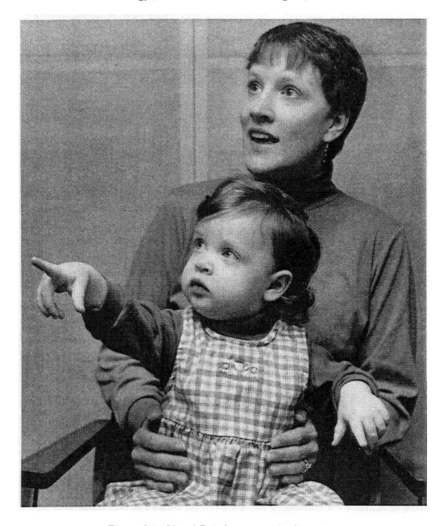

Figure 5-6. Visual Reinforcement Audiometry.

conduction audiometry, as well as speech data for each ear, physiological measurements such as ABR testing can be completed.

Behavioral Measurements

Behavioral Observational Audiometry

Infants up to six months of age are often assessed via physiological measures or Behavioral Observational Audiometry. It should be anticipated that above six months, children can be tested by measures such as

Visual Reinforcement Audiometry or Conditioned Play Audiometry. Should children be unable to proceed to these other measurement procedures, questions might be posed regarding the child's cognitive and developmental status.

Visual Reinforcement Audiometry

As was described with the infants, some older children will still need to be tested using VRA/COR procedures. It is noted that the VRA/COR equipment may be used for those children who are not yet able to complete Conditioned Play Audiometry (CPA) tasks. A skilled audiologist will be able to amass important audiological data for children who are in the "limbo" area of being too old for standard VRA testing, but not yet conditioned for standard CPA.

Conditioned Play Audiometry

One of the most important pieces of information the audiologist is searching for is thresholds for each ear, that is, ear-specific data. At the earliest possible point in time, the audiologist will be determined to make use of either insert earphones (see Figure 5.7) or standard headphones. Even if the audiologist must continue to use the VRA equipment as reinforcers, getting separate ear thresholds is most important, as the implications for amplification, probe-tube real ear measurements, etc. are contingent upon right and left ear data.

In Conditioned Play Audiometry (CPA), the child is required to perform a motoric task in response to the presentation of pulsed or steady state tones. Perhaps the most classic CPA materials used are blocks being dropped in a bucket (see Figure 5.8). It is important, however, that a variety of CPA materials are available. Some examples of materials this audiologist has made use of include: rings on a spindle, marbles on a track, marbles into a bud vase of water, puzzle pieces into a puzzle frame, cars down a slide, etc. The challenge for the audiologists is to keep the child interested. Unfortunately, some children think that once they have gone through the first group of materials (for example 15 blocks), their work is finished. It is important not to suggest to the child that all they will be doing is playing with these finite number of blocks. Threshold determination will be most dependent on the bracketing procedure utilized and the child's reliability of responding. With the same items being recycled for the child, just the suggestion of competition whereby the child and audiologist "race" to see who drops the block

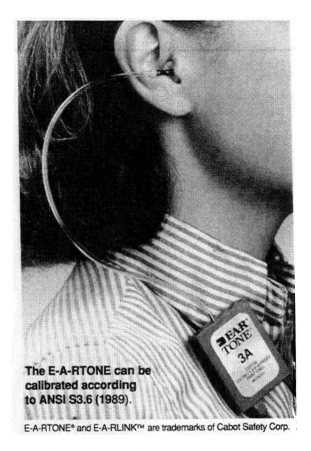

The E-A-RTONE can be calibrated according to ANSI S3.6 (1989).

E-A-RTONE® and E-A-RLINK™ are trademarks of Cabot Safety Corp.

Figure 5-7. Insert earphones (photograph courtesy of Cabot Safety Corporation, Auditory System Division, manufacturer of the E-A-RTONE 3A Insert Earphone).

in first, can extend the child's attention for several more presentations (the audiologist is, of course, reminded not to beat the child in responding to the sound presentation!).

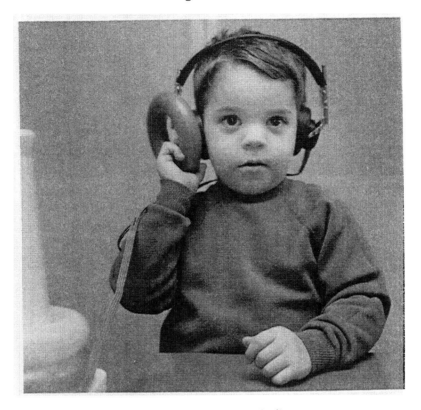

Figure 5.8. Conditioned Play Audiometry.

COMPREHENSIVE AUDIOLOGIC DIAGNOSTICS AND MANAGEMENT

The AVI Suggested Protocol for Audiological and Hearing Aid Evaluation

In response to the need to delineate recommended components of a comprehensive audiological and amplification management program for children with hearing impairments, the board of directors of Auditory-Verbal International (AVI) developed a protocol to standardize clinical practices and suggest assessment components (see Table 5-III). Its use is recommended, regardless of the communication program in which a child might be enrolled (see Appendix A).

TABLE 5-III.
SUGGESTED PROTOCOL FOR AUDIOLOGICAL AND
HEARING AID EVALUATION (AVI) 1991A).

The audiological test procedures indicated are recommended for use with children in order to ensure that maximum use of residual hearing can be achieved. A battery of audiological tests is always suggested since no single procedure has sufficient reliability to stand alone. Optimally, every aural habilitation program should have on-site audiological services, but regardless of setting, close cooperation between audiology and therapy service providers is essential. Parents should be present for, and participate in, the administration of all assessment procedures in order to include them in this aspect of the child's care.

Procedures to be Included in All Audiological Assessments, Regardless of Child's Age

- Case History/Parent Observation Report
- Otoscopic Inspection
- Acoustic Immittance: Tympanometry, Physical Volume Test, and Acoustic Reflexes. Cautious interpretation is recommended if the child is younger than six months.

For a Child 0–6 Months of Age, the Following Additional Tests are Recommended

- Auditory Brainstem Response (ABR)—Alternating click and tone and tone pips response by air conduction and by bone conduction. CAUTION: ABR should not stand alone for diagnostic purposes. Lack of response to ABR testing does not necessarily indicate an absence of usable hearing.
- Amplification and auditory learning are recommended as the first option unless special imaging (CT Scan or MRI) confirms an absence of the cochlea. Behavioral testing, amplification, and therapy are otherwise indicated before a decision of no usable hearing is made.

For a Child 6 Months to 2 Years of Age, the Following Tests are Recommended
Use Behavioral Observation Audiometry (BOA) or Visual Reinforcement Audiometry (VRA) to obtain the following:

- Detection/Awareness of voice and warbled tones from 250–6000 Hz in the sound field and/or 250–8000 Hz under headphones.
- Startle response in sound field, under headphones, and by bone conduction.
- Evaluation of auditory skill development.

For a Child 2 to 5 Years of Age, the Following Tests are Recommended
Use VRA or Conditioned Play Audiometry (CPA) to obtain the following:

- Responses to pure tones from 250–12,000 Hz by air conduction, and bone conduction from 500–4000 Hz with masking (at $3^{1}/2$ years+).
- Speech Awareness Threshold (Speech Recognition Threshold, if language development allows) using Ling Six Sounds (/m/, /u/, /i/, /a/, / ʃ /, /s/), body parts, speech perception tasks, or formal tests such as the WIPI.

For a Child 5 Years of Age and Older, the Following Tests are Recommended

Use CPA or standard audiometry to obtain the following:

- Air and bone conduction, Speech Recognition and Speech/Word Identification.

TABLE 5-III (Continued)

Amplification Assessment

Electroacoustic Analysis of Hearing Aids Should Be Performed

- On day of fitting
- At 30–90 day intervals at user volume as well as full-on volume.
- Whenever a hearing aid is repaired. In addition, do a close check of internal settings.
- Whenever parental listening check or behavioral observation raises concern.

Sound Field Aided Response

- Parents and therapists can prepare the children by teaching them to respond consistently to voice and the Ling Six Sounds.
- Aided measures should include: Speech Awareness or Recognition, Word Identification at 55 dB HL in quiet, and, if possible, in noise; response to warbled pure tones from 250–6000 Hz wearing binaural hearing aids, or monaural measures to complete responses at each ear.

CAUTION: It is important that the aided results be evaluated in relation to the unaided audiogram. Recommended aided results for the "left corner" audiogram with optimum amplification should be in the 35–45 dB HL (ANSI) or better range at 250, 500, 1000 Hz.

Probe Microphone (Real Ear) Measures Should Include

- Unoccluded measurement of External Ear Effect as well as full occlusion with the hearing aid OFF to measure insertion loss.
- Insertion gain measured with hearing aid at customary settings to verify appropriate gain and output levels and to compare change in settings.

CAUTION: Many of the existing formulae may underestimate the gain required by children with severe to profound hearing impairment.

FM Systems

- When FM systems are in use, they should be evaluated at the time of the complete audiological and hearing aid assessment using the same format described for amplification.

Frequency of Assessment (Aided and Unaided)

- Every 90 days once diagnosis is confirmed and amplification fitted, until age 3.
- As early as possible, but at least by age 2, a complete unaided and aided audiogram should be obtained (preferably under headphones, but at least in the sound field).
- New earmolds may need to be obtained at 90 day intervals or sooner until age 3–4 years in view of the typically rapid growth rate at this time.
- Assessment every 6 months from age 4–6 years is appropriate if progress is satisfactory.
- Above age 6 years, assessment at 6–12 month intervals is appropriate with earmolds at the same intervals.

TABLE 5-3 (Continued)

• Immediate evaluation should be scheduled if parents or caretakers suspect a change in hearing or hearing aid function.

CAUTION: Modifications of this schedule are appropriate when middle ear disease is chronic or recurrent, and/or when additional disabilities are present.

Reports

Reports should be supplied promptly upon receipt of written release and sent to parents, therapists, physicians, and educators. Reports should include:

- Test procedures and reliability assessment.
- The complete audiogram with symbol key, calibration standard, and stimuli used.
- Hearing aid identification or make, model, output and volume settings, compression or special feature settings.
- FM system identification and settings.
- Interpretive information regarding relationship of audiological findings to acoustic phonetics, especially with respect to distance hearing and message competition.
- Analysis of auditory behaviors and development of the listening function.

It should be noted that for children with sensorineural hearing loss, aggressive medical and audiological management of middle ear problems should transpire. The addition of the conductive hearing loss on top of the existing sensorineural hearing loss leads to an increased communicative deficit and, therefore, must be attended to quickly and proactively.

Case History/Parent Observation Report

It is the belief of this author that parents are the best diagnosticians. In fact, mothers are typically the first to notice a problem with their child's hearing (Haas & Crowley, 1982; Shah, Chandler, & Dale, 1978).

In early diagnostics, the use of a case history form is advocated, so that the audiologist and other professionals have documentation regarding a host of factors which may be relevant in the identification and management of a child with a hearing impairment. It is advisable for the written questionnaire to be completed by the family prior to the audiologic appointment. Basic identifying and demographic information is initially determined. It is advisable for an open-ended question be provided which asks the parents to state in their own words what it is about their child's hearing which concerns them. Questions about the child's communicative behavior can next be posited. Inquiry regarding age of onset, progression, and severity of the hearing impairment should be asked. Details concerning the child's middle ear history are important, including the number, at what ages, duration, and treatment history of the middle ear problems. Other important broad areas of questions should include (1) medical history, (2) history of pregnancy, (3) birth and delivery history, (4) physical developmental history, (5) speech and language history, (6) educational history, (7) family history, and (8) special education intervention services. Should the child already be using amplification, details should be clarified regarding the make and model of the hearing aids or FM system, date first amplified, hours of use per day/consistency of amplification, and any previous amplification devices used.

In practice, the written case history can be an invaluable source of information. However, in addition to the formal questionnaire, it is a common practice for the audiologist to also pose additional questions to the parents, as well as ask questions for clarification of responses provided on the written document.

Otoscopic Inspection

The audiologist should always make use of an otoscope to initially evaluate the status of the child's external ear (see Figure 5.9). The verification of the absence of cerumen (wax) and a determination of the status of the tympanic membrance is advocated. Although not in a position to diagnose, the audiologist can certainly determine if the eardrum is retracted, inflamed, etc. A prompt medical referral for either the evaluation of the abnormal appearance of the tympanic membrane and/or wax build-up, would be responses of choice.

Acoustic Immittance

Acoustic immittance is a term referring to a series of tests of the middle ear status. Acoustic immittance does not test a person's hearing per se, but rather the functioning of the middle ear. The primary

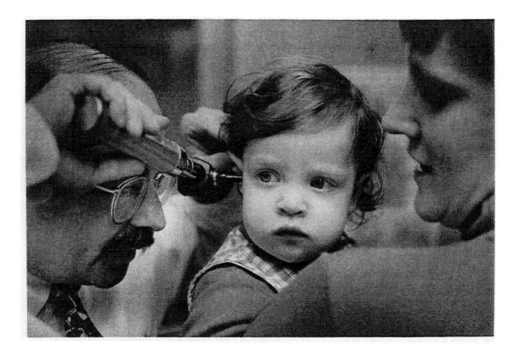

Figure 5.9. Otoscopy.

acoustic immittance test components are *tympanometry, static compliance,* and *acoustic reflex measures* (see Figures 5.10).

Tympanometry is a measurement of acoustic immittance of the tympanic membrane (t.m. or eardrum) as air pressure changes. A tympanogram is a graphic representation of how the eardrum moves, in response to changes in air pressure presented into the external ear canal.

To perform tympanometry, the audiologist or physician places a probe tip through which air flows, into the child's ear canal. The amount of air pressure in the ear canal is changed mechanically by the tympanometer equipment. As the air pressure is varied in the outer ear canal, the equipment records the movement of the tympanic membrane. No response is required by the child during tympanometry, although he/she must cooperate by sitting quietly for a few seconds while the testing is being conducted.

The tympanogram reflects air pressure on the horizontal axis and compliance (movement of the tympanic membrane) on the vertical axis. The peak pressure point on the tympanogram provides information to the audiologist regarding a middle ear pressure measurement as well as a compliance figure.

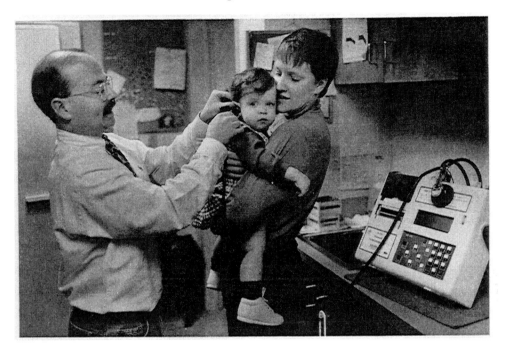

Figure 5-10. Acoustic immittance testing.

There are three major types of tympanograms (see Figures 5.11 & 5.12). A Type A tympanogram is suggestive of normal middle ear pressure and normal compliance of the tympanic membrane. A normal middle ear will provide a Type A tympanogram. A Type B or "flat" tympanogram is noted when there is no measurable tympanometric peak pressure point and minimal to no compliance of the tympanic membrane. This finding may be associated with middle ear fluid being present in the middle ear space (which is typically air-filled). When there is a tympanometric peak pressure point which is negative (for example, -150 mm H_2O or -150 daPa), a Type C tympanogram is noted. Type C tympanograms may be associated with Eustachian tube dysfunction. Children with Type C tympanograms may be commencing the development of middle ear effusion or are recovering from the presence of middle ear fluid build-up.

Static compliance is a number reflecting the mobility of the tympanic membrane.

Acoustic reflex measurements are made by delivering pure tones through a probe tip to the client's ears. The client must sit quietly for this test. The acoustic reflex measures are typically completed at a

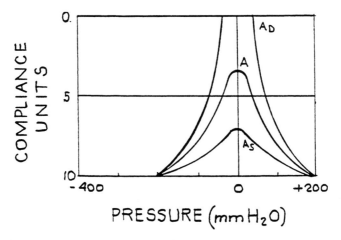

Figure 5.11. Tympanometry classification according to Jerger (1970).

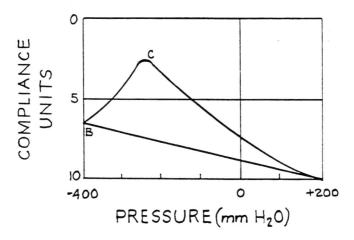

Figure 5-12. Tympanometry classification according to Jerger (1970).

variety of frequencies. Ipsilateral acoustic reflexes are for the probe tube ear and contralateral acoustic reflexes are for the ear opposite the probe tube ear. The acoustic reflex is normally elicited at approximately 60–70 dB above a person's hearing threshold. Because of the limits on how intense a sound the tympanometer can produce, many children with significant hearing losses will not demonstrate measurable acoustic reflexes. The presence or absence of a response by the stapedius muscle in the middle ear can assist the audiologist in estimating hearing threshold levels and is particularly helpful in determining whether or not the person shows abnormal sensitivity to loud sounds—a condition called recruitment. Caution must be taken in setting the output of the client's amplification system such that sounds are not made too loud for him/her by the hearing aid or FM system.

A physical volume measure is often calculated during acoustic immittance testing. The audiologist can interpret the volume measure and refer the client to a physician if the physical volume test measure suggests a perforation of the eardrum or if a Pressure Equalizing (PE) tube is no longer open (patent). For the former, a larger than normal volume would be noted, and for the latter, a small or normal volume measure is demonstrated.

"Standard" Audiometry

A comprehensive diagnostic audiology program for children with hearing impairments should of course address the comprehensive assessment of unaided and aided hearing, assess the electroacoustic functioning of the amplification system(s), and monitor middle ear status. In addition, however, the overall communications program should include the additional areas listed in Table 5-IV.

TABLE 5-IV.
COMPONENTS OF A COMPREHENSIVE AUDIOLOGIC
(RE)HABILITATIVE PROGRAM

1. Amplification
2. Audiologic Management
3. Auditory Learning (see Appendix B)
4. Speech Services
5. Language Services
6. Academic Services and Curriculum
7. Inclusion (School-based issues)
8. Classroom Modifications
9. Psycho-Social Support Services
10. Special Services (for example, interpreters, note-takers)
11. Related Services (for example, PT, OT, vocational)
12. Counseling

The reader is referred to the ASHA Definition of and Competencies for Aural Rehabilitation (1984), as well as a listing of services for public school, hearing-impaired children developed by Brackett and Maxon (1986) for additional information regarding the multitude of services to be considered in the comprehensive intervention program for these children.

Standard audiometric information, such as the unaided and aided audiograms, serve as the basic information for children with hearing impairments. Cumulative data sheets with audiometric results from serial assessments of unaided and aided thresholds are especially helpful in evaluating auditory functioning (Figures 5.13 & 5.14).

THE HELEN BEEBE SPEECH AND HEARING CENTER
Cumulative Record of Air Conduction Thresholds

Client Name _____ File Number _____

DATE	RIGHT									LEFT									Audiologist
	250	500	1000	1500	2000	3000	4000	6000	8000	250	500	1000	1500	2000	3000	4000	6000	8000	

Figure 5-13. Cumulative record of unaided air conduction thresholds.

Thresholds on the audiogram, however, only demonstrate an auditory response at the level of detection (presence or absence of sound). It is important to ascertain how the child functions at the levels of discrimination (perception of same versus different), identification (recognition), and comprehension (Erber, 1982).

Ling Sound Test

The Ling five sound test (see Figure 5.15) (plus sixth sound /m/, recently added), should be routinely used to determine the child's detection or identification/recognition of the sounds /m/, /a/, /u/, /i/, / ʃ /, and /s/. These sounds span across the frequency range and allow the clinician to judge basic auditory abilities. The six sounds can be easily presented in a quick fashion, in order to obtain a baseline of auditory-only responses. Once the baseline has been established, should subsequent measures indicate a change in responses, the clinician must investigate if middle ear or amplification status is negatively influencing the child's auditory abilities. Responses to the Ling sounds should be

THE HELEN BEEBE SPEECH AND HEARING CENTER
Cumulative Record of Air Conduction Thresholds

Client Name_____File Number_____

DATE	AIDED SOUNDFIELD									HEARING AID TESTED WITH	Audiologist
	250	500	1000	1500	2000	3000	4000	6000	8000		

Figure 5-14. Cumulative record of aided thresholds.

noted at varying distances (see Figure 5.16), as well as threshold data measured via monitored live voice in the test booth.

A variety of additional speech audiometric tests and speech perception protocols exist that can also be administered to measure auditory functioning (see Table 5-V). The measures to be selected will depend upon the child's auditory skills, age, and receptive vocabulary, among other factors.

Speech Awareness and Recognition Thresholds: SATs and SRTs

A basic threshold measurement should be obtained using speech stimuli. The stimuli used will be influenced by the child's age. For young children, the examiner might use "buh buh buh," calling the child's name, or the "Bronx cheer" ("raspberries") presented via monitored live voice to verify the "loudness" or intensity of presentation. The audiologist should establish the softest level that the child can repeatedly respond to the speech stimuli. This level is referred to as a Speech Awareness Threshold (SAT). The SAT may be established in sound field for the youngest children and for each ear if insert earphones or headphones can be used.

Using spondee words as the stimuli (two syllable words with equal

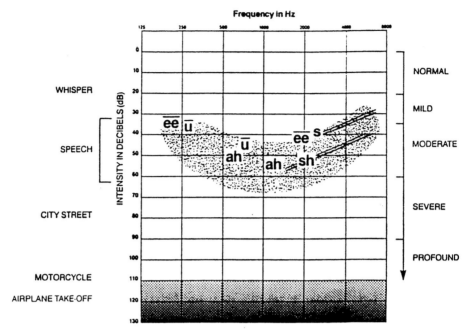

Figure 5-15. "Speech banana" with relative speech levels of the acoustic components of the Ling Five Sounds, spoken at two yards. The Ling Sounds are used as a subjective test to check a child's hearing aids and listening performance. (Reprinted with permission from Pappas, 1985).

stress on each syllable, for example, baseball, hot dog, ice cream), a threshold level can be established, referred to as a Speech Recognition Threshold (SRT). For some children a picture board with approximately 12 spondee words might be used (see Figure 5.17). For others, actual toy examples of the spondee words are effective for obtaining the SRT.

Both the SAT and the SRT measures should be evaluated in view of the low frequency thresholds on the audiogram. For some practitioners, the SRT is compared to the Pure Tone Average (average threshold level for responses at 500, 1000, and 2000 Hz) as a measure of intertest reliability. Both the SAT and SRT measures are influenced primarily by low frequency acoustic energy.

Speech Perception Measures

For some children, especially new listeners and those with significant hearing losses, the audiologist should consider speech audiometric measures which focus on suprasegmental ("pitch"/frequency, duration, and "loudness"/intensity), as well as segmental (specific speech sounds) features. If the child is unable to complete a task by identifying the specific

LING SIX SOUND TEST

CHILD'S NAME_____ DATE_____

	RIGHT EAR	LEFT EAR

AMPLIFICATION (MAKE/MODEL)_____ _____

VOLUME SETTINGS   _____ _____

SETTINGS   _____ _____

SERIAL #   _____ _____

DISTANCE FOR DETECTION OF SOUNDS

SOUND	1 FOOT	3 FEET	6 FEET	9 FEET	12 FEET
/U/ OO					
/ɑ/ AH					
/i/ EE					
/ʃ/ SH					
/s/ S					
/m/ M					

Figure 5-16. Record of auditory responses for the Ling Six Sounds at varying distances.

segmental features of the stimuli, he/she may be successful at recognizing stress patterns. Examples of speech perception protocols that this author has found especially meaningful in evaluation of listeners who have difficulty with "standard" speech measures, include the GASP!, CAT, ANT, and the Early Speech Perception (ESP) Test (described below).

The ESP has a low-verbal and standard version. Subtest 1 evaluates pattern perception by having the child identify monosyllable versus spondee versus trochee (two syllable word with unequal stress on each syllable) versus three syllable words (see Figure 5.18). The child's accu-

TABLE 5-V.
AUDITORY AND OTHER SPEECH AUDIOMETRIC/PERCEPTION
MEASUREMENTS TO ASSESS AUDITORY FUNCTIONING

Threshold data with Ling 6 sounds (/a/, /u/, /i/, / ʃ /, /s/, /m/)
Ling 6 sounds at varying distances
Speech Awareness Threshold (SAT)
Speech Recognition Threshold (SRT)
Early Speech Perception Test (ESP) (Moog & Geers, 1990)
Auditory Numbers Test (ANT) (Erber, 1980)
Children's Auditory Test (CAT) (Erber & Alencewicz, 1976)
Glendonald Auditory Screening Procedure (GASP!) (Erber, 1982)
Sound Effects Recognition Test (SERT) (Finitzo-Hieber, Matkin, Cherow-Skalka, & Gerling, 1977)
Auditory Perception of Alphabet Letters Test (APAL) (Ross & Randolph, 1988)
Word Intelligibility by Picture Identification (WIPI) (Ross & Lerman, 1971)
Northwestern University—Children's Perception of Speech (NU–CHIPS) (Elliott & Katz, 1980)
Test of Auditory Comprehension (TAC) (Trammell, 1981)
Speech Perception Instructional Curriculum and Evaluation for Children with Cochlear Implants and Hearing Aids (SPICE) (Moog, Biedenstein, & Davidson, 1995)
Minimal Auditory Capabilities Battery (MAC) (Owens, Kessler, Raggio, & Schubert, 1985); (Owens, Kessler, Telleen, & Schubert, 1981)

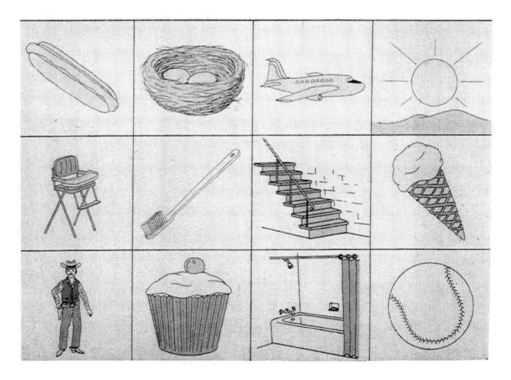

Figure 5.17. Spondee picture card.

racy at exact word identification and stress pattern identification is assessed. The next two measures on the ESP evaluate word identification skills. Subtest 2 evaluates ability to correctly recognize spondee words and finally subtest 3 investigates ability to identify monosyllabic words, all beginning with /b/. With the low verbal version of the ESP pattern perception training is first completed. Following training, both the pattern perception test (all four stress patterns) and the word identification measures (spondees and monosyllables) make use of toy objects in establishing the child's ability to identify words and stress patterns.

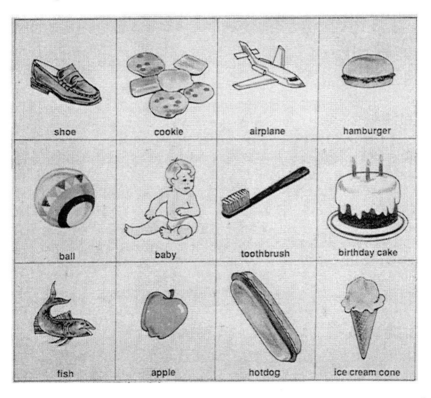

Figure 5.18. Early Speech Perception (ESP) Test—Subtest 1 picture card developed at Central Institute for the Deaf.

In all speech audiometric measurements, it is important that the presentation level is recorded and that the child's aided (with amplification) or unaided status during testing is noted.

Word Recognition Measures

Both the Word Intelligibility by Picture Identification (WIPI) and NU–CHIPS are two common word recognition measures for children.

These tests can be administered in the aided and unaided condition. In the unaided condition, scores can be determined for both the right and left ear separately. With amplification, the testing will be conducted through the loud speaker. The angle of measurement (degree azimuth of client to speaker), presentation level, presence or absence of noise (record signal-to-noise levels as appropriate), etc., must all be reported.

With the WIPI and NU–CHIPs, picture plates are used and the child is asked to identify (typically by pointing), the item presented in a carrier phrase such as "Show me _____" or "Point to _____." The intensity of the presentation does not vary (this is *not* a threshold measurement). Scores are usually reported in percentage correct. Should a test assistant be in the test area with the child and the examiner is not in position to see the child's selections, the assistant should be encouraged to tell the examiner the item the child points to versus stating "correct" or "wrong" or only reporting to the examiner when there is an error. Children are amazingly adept at knowing when they are making errors and such negative feedback should be minimized.

Conclusion

A variety of testing procedures may be utilized in order to amass a comprehensive picture of the child's hearing abilities. By following the AVI Suggested Protocol, the child with a hearing impairment will be appropriately evaluated and managed, in order that he/she has the potential to learn to listen in order to learn spoken language.

Chapter 6

SENSORY AIDS

DONALD GOLDBERG

INTRODUCTION

For children with hearing impairments, hearing aids, FM systems, cochlear implants, and/or other sensory aids are their "ears." The consistent use of appropriately fitted and functioning equipment, including earmolds, cannot be overemphasized as a most critical component of an early intervention program following the principles of the Auditory-Verbal Approach.

In view of the fact that for school-age children, hearing aids and FM systems are often not functioning (e.g., Busenbark & Jenison, 1986), an aggressive amplification management program is required in the overall intervention program. Personal experience has revealed in many cases, less than regular audiological evaluations, inadequate assessment components (for example, limited or no speech perception measurements and missing real ear measurement data), poorly fitting earmolds, inappropriate amplification systems and settings, and an overall lack of case management in the areas of audiological and amplification assessment and follow-up. If the child's earmolds, hearing aids, FM system, and/or cochlear implant are their "ears," it is imperative that the child have a well-fitted and functioning amplification system. The ideal intervention program will pay significant attention to, and be respectful of, the issues involved in pediatric amplification and audiological management.

The purpose of this chapter is to provide a discussion of sensory aids, including, hearing aids, FM systems, other auxiliary aids, tactile devices, and cochlear implants. In addition, a description of a comprehensive amplification evaluation and management plan will be provided.

HEARING AIDS

A hearing aid is an electronic device that amplifies sound. Hearing aids consist of four basic components: a microphone, amplifier, receiver, and battery. The microphone functions to pick up the signal and change the acoustic signal into an electrical signal. The amplifier "amplifies" the electrical signal from the microphone. Next, the receiver converts the amplified electrical signal back into an acoustic signal. The battery serves as the power supply for the hearing aid.

A variety of input selection controls are typically present on a hearing aid. Switches often include an off (O) switch and a microphone (M) switch which turns the hearing aid on. Sometimes the hearing aid does not have an off switch and therefore the battery compartment must be opened to turn the hearing aid off. A telephone (telecoil or T switch) may be present. When the hearing aid is set on T, a magnetic induction field is activated for the enhanced reception of certain signals, most notably the telephone. The option of a combination switch (M/T or +) should be strongly considered for all pediatric fittings (see FM section below). In addition to the combination setting option, all pediatric dispensers should request the option of a tamper resistant battery compartment in order to decrease the possibility of the accidental ingestion of a battery by a young child.

Most hearing aids have a volume or gain control wheel. Often the wheel has numbers (e.g., 1–4) printed on the wheel, indicating increased volume at higher numbers. In general, because of distortion concerns, a hearing aid should not be worn at the highest volume wheel setting.

A tone control setting will allow the audiologist to vary the frequency response of the amplification device. A potentiometer to vary the tone setting is often found under a "trap door" on the case of the hearing aid. A low frequency tone control setting attenuates the high frequency signal. Conversely, a high frequency tone control setting attenuates the low frequency setting. Shaping the frequency response of the hearing aid is often possible with tone control settings which are graduated.

The maximum sound output of the hearing aid is varied via an output control, typically controlled by a potentiometer, again, often hidden under a "trap door" on the case of the hearing aid.

There are four basic models of air conduction hearing aids: body, eyeglass, in-the-ear, and behind-the-ear (BTE or post auricular). The first three models of hearing aids are infrequently dispensed for children, with BTE hearing aids being most commonly fitted (see Figure 6.1).

Today's programmable hearing aids have filtering capabilities which far exceed the flexibility and range of traditional hearing instruments (Microsonic, 1994). In most programmable hearing aids, an improved

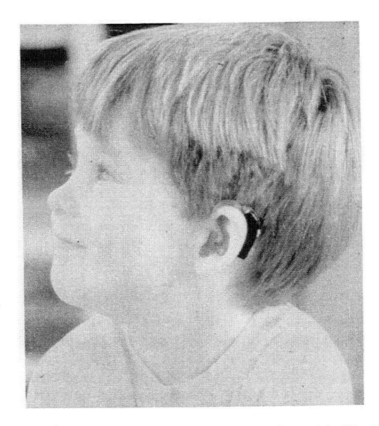

Figure 6-1. A Behind-the-Ear hearing aid (Courtesy of Oticon Inc. and the Tripod School).

signal-to-noise ratio is promoted via computer programming. Digitally programmable hearing aids allow the audiologist to electronically modify the frequency response, output, and in certain instruments, the release time, compression ratio, and crossover frequency in multiple, independent bands. In addition, the programmable nature of the device allows for increased flexibility in fitting, both in terms of varied programming for different acoustic environments (e.g., lecture, versus one-on-one, versus classroom settings), as well as adaptability when additional audiologic data is amassed (see Figures 6.2 and 6.3).

FM SYSTEMS

It is a very common finding that our school classrooms, preschool and daycare settings, as well as our homes, have a degree of noise which can seriously interfere with the optimal transmission of important signals

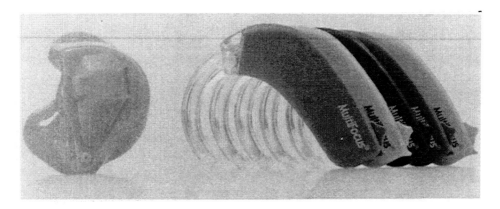

Figure 6-2. Oticon MultiFocus programmable hearing aids (Courtesy of Oticon Inc.).

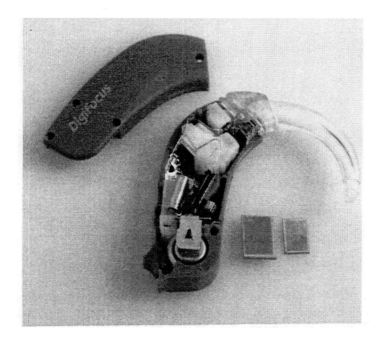

Figure 6-3. Oticon DigiFocus fully digital hearing aid (Courtesy of Oticon Inc.).

such as the teacher's or parent's voice and other students' questions and contributions from class discussions. In addition, it would be fairly rare for the teacher or even the parent to always provide a signal from 3–5 feet from the child/student in order that his/her personal amplification system can do its most effective job.

Because of these assorted conditions, the child's listening environment (home or classroom) may need to be modified to some degree to aid in the child's reception of sound stimuli. Some of the areas for modification include the use of acoustic ceiling tiles, carpeting, window coverings, etc.

In addition to these items, noted above, many audiologists commonly recommend the use of a personal FM or auditory trainer system. With these systems, the teacher or parent wears a microphone (positioned approximately six inches from his/her mouth) and a transmitter. The student wears a receiver unit. This receiver unit is typically "connected" to the child in one of three ways. One method is for the receiver to be directly coupled via a cord, to earmolds or receiver units worn at or in the child's ears. A second method is for the receiver to again be coupled via a cord which connects directly into the child's own hearing aids [referred to as Direct Audio Input (DAI)]. The third method, often the choice of older students with hearing impairments, is for the individual to continue to wear his/her own hearing aids. In addition, the student can wear a loop (teleloop) around his/her neck (often hidden under a blouse or shirt). Provided the student has a T-switch (telecoil or telephone switch) on his/her hearing aids, the teleloop worn around the neck sets up an induction field for the reception of the teacher's voice. The obvious advantage here is that the children do not have a conspicuous cord leading from their receiver to their ears.

In the last few years, revolutionary FM systems have been developed (see Figures 6.4, 6.5, 6.6 & 6.7). In the newest FM systems, the FM is combined into the case of the hearing aid receiver units, each with its own antenna. The parent or teacher must continue to wear a microphone and transmitter; however, the child has a self-contained unit which can serve as hearing aid, hearing aid combined with FM system, or FM system only.

With the exception of a "spelling bee" or lecture situation, this audiologist advocates that the child's hearing aids or FM system receive the combined hearing aid *and* FM signal. With the combined setting option, children can auditorily self-monitor their own voice, hear signals picked up near the microphone of their own personal amplification, as well as receive the signal from the microphone of the FM transmitter unit. The need for a combination setting on children's hearing aids (M/T or + settings) should be considered *at the time* of the initial dispensing of the amplification device, versus waiting for the potential recommendation of

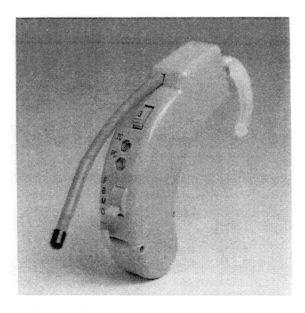

Figure 6.4. AVR Sonovation Extend-Ear BTE FM Hearing system (Courtesy of AVR Sonovation).

an FM system after the child has learned to listen through his/her personal hearing aids. In addition, the option of Direct Audio Input coupling capability should be routinely ordered for all pediatric amplification fittings.

OTHER AUXILIARY AIDS

Briefly, it should be pointed out that in addition to hearing aids and FM systems, there is a host of auxiliary aids which should be considered for the pediatric population. Some auxiliary aids can be used independently; others are utilized in conjunction with the child's hearing aids.

Various alerting devices and systems are available which signal the presence of sounds such as the ring of the telephone, a fire or smoke alarm, a knock at the door, or an alarm clock. Some alerting devices are auditory, others make use of flashing strobe lights, and some may use vibration (e.g., a waking device placed under a pillow or mattress). As can be imagined, some alerting devices are specifically developed as emergency devices.

In the area of telephone aids, some units use amplifiers (portable or built into the handset); others use frequency transformation for the ring

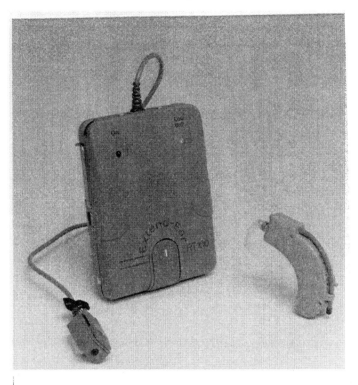

Figure 6.5. AVR Sonovation Extend-Ear BTE FM Hearing System (Courtesy of AVR Sonovation).

of the telephone and/or the frequency response of the signal. Text telephones (TT), formerly referred to as Telecommunication Devices for Deaf People (TDD), permit telephone communication without talking. With TT, callers place the telephone receiver on the TDD "cushions," type in a message, and send it over the telephone wire to another TT. On the LED readout display, computer screen, or paper printout, the message is depicted. In some instance, the user might make use of a relay system (now mandated in each of the 50 United States), whereby an operator receives the typed message and transfers it to another party via a voice telephone. The voice message from the second party can then be typed back to the first user with the assistance of the third party relay operator.

Personal and group listening systems are also available which are designed to carry sound from the speaker (or other sound source), directly to the listener and to minimize or eliminate environmental noises. Audio loop and infrared systems are two examples of such

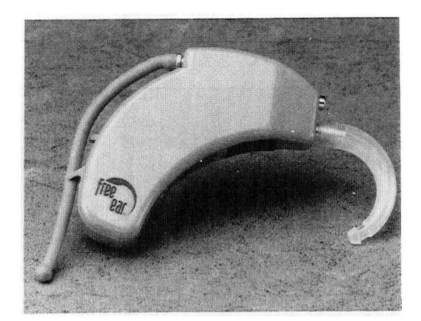

Figure 6.6. Phonic Ear FreeEar BTE-FM system (Courtesy of Phonic Ear).

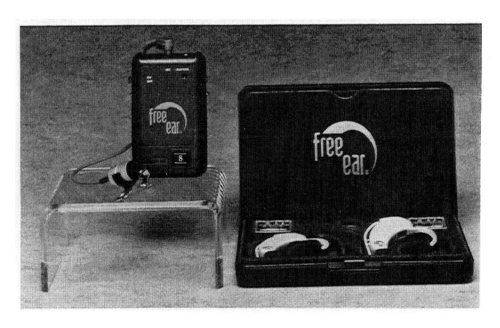

Figure 6.7. Phonic Ear FreeEar BTE-FM system (Courtesy of Phonic Ear).

systems. The infrared system, in particular, has application for television viewing, with the provision of excellent sound quality.

Finally, captioning is an option for some individuals. With open or closed (may require a special adapter or decoder box) captioning, a visual representation of the spoken words is depicted on the screen to be read by the person with a hearing loss. The captioning is similar to subtitles for a foreign language film. Today, numerous television broadcasts, along with many movies are captioned for persons with hearing impairments.

With each of the auxiliary aids described above, it should be realized that their use can help establish the independence of the child with a hearing impairment. This is an important goal which can be facilitated with the use of auxiliary aids.

TACTILE DEVICES

As described by Flexer (1994), tactile communication devices analyze sound into frequency bands and convert the frequency bands into signals that are felt on the skin as vibrations from electrical impulses. Typically, tactile devices are worn on the sternum, abdomen, neck, knee, or fingers. A recent multichannel tactile aid described by Osberger (1990) is the Tactaid 7 by the Audiological Engineering Corporation (see Figure 6.8).

Tactile devices should be considered for individuals with minimal to no useable residual hearing. These devices are sometimes utilized for persons being evaluated for cochlear implants. Research, however, has indicated that the performance of even the highest functioning tactile-aid user is below the performance levels demonstrated by multi-channel cochlear implant users (see Osberger, Maso, & Sam, 1993).

COCHLEAR IMPLANTS

Cochlear implants in children with hearing disorders are one of the most exciting and dynamic developments in the fields of medicine, engineering, audiology, speech-language pathology and education today (see Chapter 7). For children who present with bilateral, profound degrees of hearing impairment, who do not obtain significant benefit from conventional amplification (hearing aids and/or FM systems), a whole new world of sound becomes available through the cochlear implant. Provided candidacy issues are comprehensively evaluated and

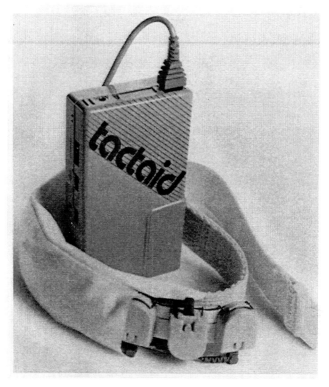

Figure 6.8. Tactaid 7 (Courtesy of the Audiological Engineering Corporation).

qualitative follow-up programming is implemented, children with hearing impairments who receive cochlear implants are then in a position to listen and learn (or continue to learn) speech and language. The key, however, is to tap into the rich perceptual bounty the cochlear implant can provide, ideally via the Auditory-Verbal Approach.

EARMOLDS

An earmold is an individually fabricated ear insert that channels the sound reproduced by the hearing aid or FM system through the ear canal to the eardrum (Microsonic, 1994). The following earmold objectives have been outlined:
- provides a satisfactory acoustic seal
- couples the hearing aid to the ear acoustically
- retains the hearing aid on the pinna (auricle)
- modifies acoustically the signal produced by the hearing aid

In addition, the earmold must be comfortable to wear over time, and be aesthetically acceptable to the client (Microsonic, 1994).

The earmold is typically fabricated by an earmold manufacturer following their receipt of an ear impression. For children with hearing impairments wearing hearing aids, they will have numerous experiences having ear impressions made. Technically the process is not complicated; however, for small, young children, the experience and expertise of the audiologist is often critical.

The audiologist will first examine each ear with an otoscope. Next a cotton or plastic block attached to a string is placed in the ear canal, often with an illuminated instrument which can guide the pushing of the block into the canal. For high gain hearing aids, the ear impression and subsequent earmold must reflect a long canal portion, therefore, the block should be situated beyond the second turn of the ear canal. After the blocks are placed in each ear, the audiologist will typically mix powder and liquid materials, inserting the compound into the ear canal and concha of each ear with a syringe. A hand-mixed silicone impression material delivered to the ear through an acrylic syringe is also an option. It is important that the child remain still throughout the process and that the impression material does not have any gaps or unfilled portions in the canal or bowl of the ear. After the impression material is placed in the ears, this audiologist will request that the child produce several sounds or at least move his/her mouth normally while the material is setting. As the earmold should accommodate speech production and mouth movements, it would be potentially problematic to make the impression without allowing the material to accommodate some mouth movements during the setting time period.

For children fearful of the ear impression process, this audiologist has enlisted the help of the child in pretending to make an ear impression on a stuffed animal or doll. With the child and audiologist each taking turns, the child becomes aware of what the audiologist will next be doing to his/her ear (keep in mind that the child will not be wearing his/her hearing aids and therefore is at a further disadvantage during this process). Often the child will be more willing to have his/her turn at additional taps of the block into the ear canal or staying still as the impression material is syringed into the ear, if he/she has just performed the same step on "Mr. Bear!"

The amplification produced by the hearing aid is modified by the tone or earhook of the hearing aid, the tubing, and finally the earmold (and its tubing). For children with hearing impairments wearing hearing aids, the earmolds *must* fit well or feedback will occur. The unfortunately common practice of lowering the volume or gain control of the hearing aid when there is feedback is WRONG! The earmold(s) instead must be remade so that they fit more tightly and there is no sound escape to be reamplified and create feedback.

Earmold acoustics can be changed via acoustic options such as venting (attenuates or reduces low frequency amplification), damping (via lamb's wool, dampers or filters, inserts, or damped earhooks on the hearing aid) which smooths the frequency response in the mid-frequency range, especially 1000–3000 Hz, and horn effects. For many children with significant hearing impairments, their worst hearing thresholds are in the high frequency range. The "belling" of the earmold and/or tubing will provide the enhanced delivery of high frequency amplification, without degrading the mid and low frequency gain (see Figure 6.9).

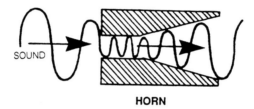

HORN

Figure 6.9. Horn effect (Courtesy of Microsonic, Inc.).

"Acoustically tuned" earmolds include, among others, Killion molds (e.g., Killion, 1976; Killion, 1981), Libby horns (e.g., Libby, 1981), and Continuous Flow Adapters (CFAs) (Schlaegel & Jelonek, 1991) (see Figure 6.10).

AMPLIFICATION EVALUATION AND MANAGEMENT

Electroacoustic Analysis

At the time of each audiologic evaluation, each time a hearing aid is repaired, whenever a parent or professional questions the functioning of the hearing aids, and ideally on a monthly basis, the hearing aids and/or FM system should be subjected to an electroacoustic analysis (EAA). Special equipment has been developed to assess the functioning of the amplification device, to be compared to the manufacturer's specifications for that particular instrument. The principal measurements include the following:

A. information regarding the gain and output of the unit

AUDIOGRAM #4

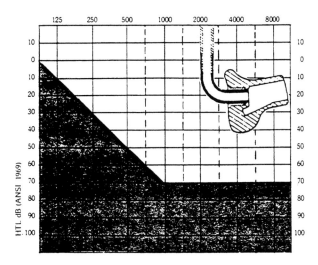

Figure 6.10. Acoustically-tuned Continuous Flow Adapter (CFA) earmold (Courtesy of Pacific Coast Laboratories, Inc.).

- maximum Saturation Sound Pressure Level (SSPL) 90 or maximum power output (MPO)
- High Frequency Average (HFA) SSPL 90
- HFA Full on Gain (FOG)
- Reference Test Gain (RTG) to simulate the "user position"
B. distortion percentages
  - Total Harmonic Distortion (THD) at 500, 800, and 1600 Hz
C. information regarding the internal "noise"
  - Equivalent Input Noise (EIN)

When a hearing aid is run electroacoustically, ANSI standards for evaluating the device require that the internal settings or potentiometers be set (if necessary) to allow for maximum power and the widest frequency response. It is important that the fitter reset the hearing aid's controls back to the original "user setting" following the completion of the EAA, should the potentiometers have been disturbed.

Because the responses obtained through hearing aid test sets are not exactly what will be found in the real ear (Microsonic, 1994), it is recommended that EAA be completed at the user's typical internal settings, as well as coupled to his/her own earmold versus the standard 2cc coupler provided in the test box. These measures will be more representative of the functioning of the hearing aid and earmold. Finally, the use of probe tube or real ear measurements (described below), should routinely be completed as well.

Aided Measurements

Testing with amplification is a most important component of the diagnostic assessment for children with hearing impairments. Regular testing in the unaided condition is, of course, important, but knowing that the child with a hearing loss is wearing amplification throughout his/her waking hours, the testing to verify aided results is most critical.

Real Ear/Probe Tube or Microphone Measurements

The amplification evaluation might best begin with the electroacoustic analysis of the hearing aid to verify appropriate functioning. Next, real ear measurements should be completed. The technology of real ear measurements allows the audiologist to evaluate the hearing aid fitting through the use of a thin, soft, silicone tube that is inserted into the ear canal while the hearing aid and earmold are in place (Flexer, 1994) (see Figures 6.11 and 6.12). Feigin and Stelmachowicz (1991) noted that the inspection of the real ear measures obtained provide the audiologist with information regarding the aided response and amplified signal intensity in the child's ear canal.

Follow-up amplification measurements

As a verification of the real ear measurements, follow-up testing should be completed in the sound field. Aided thresholds for the frequencies 250 through at least 4000 Hz should be obtained, typically using warble tones or narrow band noise (NBN). In addition to the aided thresholds, aided speech audiometrics must be completed. As always, depending on the age of the child, aided SAT, SRT, Ling threshold data, and word recognition measures may be attempted. Should the child be making use of an FM system; measurements are needed in the hearing aid only, hearing aid combined with the FM system, and FM system alone conditions.

EMPOWER THE PARENT!

A PARENT IS WORTH 10,000 SCHOOLMASTERS — A Chinese Proverb

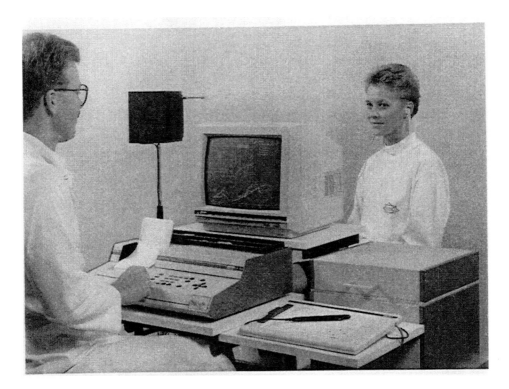

Figure 6.11. Real ear measurement on an adolescent (Courtesy of Madsen Electronics).

Parents can become extremely knowledgeable about the audiologic and amplification needs of their child. With parent education, the most important advocate for the child—THE PARENT—is enabled and empowered to make audiology the foundation of a successful auditory-verbal program. It is hoped that the information provided in these chapters on audiology has assisted in establishing such a foundation for *THE* critical change agents for children with hearing impairments—their parents!

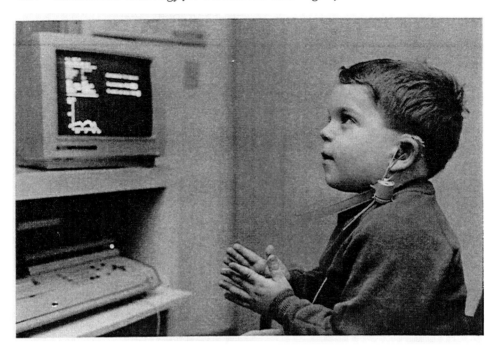

Figure 6.12. Real ear measurement on a preschooler.

Chapter 7

COCHLEAR IMPLANTS: AN AUDITORY–VERBAL PERSPECTIVE

NANCY S. CALEFFE-SCHENCK

The availability of cochlear implants has provided another option to parents who are committed to the development of their deaf child's auditory potential to the fullest extent possible. This chapter will discuss the process of receiving a cochlear implant and the application of this technology in teaching children who are profoundly deaf to learn spoken language through listening.

THE MULTICHANNEL COCHLEAR IMPLANT

Graeme Clark, at the University of Melbourne in Australia, is credited for the development of the Nucleus 22-Channel cochlear implant from research he conducted in the 1970s. It is now worn by 80 percent of children implanted worldwide (Clinical Bulletin, 1990). In 1990, the United States Food and Drug Administration (FDA) approved the Nucleus 22-Channel cochlear implant for use with children in the United States. Currently it is the only cochlear implant approved for children in the United States.

How the Device Works

The Nucleus 22-Channel cochlear implant system consists of three major parts. The internal or implanted unit consists of the receiver/ stimulator which is attached to the electrode array. The external components include the speech processor and the headset. The speech processor is the approximate size of a pocket calculator and serves as a mini-computer which is uniquely programmed for each child. The headset includes a directional microphone which is worn behind the ear like an ear-level hearing aid, a transmitting coil with a magnet in the center, which is placed on the head over the implanted receiver/stimulator, and two cables that connect the microphone, speech processor, and transmitting coil. Figure 7.1 shows these components.

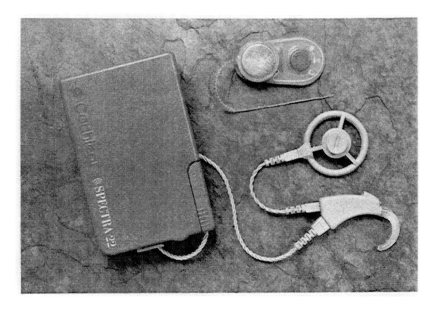

Figure 7.1. The components of a Nucleus 22 channel cochlear implant. Courtesy of Cochlear Corporation.

Sound is received through the microphone and sent via a cable to the speech processor. The speech processor, which has been individually programmed for a particular child, selects specific characteristics of the sound and electrically encodes them. The coded message is sent via a cable to the coil where the code is transmitted through the skin by radio frequency to the receiver/stimulator. The message is decoded and passed along the electrode array. Up to 20 different places along the basilar membrane in the cochlea are stimulated at different times according to the frequencies of the sound which was originally received through the microphone. The message goes to the auditory nerve and on to the brain where auditory sensations that vary in duration, pitch and intensity are interpreted by the listener. This entire process happens almost instantaneously (Teacher Guide, 1994). Figure 7.2 depicts the process by which the Nucleus 22-Channel cochlear implant produces hearing sensation.

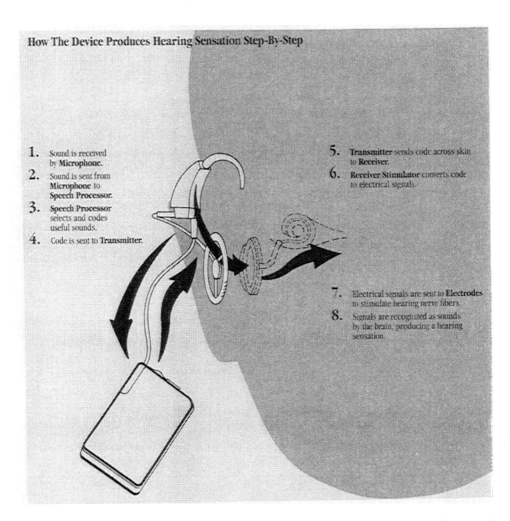

Figure 7.2. Schematics of how the Nucleus 22 channel implant processes sound. Courtesy of Cochlear Corporation.

THE TEAM APPROACH
WITH COCHLEAR IMPLANTS

A strong team approach is critical throughout the entire cochlear implant process, from candidacy through therapy and education. Each team member is important for providing information in a particular area of expertise, as well as being able to consider the "whole" child. Each team member must ask and answer the questions: How can we predict (during candidacy) and assist (postimplantation) in a child's functional use of the cochlear implant?

Team members important to the process are parents, otologist, audiologist, speech/language therapist, psychologist, auditory-verbal therapist (or a professional knowledgeable and experienced in auditory development), and educator. If a child has sensorimotor integration delays, an occupational therapist also joins the team. Professionals who provide services to the child and family outside of the cochlear implant center (e.g., school teachers and therapists) should be included as team members from the beginning. Communication among team members must be consistent, honest, and supportive for the benefit of the child and his family.

Parents must be considered as their child's primary case managers. They need to make informed decisions and be effective and positive advocates. Critical to the process is a sense of mutual respect and trust among parents and professionals on the team.

CANDIDACY: VARIABLES IN PATIENT SELECTION

Determining whether a child is a candidate for a cochlear implant is one of the most challenging aspects of the cochlear implant process. A number of variables related to the individual child contribute to differences in performance with the cochlear implant. These variables must be considered seriously by the cochlear implant team.

Staller et al. (1995) reported on the long-term, five-year performance of children with the Nucleus 22-Channel cochlear implant. The device itself provided a range of benefits to different children, from excellent benefit to little or no benefit. Reported differences among these children were related to age at implantation, educational settings, and communication modes.

Many variables are important, and they must be considered as a group rather than individually. One strong indicator alone (e.g., degree of hearing loss) does not define a proportionally strong candidate.

Degree of Hearing Loss

During FDA pediatric clinical trials conducted in the United States prior to 1990, children were considered cochlear implant candidates only if they had bilateral profound-to-total sensori-neural hearing loss.

They needed to demonstrate little or no benefit from hearing aids. Their scores on speech perception testing needed to be virtually zero on open-set measures and/or chance scores on closed-set assessments (Beiter, 1991).

Sometimes children with profound hearing impairment who had been trained in an Auditory-Verbal Approach did not fall within these guidelines. They had learned auditory self-monitoring and identification in spite of their profound deafness. Yoshinaga-Itano (1988) found that children trained in the Acoupedic (or Auditory-Verbal) method had an aided mean speech discrimination score of 71.6 percent with mean unaided pure tone averages of 92.4 dB HL for the right ear and 92.2 dB HL for the left. They were able to perceive subtle differences in acoustic signals and to understand single words without the use of visual cues, such as lipreading, cued speech, fingerspelling, or signing, even when technological advances provided by the cochlear implant had not been available to them.

The degree of deafness criteria is beginning to change. Yaremko (1994) discussed the results of 24 children who had achieved good speech and had open-set listening using hearing aids prior to implantation. She stated that these children have performed well with their implants. Chute (1995) discussed the trend toward the inclusion of children with some residual hearing in the selection criteria for implantation. More specifically, Adam and Fortier (1994) consider children as cochlear implant candidates if they are unable to hear formant information in frequencies above 2000 Hz.

If it is shown that the cochlear implant has the potential to provide more auditory information than that available with standard amplification, a recommendation may be made for the child and his family to continue through the candidacy process.

Use of Amplification

A child is referred as a cochlear implant candidate after he has completed a trial period with hearing aids or a frequency transposition aid. A trial period must include more than simply wearing amplification. A child must be fit with appropriately powerful amplification which is worn during all waking hours. The child and family must be involved in a therapy and/or educational program which emphasizes listening and talking. Parents need to be well-informed.

The team can assess the child's potential benefit from a cochlear implant versus amplification only when these conditions have been met. Yaremko (1994) found that the best results with implants appeared to be achieved in children who have been excellent hearing aid users and who have benefited from auditory training.

Age at Implantation

At this time in the United States, children must be two years of age before being implanted with a cochlear implant. The candidacy process may begin prior to this age, so that if a child is considered to be an appropriate candidate, implantation is done soon after the second birthday. In a few other countries, children are being implanted under the age of two years (Dahm et al., 1994).

The benefits of implanting children as early as possible is indicated in the research. Waltzman (1994) found that children implanted between the age of two and three made greater and more rapid progress in the development of auditory perceptual skills than children implanted in an older age group. Osberger (1995) found a trend for higher postimplant performance in children who were implanted at an earlier age of 2 to 4 years versus those who were implanted older than 4 years. Staller et al. (1994) reported that a larger proportion of children implanted before the age of six years reached higher levels of performance than children with the same amount of implant experience who were implanted later in life.

Age at Onset of Deafness

The majority of children who are cochlear implant candidates were deaf at birth or were deafened prior to two years of age (Osberger, 1995). Research now indicates that these children can be good candidates, assuming that other variables are strong (Parisier and Chute, 1994; Osberger, 1995).

Duration of Deafness/Years of Listening

Duration of deafness has been investigated in relationship to children's performance with a cochlear implant. A more identifying variable might be years of listening, or years of auditory-verbal therapy or auditory-based education. Rather than looking at how long a child has been deaf, we may need to consider how long the child has used audition and spoken language as a way of life.

Children or teens who have a lengthy duration of deafness, and who have used consistent and appropriate amplification in conjunction with a strong auditory-based therapy program and/or education may be good candidates provided that other variables are strong (Denver Ear Institute, 1995). A spoken language base should be present, even if it was acquired using impaired hearing, since speech development is a primary reason for implanting a child.

Support Services: Education and Therapy

Children being considered for a cochlear implant must be enrolled in an educational program which emphasizes the development of auditory skills (Teacher Guide, 1994) and one which provides abundant opportunities for interactions with children and adults using spoken language. Several researchers support the importance of an appropriate educational placement (Moog and Geers, 1991; Boothroyd, 1991; Ross, 1994). In order for a child to reach the more complex levels of auditory processing and understanding, the child must rely on the implant for communication.

Psychological Issues

Every child who is being considered for a cochlear implant is seen by a psychologist for an assessment of cognition and learning styles. The psychologist also continues the discussion with the parents and the child, if appropriate, about their expectations from the implant. The psychologist contributes to the team by noting any observations or results of testing which indicate cognitive delays, social/emotional issues, or additional handicaps which may impact negatively on the use of the implant. However, child psychological predictors of implant outcomes have not been clearly identified yet (Knutson, 1995).

Some parents express that their primary reason for wanting the implant is to allow their child to hear environmental sounds. This level of use of the implant is not optimal, and may result in the child becoming a nonuser. If the child does not learn to process spoken language, he may feel that sound is an intrusion into his world rather than an enhancement. Peer pressure and cosmetic concerns may take priority over wearing the device (Tonokawa, 1994). Nonuse is costly to everyone involved: the child, parents, professionals, and society.

It is our responsibility as parents and professionals to implant and support the children who will use the device optimally so that nonuse is minimal.

Parent Support and Commitment

Diagnostic therapy during the candidacy process provides an opportunity for the cochlear implant professional team to interact and work closely with the parents prior to a candidacy decision. Parents' understanding and acceptance of their role in helping their child to utilize the auditory information provided by the cochlear implant is absolutely essential.

There are additional responsibilities related to the cochlear implant. It is advisable to discuss and provide in writing to the parents a list of expectations with a parallel list of what the parents can expect to receive from the professionals at the cochlear implant center. Children with implants need to return to the implant center for reprogramming of the speech processor and for annual audiological and speech/language evaluations. Equipment must be maintained in good working order and may need to be upgraded, as current technology becomes available. Auditory-Verbal or other appropriate therapy and home carryover continues long after the device is implanted. Team and/or educational meetings remain as vital components to the team process.

Cohen (1994) wrote an editorial on the ethics of cochlear implants in young children. He summarized the importance of the parents and the professionals by stating that the use of cochlear implants for the young deaf child requires years of training, habilitation, and devotion by teachers, speech pathologists, and parents. Parents must be willing to spend time daily in speaking with their child, listening to him, and helping him to practice both hearing and speaking.

The candidacy process may be time-consuming and take a great deal of effort and coordination. However, the time and energy commitment continues long after a decision to implant is reached. The candidacy stage should be thought of as an introduction to a process, rather than a means to an end (Franz, 1995).

SURGERY

Orientation

The child is prepared for surgery by looking at a model of the receiver/stimulator which will be implanted and by meeting other children who have been implanted. The child and family are taken on a tour of the hospital to see where to check-in the morning of the surgery and to view where they will wait until it is time to go into the operating room. Typically, at least one familiar person from the cochlear implant center accompanies the child into the operating room and stays with him throughout the surgery.

Surgical Procedure

The cochlear implant is surgically implanted into the inner ear. The surgical procedure involves three separate parts. One part is making the seat for the receiver/stimulator in the mastoid bone behind the ear. The second part is removing the bone of the mastoid to get access to the inner ear. The third part is inserting the electrode array into the inner ear (Kelsall, 1995). Residual hearing in the ear is destroyed during this process. Figure 7.3 depicts the placement of the electrode array in the cochlea.

The surgical procedure is not considered dangerous or particularly painful (Issues and Answers, 1994). There have been few serious major complications and relatively few minor complications (Cohen and Hoffman, 1991). It is reported that 2.2 percent of adults and children worldwide who have been implanted with the Nucleus system have had an implant malfunction after a period of successful use (Staller et al., 1994). In the case of internal device malfunction, a new device can be implanted with relative ease (Cohen and Hoffman, 1991).

PROGRAMMING

Preparing the Child for Programming

Children are prepared for programming by play activities which have been used during therapy sessions and at home prior to this time, using

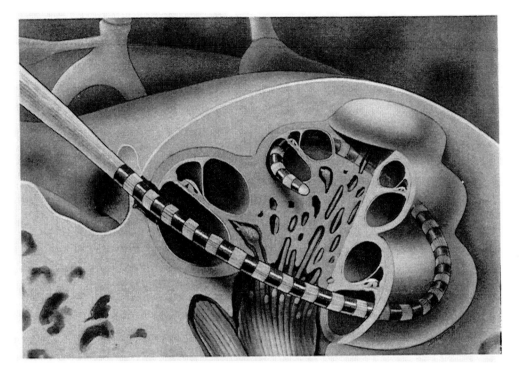

Figure 7.3. The placement of the electrode array in the cochlear. Courtesy of Cochlear Corporation.

hearing aids, a frequency transposition aid, or an FM system. If the child has no residual hearing, a vibrotactile aid may be used. The concepts of presence and absence of sound and softness and loudness are taught.

Threshold levels, or T-levels, are set using conditioned play audiometry techniques. Some favorite activities are: Adding parts to Mr. Potato Head; building a nesting cup tower; adding beads to a yarn necklace; and pushing a Popsicle® puppet into a play dough mound.

Comfort levels, or C-levels, are demonstrated by the child by either indicating to the audiologist to "stop" when the sound is perceived as loud, or by behavioral observations by the adults of the child's facial and bodily expressions.

Children also need to learn the concepts of same and different as they relate to loudness, and higher and lower as they relate to pitch. A child may need to wear the implant and be involved in an auditory-based therapy program before mastering these concepts.

Initial Stimulation

Four to six weeks after surgery, the child is accompanied by his parents/caregivers to the cochlear implant center to have the speech processor programmed. This is called "initial stimulation" and can be a very exciting time for the child, family, and professional team because it is the first time the cochlear implant is activated to deliver sound to the child. It may be a challenging time for the child and his family. Sometimes the child is uncertain of the sensation of hearing and does not know how to interpret the stimulation. Parents may have unrealistic expectations of their child suddenly being able to hear, in spite of extensive counseling which was done with them concerning the lengthy process of learning to process sounds. For these reasons it is advisable to have a "low key" approach to initial stimulation.

It is important to have two professionals working together during initial stimulation and reprogramming sessions with young children. Two professionals are used for confirmation of behavioral observations. In addition, one professional keeps the child focused on the activity while the other presents the computer-controlled test stimuli. The parents are present to better understand the process, to provide input on observations, and to be supportive to their child.

Typically, initial stimulation is done over a two- or three-day period. During this time, two different levels are set for each active electrode. These levels are T-levels which are the levels at which the child first detects the sound, and C-levels which are the levels that are comfortably loud for the child. These values set the child's electrical dynamic range which is the difference between the C-level and the T-level for each electrode.

Once T-levels and C-levels are determined, the audiologist will sweep through the electrodes, or balance the electrodes if the child is a sophisticated listener. Sounds for each electrode are presented one after the other at comfort levels or quieter. The child indicates through expressions, gestures, pictures, or speech if the sounds are the same or different in loudness. Sweeping or balancing is done to check that adjacent electrodes are set at equally loud levels. This enhances the quality of the sound the child receives, so that it is perceived as more "even."

The child's individualized MAP is then created. At this time the microphone and processor are activated to detect sounds and voices in the child's environment, and the child is "on the air."

After the child has had a rest or break, a therapy session should be conducted to assess the appropriateness of the MAP and to coach the parents on activities to incorporate at home. It is important for families and professionals to stay in close contact during the first few weeks following programming.

Reprogramming

Generally, the child is rescheduled to return for reprogramming of the speech processor within two to four weeks after initial stimulation. T-levels and C-levels typically change, so these are reevaluated and set appropriately. During the first year after receiving the implant, children are seen on a regular basis as recommended by the audiologist, with input from the child's therapist and parents. After the first year, all children should be reprogrammed at least once or twice yearly, depending upon the child's needs, as indicated in therapy, at school, or at home. Figure 7.4 illustrates a reprogramming session with a child.

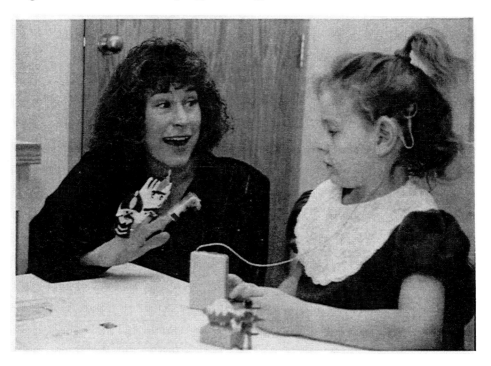

Figure 7-4. A reprogramming session. Courtesy of Cochlear Corporation.

Parents, teachers, and therapists should recommend reprogramming when the child's auditory skills appear to diminish. This would include, but not be limited to, auditory changes in detection of phonemes and sounds, distance hearing, self-monitoring of speech, voice quality and articulation, and processing and memory. If a child is not remapped at appropriate intervals, the quality of the auditory signal is less than optimal. This violates a basic principle of the Auditory-Verbal Approach, which is, that a child is fitted with the most appropriate form of amplification or technology available.

THERAPY FOR CHILDREN WITH COCHLEAR IMPLANTS

Children do not learn to listen simply by receiving a cochlear implant. Although the device provides excellent detection of environmental and speech sounds over a wide frequency range, children must learn to process this auditory information and incorporate it into spoken communication. Children and their families must be supported by being enrolled in a therapy program which focuses on:

(1) The development of spoken language through listening;

(2) The active involvement of parents, primary caregivers, and teachers; and

(3) The integration of audition into daily activities where a rich and accessible auditory environment is maintained.

Auditory-Verbal Therapy

The principles of an Auditory-Verbal Approach include teaching a child to incorporate listening into his total response to the environment (Pollack, 1985). It includes the integration of audition and speech, which is necessary for listening to become a way of life for a child with a cochlear implant. This practice has been shown to be an effective therapy approach for children with cochlear implants (Tyler, 1990; Bertram, 1994).

Therapy for children with cochlear implants is not significantly different than for children with amplification. Children with implants start at the beginning stages of auditory development, auditory awareness and attention, and continue in a logical progression until they learn to process and understand auditory information. Children with implants may progress at a faster rate than children with similar unaided degrees of hearing loss who wear hearing aids, and may also pass the levels of speech perception attained by these children (Osberger, 1993).

There are a few differences in hearing aids and cochlear implants of which parents and professionals should be aware:

(1) The awareness of high frequency sounds may be more available to children with implants. Detection and discrimination of high frequency consonants such as s, z, f, v, sh, and zh are often easier for a child with a cochlear implant than with hearing aids. High frequency tones in the sound booth are more easily detected.

(2) Localization is different with an implant, because only one microphone is used rather than the two microphones.

(3) Distance hearing may be better with an implant.

(4) Subjective listening checks are not possible with implants; however, objective testing can be done by the audiologist at the cochlear implant center to determine the integrity of the electrodes, the electronic components, and the brain responses of the child who is wearing the implant (Shallop, 1995).

OUTCOME STUDIES RELATED TO SPOKEN COMMUNICATION

A child's progress with the cochlear implant should be monitored on a regular basis. The results of this testing is often reported in outcome studies to quantify the effectiveness of cochlear implants for children. Recently, the impact of communication mode (oral versus total communication) on the auditory and verbal development of children with cochlear implants has surfaced in the literature. Barnes and Franz (1994) reported on 15 children with the Nucleus 22-Channel cochlear implant. They stated that those who are totally immersed in an oral language environment immediately after initial stimulation have made the transition from total communication to oral communication more easily than those children who returned to total communication settings.

Speech Perception

Speech perception testing assesses a child's ability to discriminate or understand speech without the use of visual cues. The tests vary in difficulty based on test format and difficulty of test items.

Test formats vary by having closed-set versus open-set answers. In a closed-set format, objects, pictures, or written words are provided, and the child identifies the answers by pointing, verbalizing, or signing. In open-set measures the child is required to repeat or sign word(s) or answers to questions. Tests are administered using live-voice or tape-recorded speech.

Difficulty of test items is controlled by differences in duration, stress, number of syllables, segmental features, vocabulary, memory, comprehension, and signal to noise ratios.

Recent outcome studies indicate that many children with cochlear implants improve in their ability to understand speech (Staller et al., 1991; Osberger et al., 1991; Osberger, 1993).

Researchers have reported that children enrolled in programs emphasizing oral communication tend to perform at higher levels on more difficult speech perception tasks than children enrolled in total communication programs (Staller et al., 1994; Tonokawa, 1994).

Speech Intelligibility

Speech intelligibility is how understandable a child's speech is to naive listeners. Studies have indicated that cochlear implants provide auditory information which assists children in the development, production, and use of speech. Speech intelligibility has improved after implantation (Tobey and Hasenstaab, 1991; Tobey et al., 1994; Grogan et al., 1994; Nicholas, 1994).

Individual differences in the intelligibility scores of cochlear implant users have been associated with mode of communication. Children who use oral communication have demonstrated significantly better speech intelligibility than children who rely on total communication (Osberger et al., 1994; Kirk, 1994; Moog and Geers, 1994).

Language

Cochlear implants can contribute to the growth of a child's spoken language abilities. Studies have shown that children improve in spoken vocabulary, syntax, and overall communicativeness when educated in an oral environment (Geers and Moog, 1994; Nicholas, 1994).

SUMMARY

The multichannel cochlear implant has provided a viable option in providing sound to children who are profoundly deaf. It is not an appropriate option for all children who are deaf. It is an excellent option for children who meet the candidacy requirements and who have the parental and professional support discussed in this chapter and book.

Chapter 8

THE DEVELOPMENT OF
A LISTENING FUNCTION

The main goal of an Auditory-Verbal Approach is the integration of hearing into the personality of the so-called deaf or hard-of-hearing child. Therefore, treatment is concerned first and foremost with developing hearing perception.

If hearing is to be integrated into personality, the infant must wear two hearing aids or a cochlear implant throughout his waking hours. He must then be stimulated in such a way that a *listening function* is developed, regardless of his degree of loss or chronological age. Indeed, he may be said to have a *hearing age*, dating from the purchase of his own hearing aid. That is, if he is two years old chronologically when he is fitted with an aid, his *hearing age* is only one day.

Watson (1961) stated that there are optimum maturational stages for development of speech and language through which hearing children pass in the course of their development. The closer in time to normal that the hearing-impaired child can be enabled to reach these stages, the more likely is his linguistic ability to make good progress.

It is also true that the closer we follow the normal *pattern* of development, the better the results will be. Nature proceeds in an orderly sequence. It is therefore of the greatest importance to study the *normal* development of a listening function. A useful chart has been composed by Ruth Griffiths in her book, *Abilities of Babies* (1954).

NORMAL DEVELOPMENT OF A LISTENING FUNCTION

A. Prenatal

It is assumed that awareness of sound, either as vibration or through bone conduction, and particularly awareness of the maternal heart beat, or "lubdub" rhythm, which Bluemel (1959) has conjectured to be the source of the two syllable babble, begins *in utero*. It is interesting to note

141

TABLE 8-I
HEARING AND SPEECH SCALE
FIRST YEAR

First Three Months
1. Is startled by sounds
2. Is quieted by mother's voice
3. Makes murmured sounds, other than crying
4. Listens to a soft bell near him
5. Makes definite cooing noises, one syllable
6. Searches for sounds with eye movements
7. Listens to music
8. Makes two or more different sounds

Second Three Months
1. Searches for sound with head movements
2. Laughs aloud
3. Turns his head deliberately to the bells
4. Listens to a tuning fork
5. Coos or stops crying on hearing music
6. Talks or babbles to persons
7. Manipulates the hand bell
8. Makes 4 or more different sounds (separate single sounds or syllables)

Third Three Months
1. Responds when called
2. Uses two-syllable babble
3. Shouts for attention
4. Listens to conversation
5. Uses singing tones
6. Uses babbled phrases of four or more syllables
7. Says "mama" or "dada" etc. *One* word clear
8. Listens to a stopwatch

Fourth Three Months
1. Shakes head for *No*
2. Now says *two* clear words
3. Uses short meaningful babble, like sentences
4. Rings the bell
5. Reacts to music vocally
6. Babbled monologue when alone
7. Says *three* clear words

Courtesy of Griffiths, Ruth: *Abilities of Babies.* London, U. of London, 1954.

that congenitally deaf children experience difficulty in reproducing a two-syllable babble and usually babble unrhythmically—*ababababababa*, before training.

TABLE 8-II
HEARING AND SPEECH SCALE
SECOND YEAR

First Three Months
1. Tries to sing
2. Looks at pictures for a short while
3. Knows his own name
4. Likes nursery rhymes and jingles
5. Uses 4 or 5 clear words

Second Three Months
1. One object in the box is identified when named
2. Uses 6 or 7 clear words
3. Makes long babbled conversations, with some words clear
4. Enjoys a picture book
5. Two objects in the box are identified
6. Uses 9 clear words

Third Three Months
1. Four objects in the box are identified
2. Vocabulary — 12 clear words
3. Picture vocabulary — one picture named
4. Uses word combinations
5. Picture vocabulary — Two pictures named

Fourth Three Months
1. Listens to stories
2. Vocabulary — 20 words clear
3. Names 4 toys
4. Uses sentences of 4 or more syllables

Courtesy of Griffiths, Ruth: *Abilities of Babies.* London, U. of London, 1954.

B. First Three Months: The Development of Auditory Awareness and Attention

Postnatally, it will be seen from the chart that an increasing number of responses to sound occur during the first three months of life. The newborn is aware of sound and is characteristically startled by loud noises, so that Moro's Reflex is seen. He is confronted by a complexity of sounds which are meaningless to him (environmental noises and vocal sounds) but he appears at first to take little notice unless they are very loud.

Because a normal neonate has hearing, and is stimulated by sound all the time, he begins to listen with varying degrees of attention, and after much repetition within a limited environment, he begins to understand the source of these sounds and they become meaningful to him, for example, the noise made by the bottle, and his mother's voice.

The normal neonate's first responses, then, are to gross sounds, such as the vacuum cleaner, loud rustle of paper, door banging, and so on. If a baby is being held near the telephone when it rings, and is not deeply asleep, he will almost jump out of one's arms at the sound. Sound responses are so obvious that the absence of them will probably indicate a most profound hearing loss, but they may indicate the presence of other problems.

As the weeks go by, the baby learns that these sounds do not threaten him and are not followed by any experiences meaningful to him, so his responses are gradually inhibited, and we see that it is possible for him to ignore much of the noise in his environment unless it is significant to him at that time, or new, or perhaps a little bit different and intriguing. (This is surely a protective device, for he would be driven mad if he reacted to every sound he heard!)

At first, when he hears a loud sound, a baby reacts by jerking, blinking, or other muscular movements such as raising his eyebrows, frowning, and mouth twitching. There may be a change in his breathing pattern. During the first three months, these reactions will be observed more frequently to *quieter* sounds. These are essentially reflexive responses to hearing, but gradually the normal baby begins to *pay attention*, that is, to *listen*, sometimes as soon as he has learned to nurse satisfactorily. One may detect a certain bodily tension during a sustained noise, or even slight eye movements, as if he is searching for the sound. If it is loud enough, he will stop crying, at least momentarily.

Experienced mothers know when a baby has a "fussy" period, usually in the late afternoon or early evening, that music from a music box or radio seems to be pleasing and has a calming effect. Brazelton (1974) has described how babies will move their bodies or limbs in rhythm with music or the human voice.

By six weeks of age, a baby may respond to being called by a quiet look or a pleasurable waiting attentiveness, as if he already recognizes his mother's or caretaker's voice. By two to three months of age, he will begin to laugh in response to his parents' laughter or when jiggled about. At the same time, he is becoming increasingly vocal, engaging in an "answering type conversation" with much bodily straining as he tries to vary the tonal range or make various sounds with tongue and lips. One sound often heard is a hearty crow of glee, another seems to be a guttural sound of impatience. Some young infants vocalize when they eat cereal, a prespeech activity which lends support to the "Chewing Theory" of the origin of speech (Froeschels, 1941).

As soon as a baby develops attention to sound and begins to listen, he learns that there are all kinds of sounds: loud, quiet, rhythmic, noisy, percussive, male, female, and so on. He is also hearing himself—his own bodily noises, crying, and other vocal sounds.

At first he reacts only to those sounds which are close by, but gradually he develops *distance hearing*. For example, one baby was startled by the sound of the dog barking in close proximity, but ignored the thunderstorm outside. A few weeks later, he began to be startled by outdoor sounds. Another baby recognized the sound of the dog's collar bells and smiled in that direction (Church, 1966).

By the end of the third month, a newborn has developed all kinds of auditory skills: he recognizes his mother's voice, he stops crying to listen, he enjoys playing with a few noisemaking toys, and he listens to his own sounds. *But most important of all, he has learned that sound is used for communication:* by crying or vocalizing, he gets attention and a response.

C. Second Three Months: The Development of Discrimination and Auditory Feedback

During the second three months of his life, the baby begins to turn his head to localize a variety of sounds, and he may produce sounds by playing with squeaky toys, a cradle gym, and so on.

He is now developing an *auditory feedback mechanism*—he enjoys hearing his own voice, laughing aloud again and again, vocalizing, cooing, and babbling a small number of phonemes. In general, studies of infant vocalizations have reported that vowels tend to occur proportionately more often in the earlier months, while consonants become more frequent in the later months of the first year (Smith and Oller, 1981). This is also true of children with hearing loss (Smith, 1982).

Hearing is now contributing to spatial awareness. It keeps a baby in contact with his environment at all times even when it is dark. When he is left alone he is reassured because he can hear sounds around himself.

However, the kind of environment to which a baby is accustomed influences his reactions to sound. If he is surrounded by a lot of noise from birth (children playing, radio or television turned on all day, and so on) he soon ignores sounds. If he is in a quieter environment, he retains reflex reactions much longer.

Between three and five months, it is sometimes very difficult to test a baby's hearing by observation of reflexes. Especially around five months, it seems as if all the noises to which the baby has reacted are now "old," yet he has not developed discrimination or localization to the point that other reactions can be observed. He may be more interested in visual stimuli at this point. However, Gaeth found that a baby of this age will cry when he hears a chromatic whistle. Apparently, this is a disagreeable and frightening noise to a three to five-month-old child.

The multiple listening experiences of the early months lead to a new auditory skill, that of *discrimination*, which begins with a conscious awareness of the presence or absence of sound and becomes more and more sophisticated. For example, one three-month-old raised his head to listen to a wind-up toy, then dropped it when the tune was finished and went to sleep.

Eisenberg (1970) established that neonates can discriminate sound based on discrete parameters and dimensionality, and many studies have shown that infants can discriminate between tones and between speech sounds such as b and p, perhaps as young as three or four months of age (Eilers, 1977). By six months, the infant is paying definite attention to sounds, so that he reacts differently to different tones of voice, recognizes environmental sounds, and so on. Around this age, a baby who is being held face to face by an adult will cry if he hears his mother's voice. The face he is looking into does not belong with the voice he is hearing!

Another aspect of discriminatory skill is the ability to inhibit sound: at first the world is full of confusing noises, but as they become meaningful, we are able to focus on those which are important at that point in time, and to relegate other sounds to the background; that is, to ignore them. Children with learning disabilities, however, frequently exhibit great difficulty in separating the signal from noise and are distracted by all the sounds in their environment.

Thus, by the sixth month, the newborn is "becoming human"—he has a wider range of vocal and facial expression, increased motor control, greater involvement with his entire world. He likes reciprocal vocalization play, that is, an adult or sibling echoing his sounds or making sounds in response to his sounds, and he enjoys being whistled or sung to. If he is standing, he can bounce in rhythm to music. He is also using auditory clues to orient to unseen space. For example, if he drops his rattle, he is able to find it within the limits of his visual and auditory range.

D. The Sixth Through Ninth Months: The Development of Localization and Babbling

The next important milestone is *localization.* Luria (1973) described this as the "orienting reflex" and wrote that it is associated with a whole group of autonomic features; for example, the cessation of all other, irrelevant forms of activity, and the occurrence of respiratory, cardiovascular and psychogalvanic responses. The importance of the orienting reflex is such that the formation of a conditional reflex will be slow to develop in its absence.

The *ability to localize* develops gradually and is closely linked with maturation and opportunity. It may be said to begin when a child is put into a sitting position, i.e., by the sixth month. At first the sound has to be close to the meatus, and the eyes will turn in the correct direction, or there will be a slight turning of the head. (Research in Sweden, described by Bengt Barr at an audiology workshop in 1963, has shown that localization is difficult if the head is in a fixed position. Another factor which is known to facilitate localization is binaural hearing.) Taylor (1958) found that the young baby localizes only sounds on a horizontal line running through the two ears and approximately three feet from the ears. If the sound is much above or below this plane, or above the head, it takes time for the child to find it. If it is beyond this distance, he shows that he hears it by searching or by his facial expression, but may not localize. Sound, then, appears to be found in reference to this plane. By the end of the first year, localization is not always necessary, but an infant seems to react automatically to sounds that interest him, at almost any distance within a moderately sized room, but he does not seem to react to sounds above or behind him. Indeed it may be three years before sounds made overhead are located automatically, with the exception of airplanes.

The ability to localize sounds automatically usually occurs with the ability to sit up, and is easier when the head is in motion. It also seems to require two similar ears with hearing for minimal sounds over a wide range of frequencies. It is important for many reasons, for example for safety, as in crossing the street, for security, and so on. For the young child, it allows identification of sound with object, and is thus important for perceptive and learning processes. Many objects in the daily life of a young child are characterized by the sounds they make, so the difficulties in localization will hinder the learning process. It is interesting to note that the "Bow Wow" theory of language is based upon this. The onomatopoeic word for the sound associated with the object may be the only symbol used for a long time. A child may not learn *dog;* he will refer to the *bow wow,* because the bark is the most impressive characteristic of this animal to him. (Adults continue to add new onomatopoeic words to the language, e.g., the word "buzz bomb" during World War II.)

Localization is of great importance in identification of the mother and her voice, through which the baby learns emotional tone and gains emotional security.

From the sixth to the ninth month, the child's responses to sound increase. He will respond to or shout or both when his name is called, even when the speaker is behind him, although he probably will not recognize it until he is about eight to nine months old. One mother observed that her baby responded equally to her own name, which was Lisa, and to her sister's name, which was Cara, a similar inflection and stress pattern.

He now enjoys his own voice so much that he plays vocally by singing tones and letting his voice slide from a high pitch to a low one and vice versa. Thus, he is beginning to monitor his own sounds through the auditory feedback and feedforward mechanism. Or he may become rather silent and appear to be more interested in absorbing all the conversation and sounds in his environment. It should also be noted that in the next few months there is a period of intense oral stimulation — when the speech mechanism is stimulated vigorously by sucking, chewing, swallowing, and tasting.

E. Last Three Months of the First Year: The Development of Auditory Processing

The baby is now approaching the symbolic level, when passive word understanding comes into being. It seems likely that the first few "connections" between experience (a thing, person, or event perceived) and a word symbol are made only as the result of constant repetition. But once the child understands that the sequence of sounds which he hears represents or is associated with a specific experience which he has perceived, the pattern of learning quickens. Nevertheless, it still takes up to two or three years from birth before the average normal hearing child acquires a large intelligible vocabulary; six to eight years before his discrimination, muscular coordination, and ability to imitate result in correct articulation (Edmonston, 1963), and several years more before he achieves mature syntax (Watts, 1944).

Two new auditory skills are now of great importance: auditory-memory span and auditory sequencing. It is not known when auditory memory begins, but it probably begins at birth. Three stages of memory have been proposed: (1) a complete sensory image of just occurring events; (2) an immediate or short-term memory, which contains limited information that we are able to extract from a rapidly decaying sensory image; and (3) a permanent, long-term memory with a very large capacity.

There is controversy in the literature about the "decaying of a trace" or sensory image, and some researchers feel that the important factor is the presence of irrelevant or distracting factors which will prevent a strong initial image.

For an item to be stored in long-term memory, it must be rehearsed and associated with previous information. Our immediate auditory memory span is said to be limited to seven items, plus or minus two, as in telephone numbers, but we can increase the amount of information by building together larger and larger chunks, each chunk containing more information than before. We often use rhythm and intonation (as in learning the alphabet) or other mnemonic aids to memorize and recall. Thus, memory is associated with auditory feedback and kinesthetic cues, but its development is obviously meshed with experience, motivation, and language acquisition, or knowledge of the language code. Intelligence is also known to influence memory span. Thus, while a child's memory span for digits increases from two to six digits between the ages of 2.5 and ten years, this does not accurately predict his memory for meaningful sentences. It is apparent when children are asked to repeat sentences that they tend to fasten onto the *meaning* and convey the substance of the message rather than the exact wording. Auditory recall is a very complex and active process.

In order to learn language, then, a small child has to be able to store and recall the following:

1. Auditory images of the sounds, words, and sentence structures of the language.
2. The correct sequencing of auditory vocal patterns. (For example,

he has to correct pasgetti for spaghetti and all gone Daddy for Daddy's gone, and so on.)

Auditory memory for language seems to be localized to the left hemisphere of the brain. Lesions in this hemisphere lead to a disturbance of the complex organization of auditory perception so that a person with this lesion is unable to reproduce correctly what is said to him or retain traces of it, although his ability to handle music remains unimpaired (Luria, 1973).

By his first birthday, a normal-hearing infant is beginning to use all these basic auditory skills to respond to his environment and to process language. There is always great excitement within a family when it is apparent that the infant can understand a few words, and even starts clapping when he hears a familiar jingle such as patty-cake.

THE LEARNING TO LISTEN YEAR

We see, then, that a normal-hearing child needs at least one year (or thousands of hours) of listening experiences before he tries to communicate with words. Whetnall (1964) has called the first year "The Readiness To Listen Year." Obviously, the infant who is born with, or who has acquired at an early age, a severe hearing loss, will miss most of this first listening year. A "hard-of-hearing" or hypoacusic child will have incomplete auditory experiences or "Swiss cheese" hearing, as it has been called.

A basic premise of Auditory-Verbal education is that limited-hearing children need the same foundation of listening experiences as a normal-hearing child regardless of the age at which intervention occurs.

The principle of recapitulating normal experiences has far deeper implications than learning to listen. The lack of such experiences has been given as a reason for the language deficits of the deaf child by Levine (1956). She wrote as follows:

> The normal-hearing child was a conceptualized being before becoming a verbalized being. He is exposed to verbally expressed concepts almost from birth. The baby attends to sounds and begins to perceive differences in the sounds. But most important, these differences take on special meanings. One kind of sound informs him that someone is hurrying to him, another brings to mind his rattle, still another tells him that food is on the way. Long before the child is aware of words, he is alert to the concepts contained in familiar sounds. What is more, he reacts to them mentally, emotionally, socially. When the sounds of speech come

within his range of discrimination, his previous practice in associating gross sounds with their conceptual equivalents stands him in good stead. He now associates word-sounds with the objects, activities or feelings they represent. Eventually verbal language becomes thoroughly incorporated into the very essence of his psychological existence and development. But the deaf child lacks this "conceptual feel for language" if he misses all the preliminary auditory experiences leading up to the fusion of word and concept. Eventually, the deaf child's language development takes on the character of a dictionary, full of words but without the intimate relationship to each other and to inner development. Words must be tied in to something in a child's life—an event, an activity, an emotion.

SUMMARY

In the development of a listening function, there are definite skills which are usually attained during the first year of life, and become interwoven into all our learning experiences. They are:

1. Auditory Awareness and Perception
2. Auditory Attention and Inhibition
3. Distance Hearing
4. Localization
5. Discrimination
6. Auditory Feedback and Monitoring
7. Auditory Memory
8. Auditory Memory Span and Sequencing
9. Auditory Processing

Hutchison (Auricle, 1994) suggests that these auditory skills developed during the first year fit into three psychological purposes:

1. Environmental monitoring (auditory awareness/perception, auditory attention/inhibition, localization, distance hearing, and discrimination)
2. Self-monitoring of the child's vocal activity (auditory memory and auditory self monitoring)
3. Creative organization and management of meaning (auditory memory span, and auditory processing).

Hutchison suggests an additional step, that is, auditory association (schemata linking other physiological and psychological bases of perception).

Hutchison writes that the concepts of developing an auditory function and integrating hearing into the personality of a child with a hearing loss separates Auditory-Verbal from other educational treatments.

TEACHING STRATEGIES

Development of Hearing Perception

For the child with a hearing loss, a program to develop and refine auditory skills must begin as soon as amplification is applied. A mother or caregiver may not be able to put the child "back into the crib," but she can still hold him upon her knees, thus reliving the "closeness" associated with first listening experiences. (There is also some sensation of vibration associated with the sounds.) She should know that the best fidelity obtainable with a hearing aid is at a distance approximately four to twelve inches from the microphone, so that all sound stimulation should be given close to the child at first.

The early development of hearing perception is accomplished by the following experiences:

1. Awareness of loud and quiet sounds.
2. Learning to attend, or listen to a variety of sounds at close range.
3. Learning to listen to sounds at different distances and from different directions.
4. Localizing the source of these sounds (associating object with sound).
5. Recognizing these sounds (i.e., knowing the *meaning* of them).
6. Reacting appropriately to them.
7. Imitating or using them.

Gradually, the *range* of listening must be increased in all these experiences. We begin with the child close to the sound source and, when we observe reaction, we move the child further and further away from it, or we may move the sound source further from the child.

The "core" of listening experiences includes the following:

1. Vocal play
2. Music
3. Noisemakers
4. Other environmental sounds
5. Prespeech activities
6. Speech and language.

The last two listening experiences are discussed in Chapters 9 and 10.

These experiences are most effective when they are part of the play which normally occurs in a family where babies are given a good deal of attention. When guiding the parent of a young child, it is important to emphasize that the clinic or school session is only a demonstration of what can be done. The clinician may develop a specific skill, but the parent incorporates it into the daily routine: one does not sit down and "teach a lesson." With older children, it is sometimes necessary to set aside a special time (Courtman-Davies, 1979).

Vocal Play

The stimulation of vocal play is of tremendous importance when the first hearing aids have been fitted, not only because it helps to bond parent and infant together, but because infants are attentive to the suprasegmentals of language long before they learn words.

Parents in their homes normally clown a great deal with babies: their faces assume exaggerated expressions, their voices are higher pitched and speech is slowed down in a sing-song. Diapering is a favorite occasion for tickling tummies, moving feet, blowing bubbles, or poking out tongues. Feeding involves "biting games" with fingers or hands, and blowing raspberries. "Roughhouse time" may mean knee games, being thrown up in the air, and so on. These games are usually accompanied by exclamations, mock cries, laughter, and hugs (Sutton-Smith, 1974).

Characteristically, parents of a limited-hearing child cease to play such games when they become aware that the child is not responding normally, because these vocal games depend upon feedback: the baby initiates them as often as the adults. If they are told that they have a "deaf" child, there arises in their minds a very real barrier so that they are unable to fill their roles in a normal way. They always think, "our baby cannot hear." But, if they are told that their baby *can* hear through the hearing aid and will store all the sounds entering through the aids until he is ready to use them, the barrier will go down, and each family will develop its own vocal games. Some parents need to be told that the tone and inflection of the voice are extremely important and should be pleasant and vivacious to be "feedback-productive." They can begin by echoing the sounds made by the child and gradually add new vowels, babbling, and tunes. Imitating a baby's laughter and playing laughing games are important games, too.

The following are examples of vocal play taken from diaries written by mothers of children with severe to profound losses.

> I put K. on my knees and hold her hands. I bounce her up and down, saying, "Horsey horsey, Woo woo." When I say *Woo,* I lower her over my shins and pull her up again.

* * *

> J. likes to sit on my lap and rock in a large rocker. He likes to put his head on my shoulder, then raise up quickly and yell, "Hi." He does this over and over. When he raises up I stop rocking. I say, "Put your head down," or "Lay down," and when he does it I start rocking the chair again. We do this at naptime every afternoon.

* * *

> Cindy likes to smack her lips together and laughs when I do it, too. She also clanks her teeth and does it more if I should do it, too.
>
> Last night while I was getting Cindy ready for bed I showed her the raspberries (ththpp). She laughed and put her tongue between her teeth and made a sound with her voice.
>
> Today I tried to emphasize high and low sounds to Cindy. When she asked for more I said "more" (very low) and then "more" (very high) and she did the same. We made a game of it: "more-more-more" (high) and "more" (low). She did the same and enjoyed it. She also seems to recognize the difference of high and low without her hearing aids.
>
> Cindy likes to play follow the leader at the dinner table with herself as leader. She makes different types of sounds such as bye-bye, la-la, etc. She pats her mouth with her hand while saying "ah" (Indian fashion).
>
> Sometimes when we say to Cindy, "Yummy yummy in the Tummy," she pats her tummy.

* * *

> Ricky has made some interesting advancements. He can follow rhythm exceptionally well lately. He may not say the word given but always picks up the rhythm of the word. He is trying to say "bye-bye," which comes out "I–I." He waves on command.

The next excerpt shows that this was a most important step.

> Sometimes it is hard to fill a page in this diary but this week we could rave on and on about Ricky. The other night he began to say "bye-bye" perfectly. Not only that, but he said it for his daddy. His daddy took him for a walk and he now believes that Ricky also says "bow-wow."

Calling Games

The family should begin vocal play very close to the child and gradually move further away. It is then time to begin *calling games.* Mothers do this quite naturally, calling to the child from time to time as they move about their work—"Hi, there. I see you. I hear you." Calling the child's name, saying, "Boo!" and "I love you" are a mother's way of playing calling games. What the mother is saying is not important; it is the tone and inflection of her voice that the baby is absorbing and from which he is gaining emotional security.

When a mother keeps in contact with her limited-hearing child in this way, she is helping to extend his range of listening, and most mothers report eventually that the child "hears" her when called from another room. No limitations need be placed upon a profoundly deaf child in this respect; the mother should be told to try it (i.e., calling from another room) but not feel disappointed if he does not respond from this distance.

It should be noted that gestures are not forbidden at all; indeed, many "calling games" are accompanied by gestures: "Wave bye-bye; throw a kiss; Peek-a-boo; Big boy! or So big!" (said when a baby stretches his arms up). It is sometimes necessary, however, to check parents who use an excessive amount of gestures, or who use it instead of speech, for this would detract attention away from listening. Gestures should be used where it is normal and natural to use gestures. All children use gestures to supplement their lack of vocabulary to express what they are trying to communicate. If this accompanies efforts to talk, it need not be curbed, but some children become such effective communicators with gesture language that they do not put forth much effort to talk, and this, of course, must be carefully handled. The clinician may need to go so far as to pretend she does not understand the gesture, and encourage the child to talk. This usually applies to an older preschool child who has not received early training. If an infant is given the language to accompany his gestures as they occur, the use of gestures will decrease to normal proportions.

Music

Music should be used often. A home organ, the radio, television, and audio tapes or a CD player can be heard through powerful hearing aids, in spite of unfortunate statements often made in the media that deaf children who are wearing aids only feel music through vibrations.

Strong rhythms are best at first, and the child is held and rocked to a lullaby or held and marched around the room to marching music. Infants enjoy "dancing," (bouncing up and down or side to side) and later they enjoy clapping to music, and turning round and round.

One mother wrote:

> Every evening after dinner Cindy's daddy plays the guitar and we all sing. Mona and Cindy take turns riding the rocking horse to the music. Cindy seems to like the guitar. She runs her hand across the strings and seems to like the sound.

With music it is possible to vary the loudness levels until a comfortable listening level is found. The child should later be moved further and further away from the source of the sound, thus extending his range of hearing, until it is observed that he no longer responds to the music.

Parents of a hearing-impaired baby have to be reminded to sing when holding him.

The infant of two years and up enjoys playing with the volume control of a radio or tape recorder or CD player to elicit an "Ow—too loud!" response, or "I can't hear anything" response from adults. This is a good indication of his own awareness of high or low intensities. He can also begin to indicate when it is on or off.

Noisemakers

All babies play with noisemakers: rattles, squeaky toys, cradle gyms; and playing with noisemakers is a familiar activity in clinics and schools, but for the infant who can sit up, it can be introduced in the following way:

Place two loud noisemakers (e.g., a loud horn and a loud bell) into a large, preferably brightly-colored box. Reach inside and squeeze the horn. Clap your hands over your ears to indicate that you have heard something. Smiling, say, "What's that?" Repeat sound, restraining the child from looking into the box! Again say, "Oh! what's that?" and finally, show the noisemaker.

Another way to play this game is to sit across the table from a small child and his parent to maintain good eye contact. Hide the noisemaker under the table instead of in the box. This procedure should be followed to help the child develop the following: (1) awareness of the sound; (2)

attention to the sound without visual association with the object; (3) curiosity about the sound. Then we show him the *meaning* of the sound—the sound comes from, or means, the noisemaker. Finally, we encourage him to imitate the sound.

Visual clues are not totally excluded at this point, but the emphasis is upon the facial expression, good eye contact, and upon the gestures, such as pointing to the ears, which show that the adult is hearing and reacting to sounds. The visual clues are not being used for lipreading, but to demonstrate listening, which is a rather abstract concept for a young child.

Of course, care must be taken not to startle a child who is just becoming accustomed to amplification; however, young children can tolerate a great deal of noise. Older children, especially those who have not been fitted with aids until they are three years or older, *may* present more resistance to it. Dale (1979) states that although amplification has not been successfully used with adults who have recruitment, children appear to be helped by recruitment.

The next game, which teaches awareness of loudness and quietness of sounds, has been very successful over the years with the infant who can sit up and imitate. (The "under-ones" like to play it with a wooden spoon on their high chair.)

Sit around a small table. Take two blocks and beat them on the table. Say, "Oh, what a *loud* noise!" Hold the blocks to your ears. Use an appropriate facial expression, but do not look displeased. Do this again and again. The child will now want to participate. Either let him use your blocks, or give two blocks to him, saying, "Here's a block for you. Here's another block for you." (Always verbalize every experience.) Help him make the noise if he needs help, but it is better to demonstrate and let the child participate when he wishes to. (*From the beginning, we are creating situations in which the infant imitates all that we do because it is fun to do. This leads to imitation of all that we say.*)

Be sure to intersperse activities with words of reinforcement: "Oh, what a loud noise you made!" and so forth. Now tap the table with the blocks quietly. Say, "Oh, what a *quiet* noise." Place your forefinger against your lips and say, "SH!" Repeat this again, alternating loud and quiet.

To interrupt an activity and put toys away is an important lesson to be learned. Young children seem to learn very quickly if you say, *Bye-bye,* wave, and remove the blocks. Later they will say, *Bye-bye,* and put away items for you, especially when they are losing interest!

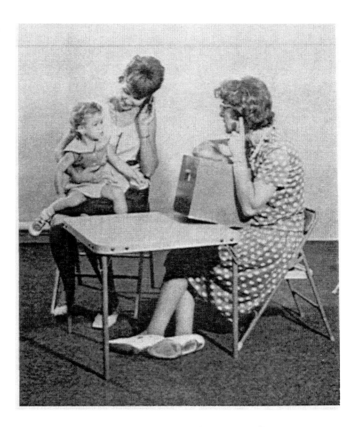

Figure 8.1. Learning to attend to noisemakers.

This lesson can be repeated with a drum, pan and spoon, and other objects. For children under four years of age, use one thing at a time because their attention span is short.

The next game is listening to and *imitating* a sound. Place two drums on a table, and after you hit one drum, encourage the child to hit the other drum. A drum can be made out of an oatmeal box or coffee can. Repeat with a loud bell, which you place beside the drum. Continue the game a few times. If the child chooses the noisemaker first, you imitate him. Use noisemakers of decreasing intensity.

Discrimination Activities with Noisemakers

First Level: Recognizing "On" and "Off"

After the child has become familiar with the sound of "pounding" on a drum, coffee can, or saucepan, rhythm and response training begins. Mother holds the child at one end of the room and pounds slowly and rhythmically on a "drum." The clinician faces them at the other end of the room. She indicates that she hears the noise, and begins marching toward them. The mother stops pounding, and the clinician stops marching, and shakes her head to indicate that she cannot hear anything. The mother begins to pound again, the clinician begins to march again, and so on.

They change places. A child over eighteen months of age will be eager to pound the drum and "make" the adult march, but he needs a little help. Many children age two and over "catch on" very quickly, and interrupt their pounding appropriately. In this way, they observe that adults or siblings respond to sound.

Other response games are as follows: (1) push a train across the floor when a whistle is blown; (2) push a car when a horn is squeezed; (3) march, dance, clap, and so forth, when music is played; (4) hold a block to your ear and drop it into a can when a sound is heard.

Second Level: Discrimination Between Sounds

The second step is listening and imitating sounds *without looking.* Begin with loud sounds. Place the drum and bell on the table. Turn the child around, or have him close his eyes, and hit the drum. Turn the child around again and say, "Which one did you hear?" Guide his hand to the correct noisemaker. *Do not let the child guess and make an error.* Repeat with the bell. It is often helpful to play this with another adult first so that the child sees the whole activity before being asked to participate. He will most enjoy making sounds and having *you* identify them!

As the child learns to recognize one sound, another new one can be added—it can be varied. The child may enjoy reaching into a large box to find the correct noisemaker.

Third level: Discrimination and Distance Hearing

The next step involves increasing the distance between the child and the sound, and is most appropriate for the child from one and one-half to three years old. Place two loud noisemakers upon a table, and two small chairs at a distance of three feet or more from the table. (Distance can be determined by the child's range of hearing in calling games.)

You, the clinician, sit down while the parent and child stand by the table. The parent rings a loud cowbell. You "overreact," clapping your hands to your ears saying, "I heard that!" The parent replaces the bell and calls your name. You *run* to the table, pick up and ring the bell. The parent claps and says, "That's right!" Then he points and says, "My turn." (Gestures are always eliminated within a short time.)

The child and parent now sit down (with backs to the table) and the game is repeated. (Chairs can be turned toward the table if the child will cover his eyes.)

The child is very amused by the *running back* part of the game. Actually it is very important, because a small child may forget what he has heard by the time he reaches the table if this game is conducted at a slow speed. The parent always guides his hand to the correct noisemaker until it is obvious that the child recognizes it.

The chairs are gradually moved farther and farther away from the table. Many profoundly deaf children develop a remarkable range once they recognize the sound. This activity is very important since it fosters the beginning of an auditory memory span.

Fourth Level: Discrimination Between Loud and Quiet Sounds

The chairs are again placed close to the table. A quiet sound is now added to the two loud sounds—a whistle, a quiet squeaky toy, the rustle of paper, and so on. The range for these may be narrower.

Fifth Level: Discrimination of Recorded Sound

For an older child, the last level involves recognizing a *reproduction* of a noisemaker. The child listens to a tape or other recording of sounds, and places a matching noisemaker upon the appropriate picture, waves it in rhythm, and so on.

One should never spend too much time on activities using noisemakers. Environmental sounds and vocal games are much more important.

Environment Sounds

Simultaneously, it is important for the child to become increasingly aware of all the sounds in his environment (paper rustling, a dog barking, water running, and so on). Normally we do not react perceptibly to most of these sounds. For example, we may hear the doorbell and leave the room suddenly, but because the limited-hearing child has not heard it, or heard it only faintly, he does not understand *why* we have disappeared. It is meaningless to him and you may think he is deaf to it. Because of this kind of experience, many "deaf" youngsters are very apprehensive and insecure, and cling to their caregivers.

A parent has to be shown how to react with a great deal of facial expression and language to all the environmental sounds, and how to attract the child's attention to them repeatedly, so that eventually he will become increasingly sensitive to them, localize, and understand them.

For example, if the mother hears the doorbell, she must say to the youngster, "Listen, I hear the doorbell," and point to her ears. (By this time it is probably being rung again.) She must pick up the child and take him to the door, again talk about hearing the bell, and should say, "Let's open the door. See who is there," and so on.

A game of door knocking with other members of the family can be played many times a day with the child and mother first knocking on the door, and then taking turns to listen behind the door and reacting to the sound. It is a good time to learn "I hear you. Hi!"

One boy (with a 103 dB average loss ISO, in the better ear) showed a total lack of response to the doorbell when he was standing directly beside the door. He was shown how to ring the bell, and the chimes were pointed out to him when someone else rang the bell. A few months later, he heard the chimes from the bedroom (a distance of 75 feet). He always reacted with great excitement, running toward the door to open it long before anyone else could reach it.

It can be demonstrated with this type of activity that a profoundly deaf youngster does not react until he knows how the sound is made, that is, until the sound is meaningful to him. Then he reacts with enjoyment over and over again and at increasing distances from the source.

The parents, then, must draw the child's attention to all the environmental sounds in this way—showing the source of the sound, talking about, and imitating it. For example: "Listen! I hear a dog. He says, 'Bow wow, bow wow.' Look, here is the dog. Listen, he is saying, 'Bow wow,'" and so forth. Or, they may hear a sound and reproduce it together as, for example, rustling paper.

Play activities can be used to make the child aware that many objects are associated with or accompanied by sound. This will reinforce real life experiences.

When sitting around a table, hide a toy dog under the table and say: "Listen! Wow wow (loudly). What's that? Listen, Mother. What do you hear? Mother joins in. "I hear wow wow. What's that?" The dog pops up over the edge of the table and jumps around with the adults saying, "Wow wow" loudly. We pet the dog and say, "Nice doggy" or Sh! Doggy," and so on.

Encourage the child to imitate the sound, but do not insist upon this at first. One of the easiest ways to initiate imitation is to cover your mouth with your hand when you make the "wow wow." Place your hand over the parent's mouth and he will imitate "Wow wow." Then the parent places her hand over the child's mouth and looks expectantly, eyes wide open and smiling, for a response. Most young children will try to imitate and are so imitative that it is rarely necessary to use the hand technique once they realize that they are expected to imitate. The sound and toy come to be associated naturally. In this way, one can also check the child's auditory memory and recall.

Other toys can be used in the same way:

- A toy duck represented by Quack-quack.
- A toy train represented by oo-oo-oo.
- A toy airplane represented by mmmmmm.
- A toy bird represented by a whistle.
- A toy cat represented by a loud meow.
- A toy car represented by brbrbr—beep! beep!
- A toy fire engine represented by eeeeeeeeee.

For a two- to three-year-old, cut out a door in a cardboard box and say:

"Knock, knock.
Ring the bell: Ding-dong!
Open the door!"

The child reaches into the box, and pulls out a toy which can be associated with a sound. For example, a toy motorbike which is pushed along the table or up and over the box, as the adult babbles b-b-b-bbbb. One should vary the vocal intensity and rhythm in all of these games.

If there are other children in the family, they can take a turn to knock on the door. Sharing and taking turns have to be learned, too.

The parent should play with toys and imitate the sounds made by them, then follow up by listening to the real sounds. For example, after playing with the car, go into a car and listen to the horn. After playing with a toy bird, try to listen to a real bird—in a pet store or in a cage. Arrange to be near a phone at a prearranged time. Have someone call and let the phone ring for some time so that you can say, "What's that?" Point to your ear. "I hear *rrr rrr*. It's the phone. It says *rrr,*" and so forth.

A mother or caregiver has to do "hometraining" activities while she is doing other chores and it is important for the clinician to develop ideas which require relatively little special equipment and which will fit easily into the every day routine. The author has found that mealtimes offer excellent opportunities to reinforce certain sounds. A young child may sit in his high chair four or five times a day. Mother can put some of his toys there, and while she is feeding her child, she may say, "Here's kitty. He says meow meow. He wants some. Feed the kitty." She smacks her lips loudly.

The following excerpts from diaries illustrate that the first reactions to wearing hearing aids are likely to be reactions to environmental sounds never before heard by the child—a point which needs emphasizing to parents, since many of them expect speech sounds to occur first!

> Jennifer responds to a knock at the door if she is listening for it. Before getting her aid, she loved to ride on top of the vacuum cleaner. Now, she hightails it for the nearest chair when it starts. Yesterday, I was dusting the piano and dropped the dust can on the keys. Jennifer nearly jumped out of her skin. She soon regained her nerve and prefers to sit on top of the piano and pound with her feet.
>
> This morning she was helping me bathe Jodie and heard the train whistle without any prompting from me and flew to the back door to wave to the engineer.
>
> She now takes a wooden spoon and without prompting, makes a soft sound—then a loud sound. She is visibly pleased with herself and practices for long periods.

* * *

> When Luann hears the dog next door, she immediately reacts and imitates him. I think this is really quite good, because there is quite a distance between them and also a fence so that she cannot see him at all—just hear him.

* * *

> When I am standing at the kitchen window watching Cindy ride her bike on the patio, and deeply engrossed in her play, I can't resist knocking on the window. Each time she looks up sharply and each time I feel the same thrill and realize how very thankful we are.
>
> I can remember worrying so about her from the time she was three months

old, and she was sitting in her infant seat in the kitchen watching me while I dried dishes. I accidentally dropped a heavy pot right near her and she didn't become startled. From that time on until we had her hearing tested clinically, we constantly tried to test her hearing at home. We snapped out fingers, clapped our hands, called her from behind, banged on doors, etc. Sometimes she turned around, and sometimes she didn't. And we couldn't be sure when she seemed to hear us whether she also saw our actions from the corner of her eye. If we banged on a pot or pan with a spoon she would react. But we could never tell any reaction for sure.

We thought, "Either you hear or you don't hear." We didn't realize that there was such a thing as a person having a loss of some of their hearing, and with the aid of a modern hearing aid being brought back into our world of sounds.

* * *

Ira shows improvement each day. One day this week he cleared his throat and was surprised to hear a sound from it. He heard the rain on the windshield wiper of the car. He hears the water in a shower, and backfire of a car on the street.

Ira was amazed to hear the sound of the crickets this morning. We were watching the television tonight and Ira heard the comedians call, "Fire, Fire." That's the first time he responded to any words over the television.

Tonight he heard the water of a river on the television and wanted to know what it was. He was also delighted to hear the horses' hoofs in a cowboy picture.

Today I was out with him and he heard the sound of the wind blowing through the trees. He immediately wanted to know what that was.

The alertness and sensitivity to sounds are markedly different in a child trained auditorily. One would never predict such results from the typical audiograms of profoundly deaf children.

Localization

As soon as it becomes apparent that the child is increasingly aware of sound, activities can be structured so that he begins to *localize* them. For example, one family played with a toy clock which had a very loud "tick tock." When their baby was familiar with this sound, they hid it behind furniture and crawled around trying to find it. Another family used a small radio.

When an infant is not able to sit up, lay him down on the floor, and kneel at his feet. Make a noise with a noisemaker in front of his face. Move the noisemaker from side to side to encourage him to turn in the direction of the sound. Move the noisemaker from his toes along the side of his body to his head, to encourage him to look down and up.

When he is able to sit up or be held in a sitting position, introduce the sound on a plane that goes through his ears at a distance from one to three feet away from either ear, or in front of him. One parent can sit in front of him and ring a bell, always directing him to "listen." Then he can move from side to side, ringing the bell. If the child does not turn his head or locate the sound, the other parent may move his head gently. The parent who is ringing the bell will move gradually further and further away until he is across the room, noticing when he seems to be getting out of range.

A similar "game" can be played using the voice to call the child's name. It is usually more effective to demonstrate this first. Mother should stand just in front of the child. Father, sitting beside the child, or with child on his knee, then calls loudly, "Mama." Mother puts her hands on her ears to indicate: "I hear that. I hear you." Next, she stands with her back to the child so that she has to turn around when she hears *Mama,* and says, "What?" Gradually she moves further and further away until she is outside the door, and a young child is, of course, very amused when she pops her head into the room when she is called. It is then time for the child to change places, and father will turn him around when his name is called. It is sometimes more effective if a reward is given to the response, such as a cookie!

Localization of environmental sounds can be taught in the same way, with the child sitting down. For example, Mother or the caregiver can leave water running and talk to the child about hearing it. Then, turning his head in the direction of the faucet, she can show how it goes on and off.

A list of "listening games" is helpful to parents, and a check sheet is helpful to the clinician.

A Listening Book or Book of Sounds

When an infant enjoys looking at pictures, a parent can be shown how to "read a book," emphasizing the sounds associated with the picture rather than the story.

> "Look! There's a doggie. Wow wow, wow wow!
> He's a nice doggie! He pants: h-h-h-h-h-.
> Ow! Don't bite, doggie," and so on.

Between two and three years of age, children enjoy making their own books. Buy a medium sized and sturdy scrapbook and help the child paste on every other page one large picture representing the toys with which he has been playing. It is best to paste only one or two new pictures each day. In "reading" this book, one emphasizes again the sounds and activities associated with the picture:

> "Look! Here's a horsey. He goes . . . (click your tongue several times). Whoa, Horsey!"
>
> "That's a candle. That's *hot!* Blow it out."

Auditory Processing of Sounds

The goal of these awareness and discrimination activities is this: Does the child realize that the *sound* has a specific *meaning?* Can he imitate it and recall it spontaneously? Place a few of the toys in front of the child and cover your mouth. If you say "Meow, meow," does he reach for the cat? If he does, a small edible reward encourages cooperation! If he does not, guide his hand to the correct toy and again make the sound *meow.*

A child may pick up a toy from the toyshelf and spontaneously make a correct sound, but this is a *conditioned* response. The ability to *choose* between toys in response to someone's directions indicates a much higher level of learning and a readiness to move on to real words.

What kind of time span is needed for the child with a hearing loss? Some children may develop these basic skills within six months; others may require eighteen months after being fitted with hearing aids. The quality of home stimulation, the age and intelligence of the child, and the degree of hearing loss are some of the factors which will influence progress.

For the clinician, it is important to apply the stimulus, shape the appropriate response, create a situation in which the response must happen spontaneously, and then move on to the next stimulus. If the response cannot be elicited after a reasonable length of time, this must be regarded as a "warning bell," and reevaluation will be necessary—of the amplification system, or the child's development in other areas.

THE BASIC DIFFERENCES BETWEEN TRADITIONAL AND AUDITORY–VERBAL EDUCATION

It will seem to the experienced reader that many of the activities and equipment described to develop hearing perceptions are not new.

Obviously, those who work with the young child teach similar vocabulary and will tend to use similar materials.

If the differences appear subtle, the purposes are entirely different. We must reconsider the basic differences between Auditory-Verbal and traditional preschool programs.

FIRST, no limits are preset according to the audiogram in an Auditory-Verbal Program. All children receive the same *foundation* of listening experiences to develop a listening function.

SECOND, the children do not receive "sessions of auditory *training.*" Their listening function develops because emphasis is placed upon listening throughout their waking hours so that hearing becomes an integral part of their personality.

THIRD, an infant's attention is never directed toward lipreading or tactile cues at the same time that the clinician is developing a listening function. His energy is directed toward listening, and the rewards and reinforcements are for listening. True, he is not blindfolded, and visual perception can take place, but only in the same natural way that it occurs during a normal-hearing child's activities. Sometimes it *is* necessary to conceal the speaker's mouth, but only when a child has become visually oriented, i.e., when he has already received lipreading training, or does not begin training until he is three to four years of age. At no time is this a multi-sensory auditory training program—the child is not directed to look first and then listen, nor to look *and* listen to the speaker, only to *listen.*

FOURTH, although the clinician provides activities which develop the necessary skills to move the child forward as rapidly as possible from level to level, this program places the onus for stimulation and repetition upon the home—the family is given back its normal role. Activities used in the clinical situation are used to demonstrate to the parent and to enable the clinician to observe the infant's responses so that proper guidance for the home-training program may be given. The author was never aware of the tremendous amount of auditory stimulation and repetition which a mother gives to a child, and which cannot be reproduced in a clinic or schoolroom, until she had babies of her own, and had observed other mothers in the pediatrician's office, the supermarket, and so on.

FIFTH, the Auditory-Verbal Program is based on the normal sequential stages of auditory-verbal development, not upon a program for the deaf. Materials are given to the parents with the understanding that they are recapitulating the early experiences of a normal-hearing child.

SIXTH, the learning environment is so structured that the child has a great deal of fun with sound, and he begins to depend upon his residual hearing. He does not know he is not supposed to be able to do these activities because of deafness! In turn, his parents talk to him as if he is hearing, which he *is* — through his hearing aids.

SEVENTH, the role of the audiologist is a primary one, making appropriate adjustments to the hearing aid and teaching the parents how to check the aids on a daily basis.

Chapter 9

THE DEVELOPMENT OF SPOKEN LANGUAGE 1: PHONOLOGY AND EARLY VOCALIZATIONS

As soon as an infant has learned to listen, that is, show awareness of and reactions to any sounds in his environment, it is time to begin intensive language stimulation.

DEFINITION OF LANGUAGE

What do we mean by language and how is it acquired by normal-hearing children? If we ask a group of parents, we will receive a variety of definitions because language does have several components which linguists have labeled as follows:

Phonology. This refers to the basic units of language called *phonemes* which enable us to discriminate *pin* from *bin*, for example, and to combine sounds into words.

Vocabulary. This refers to the meaning of words, or symbolic language, but it becomes confusing in English because one word can have several meanings, as for example, the word *fly*.

Semantics. This refers to the meaning of words when they are arranged in sentences. For example, the sentences *John hit Mary* and *Mary hit John* use the same words but have entirely different meanings. Another example: *move your chair*, and *take the chair at the meeting*.

Syntax. This refers to the development of grammar, or the rules for recombining words into sentences.

Pragmatics. This describes the intricate patterns of taking turns in dialogue, participating in conversation and anticipating the information needed by the other speaker.

Some writers describe two forms of language: the expressive form, when a person speaks, and the receptive form, when a person listens and understands. They also refer to *inner language* or the knowledge one has about one's language code which is used for thought.

Language can also involve nonverbal language, and even verbal language is accompanied by gesture, facial expressions, bodily posture and vocal intonational patterns, all of which influence the meaning as it is perceived by the listener.

But spoken language is an interactive process. Cole (Volta, 1992) gives an excellent example when she describes a typical scene. A little boy is sitting in his high chair smiling. He says "uh oh" in a characteristic rising and falling inflection and looks over the side of his chair. His mother turns around to see a piece of food on the floor. The boy's use of the sounds indicates that he has not only the motor skills for speech, but he has some cognitive knowledge about cause and effect. He knows that his mother will react to this sound and he realizes that when something disappears from sight he can look for it.

Thus, the fabric of spoken language has many interwoven strands: cognition and motor skills, together with the social-emotional aspects of the situation.

When we study the development of language, we find that the normal-hearing child can analyze and complete the basics by approximately age five, with almost no direct instruction except about 25,000 hours of listening. This amazing feat supports the idea that the normal human brain is naturally preprogrammed, as it were, to perceive patterns and structure and can learn language, providing that it receives appropriate stimulation (McNeill, 1966). It seems to be able to break each system down into the smallest combinable parts and develop rules for combining the parts.

However, a child will only use a language he experiences in his home environment. Ervin-Tripp (1971) wrote of a normal-hearing preschooler of deaf parents who was exposed to spoken language on television but did not learn to speak English because his parents used only sign language.

Children with a hearing loss are not preprogrammed to learn in a different way, and the majority will learn to speak well given the proper conditions:

1. Early detection
2. Maximum use of amplification technology
3. Relative integration of the central nervous system and normal motor development, or remediation of problems in those areas.
4. Exposure to normal spoken language.
5. Parental guidance.

THE NORMAL DEVELOPMENT OF SPEECH

Prelinguistic Activities: The Vocal Level

After the early weeks of communication through crying, a normal-hearing infant first shows self-stimulation and imitation when he begins to coo and to make more than one sound. Between the third and fifth months, he "talks" or babbles to people and will sometimes imitate single sounds or syllables. He begins to laugh and will continue to laugh if adults echo his laughter. This phase corresponds to the *vocal level* as described by Huizing (1959), Lewis (1951), and others. Between the sixth and ninth months, Huizing has pointed out, the infant is creating his own inner auditory world, and even a minimum of residual hearing in the bass part of the tone scale is sufficient to enable the profoundly deafened child to form an auditory feedback mechanism. This is a period of increased vocal play and babbling, self-initiated.

The *vocal level* is of tremendous significance. Embedded into language are the suprasegmentals: intonation, stress, rhythm, prosody, and disjuncture, which are carried by the voice and changed by duration, intensity, and pitch. This information is present in the lower frequencies and can be heard by even the most profoundly deaf with amplification. Indeed, it must be heard, for it cannot be seen. Before infants can articulate the vowels and consonants, they are making strings of vocal sounds which contribute to the development of coordination between breath control and voicing.

There have been many studies concerning the abnormality of breath control, phrasing, and voice quality of the deaf speaker, including the temporal qualities of duration, rate, and stress. Because the deaf tend to give equal stress to all syllables, they have been shown to take two to four times as long to say a sentence (Smith, 1975; Nickerson, 1975; Forner and Hixon, 1977; and Ling, 1992).

These abnormalities are caused by too much emphasis upon correct articulation taught by means of visual and tactile systems without a period of time given for vocal play, the development of auditory feedback, and auditory monitoring.

Prelinguistic Activities: The Emergence of Imitation and the Phonetic Level

The next stage might be called the *phonetic level* and includes the development of a feedforward mechanism, that is, the ability to "motor plan" and send the correct messages to the speech muscles.

Piaget (1945–1962) has described six stages of emerging imitative skills with vocal and gestural imitation development along a similar sequence:

1. Preparation through the reflex mechanisms, such as crying.
2. Sporadic imitation or vocalizations which seem to be made for their own sake rather than for distress, after stimulation of the child's voice by an adult voice, although there may be no similarity between the sounds the model and the child are making. Mutual imitation may occur if the adult imitates the exact sound or movement of the child as it occurs. However, if the adult modifies the model, the child will not modify his activities and may even stop doing anything.
3. Systematic imitation. The infant develops the ability to imitate sounds or actions *in his repertoire,* that is, not new ones.
4. Imitation of new combinations of sounds and movements already in his repertoire.
5. Deferred imitation: the child reproduces through memory.

Imitation is highly dependent upon the motivation of the infant. This means, that when an infant fails to imitate, it is exceedingly difficult to tell whether he cannot or will not (Uzgiris and Hunt, 1975).

Echolalia

After he has learned to imitate many sound combinations of his own accidental making, the infant has laid the foundation for the next step in the development of speech, *echolalia.* This is imitation of sounds which the child hears others make but which he does not himself understand, and this begins at about the ninth or tenth month. Eisenson (1938) says that during this stage the child acquires a repertoire of sound complexes which he will ultimately be able to produce at will, and which he must have before he can learn to speak, or acquire a language in the adult sense.

But echolalia is a highly complex process. We say that the child imitates sounds made by others, but what we call the *same* sounds, made for example by the father and mother, though they may be the same phoneme, are composed of phonemes which differ in pitch as well as in other characteristics, and therefore constitute very different physical stimuli. The sound that the *infant* makes, if he successfully imitates them, is of a very different pitch, which must therefore sound different to the child himself. Already at this early stage of speech development, therefore, the child is learning to recognize and reproduce the phoneme—a *pattern* which is common to the sounds made by his parents and by himself, although in other respects these sounds differ from each other.

The Three Schemata—Phoneme, Word and Sentence

Sir Russell Brain (1961) has postulated that separate *schema* must be established in the development of communication. He uses the term "schema" to describe the different levels of speech and language physiology. *Speech schemas*, when established, remain stable parts of the permanent equipment of the individual. Thus the physiological basis of the recognition of a phoneme is an *auditory phoneme schema*. However a phoneme may be uttered, we identify it at once without any process of conscious comparison with a standard. The schema is purely physiological.

Two further physiological processes which must play a part in the comprehension of spoken speech are concerned with the meaning of words. That a word exists independently of its meaning is obvious from the fact that a child can learn a word without knowing what it means. Meaning depends, first, on its power to refer to something in the surroundings or to evoke appropriate ideas. Hence, a *word schema* must possess links within the physiological bases of perception and thought. Second, the meaning of words depends upon the relationship of each individual word to those which precede or follow it in a sentence, that is, upon syntax. These two factors in meaning, which we may call the *syntactical* and the *semantic*, must be intimately related at the physiological level, because the serial order of words and their syntactical relationship influence their meaning and, conversely, meaning is reflected in serial order and syntax. So we may also have a *sentence* or *phrase schema*.

PROPERTIES OF SPEECH

Phonemes and Formants

Development of speech for communication involves learning to discriminate speech sounds, imitating them, and eliminating non-English sounds. A limited-hearing child, wearing appropriate amplification, can hear and compare his speech patterns, but if his residual hearing is absent or severely impaired at certain frequencies, how can he perceive very fine differences between the sounds? Existing data quoted by Jeffers (1966) seems to indicate that for accurate reception of all vowels and diphthongs, we would need to hear 85 to 3700 cps, but most vowels can be identified if we hear the first two formants—from 250 to 2400 cycles per second with a male voice. (A child's voice ranges from 250 cps to 3700 cps.)[1]

Figure 9.1, taken from Fletcher (1953), gives an approximation of the frequency range needed for the faithful transmission of speech sounds. The sounds are listed on intensity levels; the intensity of the sensation level decreases as one reads down the chart. As most sensorineural losses involve severe impairment above 750 Hz, it would seem that only a small group of phonemes would be heard with clarity—mainly the vowels and some voiced consonants—*l, n, m, ng, d, b, v, z,* and voiced *th.* Morley, quoting Fletcher, Watson, and Tolan, has stated that if the frequencies are cut off above 3000 cps, intelligibility is reduced by 10 percent, and above 1500 cps by 70 percent. Cawthorn and Harvey, however, feel a cutoff above 3200 cps is negligible, but above 1600 cps there is a 40 percent reduction (Morley, 1957).

Figure 9.2 shows the formant areas of vowels and consonants, with levels above ASA free-field threshold at 2 cm from the lips of the speaker (Male data from Fant in Bess et al., 1981).

Redundancy

Current research in voice science has shown that this is not the whole story. There is redundancy in speech, and a frequency range can be greatly reduced with speech remaining intelligible. Fisch (1957) describes

---

[1]For a more detailed description of formants, read *The Deaf Child* by Whetnall and Fry (1964), *The Speech Chain* by Peter Denes (1963), *Auditory Analysis and Perception of Speech* by Fant (1975) and Stoker and Ling (1992).

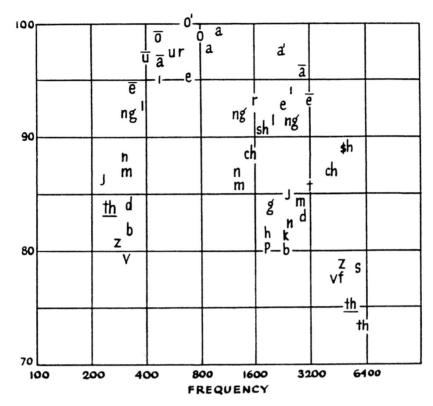

Figure 9.1. Combined characteristics of the fundamental sounds of speech. Courtesy of Fletcher, Harvey: *Speech and Hearing in Communication.* New York, Van Nostrand, 1953. (Copyright 1953 by Litton Educational Publishing.)

how acoustic wave forms can be measured and analyzed in great detail. Then the *complex wave form can be reduced to an infinitely clipped version with speech still remaining intelligible.* Haskins Laboratory has demonstrated the same kind of experiments. Natural speech has redundancy to maintain communications under adverse conditions such as noise, and it is transmitted over a communication channel of full capacity. But Shannon has shown that perfect transmission is possible over a channel of minimal capacity with elaborate terminal coding equipment (Shannon *et al.,* 1962).

Clinicians who have worked in an auditory program have found that they cannot predict from the audiogram what children will hear through appropriate aids. With intensive stimulation over a period of months, phonemes do develop normally.

The limited-hearing child can be taught the correct interpretation of

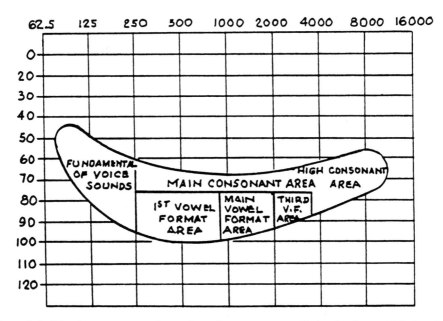

Figure 9.2. The formant areas of vowels and consonants, with levels above ASA free-field threshold at 2 cm. from the lips of the speaker. Male data from Fant as shown in Bess, F., Freeman, B., and Sinclair, S.: *Amplification in Education*, AGBA, 1981.

signals coming over a communication channel of minimal capacity. We do not really know how the human ear and brain perform this task.

The Transitions

Roger Brown (1958), in his book *Words and Things,* explains this by acoustic *and* functional attributes. The search for the acoustic invariance of English vowels is still in progress, but it is already clear that these are not formants at particular frequencies. They may be *relations between formants.* The identification in the laboratory of isolated vowels is much harder for the speaker of English than the everyday identification of vowels in context for the reason that context makes one phoneme more probable than another.

Liberman et al. (1952) showed that the following vowel "plays a critical part in the auditory perception of p and k . . . and in that event the irreducible correlate for p and k is the sound pattern corresponding to the consonant-vowel syllable."

This leads to the fact that a word is perceived as a whole, which is something different from the mere sum of its parts, and the organization

TABLE 9-I
THE CENTROIDS AND RELATIVE MEAN PEAK POWER
FOR EACH SPEECH ELEMENT

Element		3 Centroids	Relative Mean Peak Power
EE	(as in eat)	308, 2400, 3100	220
i	(as in it)	450, 2200, 2962	260
e	(bed)	550, 710, 2000	350
a	(at)	691, 750, 1900	370
AH	(calm)	825, 950, 1200	310
AW	(fall)	600, 1100	680
u	(up)	700, 1200	510
oo	(took)	475, 1000	260
OO	(too)	400, 800	260
ə	(above)	400, 800	very weak
er	(better)	500, 1500, 2200	210
Dipthongs:		Decisive characteristics from their vowel elements; the first is usually the strongest.	
AY	(as in take)		
I	(sight)		
OY	(coin)		
U	(you)		
OW	(spout)		
OH	(toe)		
b	(boat)	700-2700-3100	7
d	(down)	500-2600-2800	17
v	(very)	600-3000-3400	12
r	(red)	483-2400	210
l	(leg)	228-3000	101
m	(more)	861-1722	52
n	(no)	200-2169	36
ng	(sing)	200-2600	73
th	(there)	2 2600-4200	11
j	(jump)	as for d and z (500-2700-3100)	
g	(as in get)	1400-4000 600-	15
k	(cake)	1500-4000	13
H	(hot)	200-2600	73
ch	(cheek)	as for t and sh (1500-3000)	
p	(pat)	2800-3800	6
t	(toe)	3600-4300	15
f	(four)	3100-7000	5
th	(mouth)	3200-	1
sh	(shoe)	2200-4600	80

TABLE 9-I (Continued)

s	(sew)	4000-8000	16
z	(zoo)	2200-7000	16
3	(measure)	2600-4200	20

Compiled by Mrs. Marion Downs. From Fletcher, Harvey. *Speech and Hearing in Communication.* New York, Van Nostrand, 1953.

of these units which follow one another in time actually modifies the perception of the units themselves—an idea closely related to the Gestalt approach of Conrad (1954).

The hearing-impaired child, then, does not depend upon his residual ability to hear one formant or the other—he hears a "pattern" of sound.

Motor Kinesthetic Feedback and Perception

Sanders (1971) raised the issue of whether or not motor kinesthetic feedback plays a role in speech perception, since Liberman et al. (1967) have suggested that the distinctiveness of a speech sound is not inherent in the acoustic signal but is rather added as a consequence of linguistic experience. Several authors have suggested that speech may be perceived by reference to articulation; that is, the listener interprets the acoustic signal only after he has mimicked the articulatory pattern that he predicts gave rise to the acoustic signal he has received.

In the chapter on language development, the author describes how imitation of the word or words spoken by the clinician helps a child process what has been said (see Ch. 10).

Intensity of Phonemes

It will be seen from Table 10 that vowels are louder than consonants, and only two consonants approach the mean peak power of a vowel—*r* and *l*, sounds which develop relatively late in preschool speech. Loudness, however, is not constant because of changing stress patterns, and its value lies primarily in guiding us to select vowels as the first phonemes for auditory stimulation. There is also evidence that the intensity of a sound changes its frequency by 10 percent.

Duration of the sound also plays an important part in speech perception. For example, a twenty millisecond difference makes it possible to discriminate between *pa* and *ba*.

NORMAL ARTICULATION DEVELOPMENT

TABLE 9-II
DEVELOPMENT OF SPEECH ELEMENTS

	Age 2			*Age 3*	
w-	water		-w-	flower	
m-	mouth		-m	comb	
-m-	hammer		-n-	penny	
n-	no		-n	spoon	
h-	hot		g-	girl	
b-	boy		-g-	wagon	
-b-	baby		k-	cat	
p-	puppy		-k-	cookie	
-p-	apple		f-	fish	
d-	dog		-f	knife	
-d-	dadac		t-	teeth	

	Age 4			*Age 5*			*Age 6*
y-	yes		-d	bed		-l	bell
-ng-	swinging		r-	red		-g	big
-ng	ring		-r	car		-t-	letter
-r-	carrot		-l-	yellow		-t	hat
l-	light		-b	bib		ch-	chair
-mp	lamp		-ch-	kitchen		fl-	flying
j-	jump		-ch	watch		th-	there
-f-	coffee		sh-	shoe		-th-	nothing
s-	Santa		-sh	fish		-th	mouth
			th-	thumb		-sh-	fishing

	Age 7			*Age 8*	
v-	vase		-j	cage	
thr-	three		-v	stove	
z-	zipper		-th-	brother	
-z-	scissors		-z	nose	
-s-	whistle		-z-	measure	
-s	house				
sk-	school				
sl-	slide				
st-	stop				
sn-	snow				

Adapted from the Laradon Articulation Scale. Courtesy of Edmonston, William. Child Language Foundation, Denver.

Table 9-II, by Edmonston (1963), shows the upper limits of normal developmental patterns for phonemes. Although there is a great varia- tion among individuals, it remains true that the normal-hearing child of two to three years of age uses relatively few phonemes and needs seven years before articulation is mature and all consonant blends are correct (Poole, 1934; Templin, 1952). If one studies the earliest words used by children (*Mama, Dada, Nana, all gone, bye-bye, go, no*) another interesting fact emerges—they are made up of sounds of lower frequencies. When an infant says words like *up* and *hot,* he says only the vowel sounds at first. We also observe that the first words tend to be a consonant-vowel combination, sometimes repeated in two syllables (*Mama, choo-choo, ball, no*), or an open vowel-consonant combination, such as op for open, and app for apple.

Normal Growth in Intelligibility of Word Usage

It is interesting to compare the development of normal articulate speech with the development of vocabulary. The correctness of articulation appears to be associated both with the child's development in discrimination and his neuromuscular development. The quality of his caregiver's speech and the amount of conversation and repetition in his home must also play an important part. Irwin and Duffy (1951) found that by eighteen months, the normal-hearing infant can say between twenty and one hundred words, mostly nouns and verbs, which he uses as single-word sentences. *Speech at this age has only 25 percent intelligibility.* By the second birthday, the child should have between two hundred and three hundred words, he should be combining two words together to form sentences, and be using some other parts of speech, but his articulation will be only *66 percent intelligible.*

By the third birthday, a child has nine hundred words including nouns, pronouns, and adjectives. He is using three-word sentences and is *90 percent intelligible.* A four-year-old has a vocabulary of about fifteen hundred words, and at the age of five, he should be *100 percent intelligible.* Of course, there are children who far exceed these averages.

Linguists (Bullow et al., 1964) have been studying the development from vocal to verbal behavior in children and expect to find normal developmental patterns in the following:

1. Paralinguistic features, tone, loudness, and rhythm.
2. Phonemic units.
3. Step-by-step acquisition of speech sounds.
4. Mutual influence of mother's and child's speech patterns.

5. A consistent relationship between vocal to verbal behavior and development of other behavioral patterns.
6. Maturation and environmental influences.

Such data will be of inestimable help in guiding the limited-hearing infant.

ARTICULATION DEVELOPMENT FOR THE HEARING–IMPAIRED

Training should be planned on an individual basis, because it is best to start with the phonemes used spontaneously by the child. But since many deafened infants are relatively silent, or vocalize without babbling, we begin with the sounds which are most audible—the vowels and low-frequency voiced consonants which are also the first sounds used by normal-hearing infants. At all times one should take the cue from the child's behavior. For example, one severely deafened two-year-old child discovered she could bite her lip and she began to babble, *vvvv*. This was immediately used by her mother for auditory stimulation, although it occurs rarely in a child's first words.

At this point we are not talking about *imitation*, but input, that is, *stimulation*. Feeding the sounds into the aids so that the child will develop a strong auditory image and will develop the ability to discriminate or perceive differences between sounds is related to the analytic acoustic exercises described by Goldstein (1939).

Our purpose is to return to the prespeech or babbling level. The clinician does not *work* with a sound as in speech therapy sessions. The parent stimulates the infant with a phoneme for one or two weeks, that is, babbles it in play activities on the toes, with toys, and so on, and then she changes to another phoneme. In the same way, a normal-hearing infant can be heard to babble a sound for a few days until he discovers another one, whereupon he usually drops the first one and babbles only the new one for awhile. We may hope for and encourage imitation because it will indicate to us how the sound is being perceived by the child but we never insist upon this before moving on with the stimulation program, remembering that normal-hearing children do not imitate at our command, but store the sounds until they are motivated to use them. We must remind ourselves that a baby has a normal speech mechanism, and once he perceives a sound he will imitate it correctly within the limits set by his motor development and degree of aided hearing.

This philosophy was also expressed by Beebe (1953):

> As speech does not begin normally until the end of the first year or the beginning of the second year of life, evidently a sufficient number of hearing impressions must be accumulated until there is a kind of overflow into pre-formed pathways which stimulate the motor area of speech. One must conclude that the hearing remnants of a hard of hearing child have to be stimulated constantly and over a long period of time before spontaneous speech can develop. If the remnants of hearing are neglected the child will develop as though he were totally deaf. Later stimulation of residual hearing cannot be expected to produce the same results.

It is obvious that only a one-to-one relationship between caregiver and child effects a sufficient number of *hearing impressions.* Only within the home can a word be used *just* when it is appropriate to the needs of each child. No teacher in a classroom can do this. This is a different approach from the traditional method of teaching the deaf child to talk which includes requesting the child to look and listen, and to imitate.[1] It requires a clinician who has confidence and patience, for sometimes a great deal of *input* is given before any *output* is heard. The mother should be forewarned that she will probably do all of the work and may not see the result for several weeks, or months, when suddenly she will hear her child make this sound spontaneously. It is necessary to tell the mother quite often that the human brain is able to store up these experiences until the child is ready to use them. Once she has seen this occur, she relaxes and does not pressure for immediate results. For example, in one case the mother used the *p* sound for two weeks with no apparent results. About two or three weeks later she was driving the car and became aware that her daughter was *p-p-p-p-ing* all the way. Another mother reported that she had used the word *hot!* dramatically and frequently with no result for several weeks. One day Grandmother came to visit and was given a cup of coffee. Debra climbed up on her grandmother's lap and tried to drink the coffee, too. She yelled "Hot!"

Why is babbling so necessary when speech rarely occurs as a single phoneme except in interjections? The auditory sound schema must be clearly impressed upon the limited-hearing child before he can imitate

---

[1] There is much supporting evidence in the literature. Von Bekesy (1962) said that spontaneous attempts to talk should take precedence over correctness of articulation.

words correctly, and he needs practice in the motor skills. Normal-hearing speakers say sixteen phonemes per second, so quickly that there is no moment by moment control. The motor movements must be automatic and are checked by auditory feedback. For the normal-hearing child, this practice occurs during the early months of life, at least for many of the consonant sounds.

Observation of parents and normal-hearing children shows that the same procedure is used to teach the more difficult consonants during the preschool years. For example, the child may say, "Fank you," and his mother will say, "No, th-th-thank you."

One such incident occurred with the author's children. Her youngest son, when about eighteen months old, became aware that a response was given to a question. He had few words, but he had learned to say *No* in self-defense at an early age! Whenever a question was asked, he replied with a cheerful *No*. (This was not negativism which occurred later in a different context.) One morning his oldest brother told us that he had been awakened early by the baby and had spent time teaching him to say *Yes* instead of *No*. This proved to be unfortunate since an eighteen-month-old child cannot say *s*. So anxious was he to please that he did produce *Yeth*. This lisp remained and was incorporated into all his new words until about his fourth birthday. Then his mother began to play "The Smiling Game." Mother and child looked into the mirror casually and smiled with teeth together, and made the smiling sound, *S*. After a few weeks, she suggested casually on different occasions that he use the smiling sound; for example, "Can you say *sssssssssoap?*" At mealtime: "*Sssssssome* more?" Almost imperceptibly the lisp faded and by the fifth birthday was gone, except in the word *something*. In this case a visual cue was used initially for *correction*, because to the child's ear, *s* was associated kinesthetically with the tongue protruding between the teeth.

Stimulation Given in Meaningful Context

It must be made clear that phonemes are used in babbling activities for only a short period of time. As soon as possible, they are introduced as part of a meaningful context. For example, the *g* sound may be babbled, and then activities are planned to use the word *go*. It may be a few weeks before the child will be heard to say *g-g-g* in his play, but sooner or later he says *go* naturally and clearly.[2] The author has often heard normal-hearing babies babbling in this manner—in museums, in restaurants, and so on, and usually from a "closed position," that is, with an object or fist in the mouth. *Their* parents, however, usually take this for granted and ignore it.

All of this stimulation should be given in a *natural, contextual situation,* because babbling and making noises are insufficient conditions for the complete acquisition of oral language. Effective verbal communication, which is a goal of educational audiology, arises from precise emotional and purposive situations. Speech is best learned in a behavioral context since it must be appropriate to the situation affectively and referentially. Lewis (1963) emphasized that the rudimentary beginning of speech in infancy is the growth of a load of expressive actions toward a specific situation.

No Insistence on Early Correctness

When speech is controlled primarily by visual clues which are incomplete at best, it has been considered important and necessary for the child to be taught, carefully and correctly, the *whole* word. Indeed, traditional methods have tried to teach *all* forms of a word-speaking, lipreading, reading, and writing or fingerspelling. When speech is controlled primarily by hearing, we recognize that discrimination is a matching process which is gradually refined, and we can accept the child's attempts to match what he hears in a normal manner. It is not difficult to improve the articulation when the child is older and can help himself, but it is difficult to teach normal stress and inflection patterns later. These are acquired by hearing, during the process of trying to match what one hears. It is well known that one of the problems in teaching deaf children to talk is that they may articulate correctly and still be unintelligible to people outside the classroom or family because they lack the normal "melody" of speech.

---

[2]In their studies of normal hearing, Downs Syndrome, and hearing-impaired infants, Smith and Oller (1981) found that velar or "back" consonants dominate the earliest productions.

Speech Refinement

At what age should formal speech refinement or correction be initiated? The phoneme development chart shows that average, normal-hearing preschoolers learn phonemes gradually, so that many of them enter kindergarten with some immature or defective sounds, particularly, *r, l, s, th,* and *ch.* If a normal-hearing child requires several years to develop normal articulation, the limited-hearing preschooler must be given a similar learning period without emphasis upon correction. He must be given a period of time after he has learned to listen to perceive the differences between sounds and to imitate them naturally.

Usually his first attempts to match the sounds and syllables are either fairly accurate, or they are at least consistent with the immature speech of a normal-hearing child who also goes through a phase of learning to talk. If the limited-hearing child feels that he cannot say something, he simply does not try to do so. But later, when he really wishes to communicate, his difficulty may be observed; there are some words or sounds which he finds very difficult to match without considerable practice. If he hears a word and imitates in incorrectly, he hears this, and tries again, especially with encouragement. If he still does not approximate what he wants to say, he may try again, or he may accept his own version for the time being.[3]

Formal speech correction *by a professional person,* then, should be given at an age when the child has conscious control over his speech muscles and enjoys such activity without undue self-consciousness or anxiety. At this age he will be aware that other people are not understanding his speech. He will want them to understand him, and the motivation to improve his speech will come from within.

The correction of speech should be consistent with normal development. For example, one would expect the labial sounds and vowels to be accurate after the third birthday, whereas an immature *s* sound might be acceptable until the fifth year, or even until the second incisors have erupted. Speech development tends to correlate with the vocabulary needed. One mother became quite anxious when her daughter was four because, she said, her speech seemed to be less intelligible. The clinician pointed out that her vocabulary had greatly increased and now included many words containing the *s* sound (as in *scissors,* the tenses of verbs,

---

[3]The student is advised to read Roger Brown's *Words and Things* (1958) for the learning theories which support this approach.

etc.) and she really needed an *s*. Speech stimulation was then centered around the *s*, and eventually she was able to imitate this and incorporate it into her conversation. In fact, she delighted in saying to everyone, "Smoke a cigarette, smoke a cigar," and then, laughing, "smoke a pipe."

At the risk of belaboring the point, it must be emphasized that if a normal-hearing preschooler is not able to speak maturely until after several years of continuous normal listening, it is inappropriate to feel concern and drill a limited-hearing child a few months after he is fitted with an aid. He can be stimulated with speech sounds, he can be encouraged to match them, but he should not be hurried to the mirror to be given visual clues. Natural voice quality, rhythm, and inflection are lost when emphasis upon correct articulation is initiated too soon. It is not necessary to use drills when a young child can imitate auditorily, and drills are not very motivating even to the preschool child.

PSYCHOLOGICAL FACTORS OF SPEECH DEVELOPMENT

The Parent-Child Relationship

There is, however, far more to development of speech than perceptual and motor skills. Oralists are increasingly concerned by the failure of many deaf children to acquire adequate oral speech. One must recognize that there are many complex forces which operate for and against the development of normal speech in a child, and the same forces apply to the limited-hearing child. We must consider *why* children learn to talk in the first place (Laguna, 1963).

The Autism Theory

Linguistics offer several theories (Paget, 1943). The most interesting theory in recent years has been the "Autism Theory." Mowrer (1952) states that the child learns to talk for four main reasons. They are as follows:

1. He identifies with one person, namely an adult—his mother.
2. The sounds are mainly good sounds to him. They have been associated with relief and other satisfactions.
3. The sounds get results: he can contact; he can demand; he can use them to interest, satisfy and control his family.
4. The sounds make him like everyone else.

Sanger (1955) observed the relationships of a number of mothers and their infants over a period of many months, with special reference to the role of vocalization. One of the first things discovered was that most mothers, and particularly those who, by other criteria, seem to be *good* mothers, kept their infants bathed in sounds most of their waking hours. While caring for them or just spending leisure time with them, these mothers vocalized almost continuously, and even when other duties took them to adjoining rooms, they would commonly sing or call to the baby intermittently. Although a baby's voice does not sound exactly like a mother's voice, the similarity will usually be sufficient to cause a carry-over of some of the pleasurable qualities of one to the other and we may perhaps surmise that the production of mother-like sounds, in the form of babbling, is a first and highly useful step in the child's progression toward fully articulate speech. Because a woman's voice is more like that of an infant than is a man's voice, it is probably more efficient for women to have primary responsibility for the verbal development of children.

The most outstanding proof of this need for a close parent-child relationship in speech and language development has come from studies of the institutionalized child and the hospitalized child. Lack of this relationship has had an early and lasting effect upon these children. Goldfarb (1945) found that the child who had spent the first three years in an institution had a marked language defect in all areas which seemed impervious to environmental stimulation compared with a child who had lived in foster homes. To a lesser degree, speech and language problems have stemmed from confusion of this signal, as in bilingual homes, from dual relationships as in multiple births, from too much competition as in large families, and so on.

A basic premise of an auditory approach is that the mother is still the best model for communication. Only within the daily routine of the home can motivation, repetition, and imitation be provided as part of the child's most meaningful experiences. When parents and children are trained together, the mother becomes alert to the child's developmental needs. It is usually only after a normal infant has had many months of experience with the mother's voice as a good sound that he begins to hear it, on occasion, with implications of warning and threat. The speech learning process will have already gained sufficient momentum to be able to withstand the shock of this negative use of her voice.

The failure of many deaf children to acquire adequate oral speech may in part be explained by the psychologists' theories that learning to talk, then, is a process of unconscious identification with the mother. Speech is learned normally in a one-to-one relationship, not in a teacher-class relationship. Stengel (1947) discusses the importance of "echo reaction." If the communication between infant and mother is complete and satisfying, an infant wishes to echo what she says. If the relationship has been inadequate, the clinician may have to be a mother-substitute and prove to the child that an adult is likable and he can communicate freely with her.

Parental Anxiety About Speech

Unless hearing aids are fitted soon after birth it seems that speech development is always delayed. This is usually not of great concern to the mother until her child reaches the age of three-and-a-half or four years, when the difference between the conversation of the normal-hearing peer group and her own child becomes very apparent. She may become discouraged and overanxious unless she is acquainted with a family whose child has moved successfully through this phase and is now conversing well. Then she can take a long-term view. Parent groups thus offer great support to a young mother, and most parents who have weathered the early storms are pleased to return to the clinic and help the new parents by sharing their experiences which, of course, are far more impressive than lectures. They may also invite new parents to their homes to meet the older children.

In contrast, understanding of language develops much more quickly than expressive speech, and this is very encouraging to the young mother. For some children, speech begins to emerge spontaneously after a few months of intensive stimulation, irrespective of the degree of loss. For others, it may take a year or two. Many *normal-* hearing children do not develop speech for two or three years, but communicate by vocalization. It is, therefore, very important for the parent to relax and enjoy an infant's attempts at communication.

The enjoyment of oral communication is illustrated well by this description of a profoundly deaf two-year-old:

> Cindy's personality has changed so in these past seven months that she is like another child. Cindy was not a friendly baby and if anyone, other than me, my husband, or my mother tried to pick her up, she would scream and cry terribly.

Our new Cindy loves people, greets company, no matter who, with an enthusiastic, "Hi," loves to go visiting, calls out "Hi" to strangers on the street, lets anyone hold her, and even kisses everyone.

Cindy is such a tease. When I ask her what is my name, she points to me and says, "mah-ma." Then she gets a gleam in her eyes, she points to me and says, "MOPP." I, very indignantly, say, "What?" and she again, laughingly, points to me and says, very carefully, "maah-mahh."

I feel that language has become very much a part of Cindy. The other day she had fallen asleep in my arms. As I put her down in her crib, she part-way opened her eyes, said, "Bye-bye," and closed her eyes again.

REASONS FOR AUDITORY VERBAL SUCCESS

There seem to be several other reasons why an Auditory-Verbal Approach results in natural oral communication for the young limited-hearing child. Auditorily-educated children have the following characteristics:

1. They are learning *speech*, which is sound, through well-fitted hearing aids, and their attention is directed toward listening to sound, and toward learning to imitate and use sound.
2. They are learning speech during the critical period for speech development, that it, during infancy and preschool years, utilizing a natural developmental approach.
3. They are learning speech primarily within their homes in a community where everyone communicates with speech, and not in a teacher-class situation with a nonverbal peer group.
4. They are not being offered, at the same time, another way to think and communicate, that is, a visual or signed system.

Through an auditory approach the child is in contact with his environment at an ever increasing range. He now vocalizes constantly, perceives and imitates speech sounds, and hears and imitates inflection and rhythm patterns. The years ahead will be devoted to developing an understanding of abstract symbols through contextual clues, and the ability to acquire and use a large vocabulary in appropriate syntax.

TEACHING STRATEGIES

The infant who is using amplification consistently has now to be stimulated in two ways:

1. By a "global" input, that is, adults talking to him during all his activities as if he were normal-hearing so that he learns the melody of his language—the intonation, pitch, and so on.
2. By specific activities which lead to the development of auditory schema and motor skills.

TEACHING AT THE VOCAL LEVEL

The first noticeable result of using amplification is usually a change in an infant's vocalization: from screaming or from silence! Sometimes the child becomes very quiet during adult conversation and begins to vocalize when alone.

For most children the development of a normal-sounding, hearing-controlled voice will be greatly facilitated by a good model, because initially they are, indeed, parrots. Parents have to be reminded that "as we hear, so we speak." Some have commented that they feel their own speech has improved as a result of speaking more clearly, slowly and expressively to their limited-hearing children.

Normal inflection, rhythm, and stress are important not only for intelligibility, but because these qualities relate to the listener information of a subtle kind as compared with factual information carried by the articulation of words. This information may be the mood of a speaker: his determination or uncertainty, his sense of humor, and feelings. Frequently, the *meaning* of a word is conveyed by the inflection, especially if that word has more than one meaning, and also the meaning of the *sentence*, whether it is to be interpreted as a question or a statement. Not all communication is verbal, of course, and all of us make inferences from the speaker's bodily posture, movements, facial expressions, and dress. Nevertheless, the lack of normal voice quality creates one of the most serious barriers between the deaf speaker and listener.[4] In contrast, one of the most frequent comments made about children trained auditorily is the expressiveness and inflection of their voices. This is the result, first, of the emphasis upon *listening* to and imitating normal speakers and, second, of delaying emphasis upon correct articu-

---

[4]The author is referring to a high-pitched, strained and resonance-lacking quality, not to nasality. She has found that normal-hearing children may have similar nasality as a result of allergies and this should be ruled out first before ascribing a nasal quality to the hearing loss.

lation until the child has developed a hearing-controlled voice and is trying to say sentences or phrases spontaneously.

Inflection

In order to show the mother how to inflect her voice, the author suggests they play a vocal game at mealtime. If the baby wants more, she says, *More?* with an exaggerated and surprised inflection. Some babies take up the game and say, *More.* She says, *More?* in another inflection, and so on. One mother preferred to sing this with her child, and each new word was sung on a low note as in the following example.

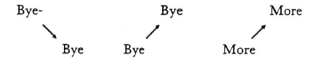

Later they played a game of imitating Daddy's low voice and sister's high voice. Another child liked vocal play when he was sitting in his high chair; for example, he threw a feather into the air and his voice slid down the scale as the feather floated down. The same vocal play can occur when bubbles are blown and they float down.

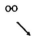

Thus, the hearing-impaired child learns inflection in a natural and amusing way. Be sure to use a lively inflected voice to counteract the monotonous quality which is characteristic of a severely deafened child. Nursery school age children will enjoy imitating musical instruments and learning songs.

The Preschool Voice

There are many activities for the older preschool child which help to develop an expressive and well-inflected voice quality once he has outgrown the early mother-child vocal games. Chewing with vocalization is excellent, and three to four-year-olds enjoy pretending to be animals, and so on. Even a two-year-old child can use a low voice for the quack-quack duck which he is moving around the table, and a high voice to represent the bird which he is flying overhead. Puppets can be used, and later, children enjoy acting out stories and nursery rhymes.

One mother suggested cutting out pictures representative of different emotions. She sat facing her daughter and said, "I have a very *sad* picture." She used a lot of emotional tone. "Do you want to see it? It's a picture of a little boy who fell and hurt his knee." Then she showed the picture. Or she said, "I have a very *happy* picture. It is a little girl who is wearing a hearing aid and she is happy she can hear." Thus she provided a good model. Mothers generally experience little difficulty in developing more pronounced inflection if the clinician has demonstrated with humor why it will be most helpful to the child.

Volume Control

Young children have notoriously loud voices and limited-hearing children enjoy shouting and hearing themselves. Soon after presenting the activities to develop awareness of loud and quiet sounds (see Chapter 8), the clinician should devise situations to encourage the use of a loud and quiet voice. Greatly enjoyed is a game first described by the Ewings called the "Wake-up Game". The child can be encouraged to use a very loud voice for the airplane going up in the air and then a very quiet voice when it flies further away, and so on.

Prespeech Skills

Blowing

Blowing is an important step toward learning the voiceless consonants and whispering. Even profoundly deaf children can hear whispering when wearing hearing aids as illustrated by the following infants, both of whom have an average loss of 103 dB, ISO level.

> We could hardly believe our eyes and ears tonight at the dinner table. I was playing games with Ricky and called his name in a whisper from the dining room to where he was sitting in his high chair. He turned around immediately and put his hands over his ears indicating he had heard his name called. We did this several times to make sure it was not a coincidence, but sure enough, he had heard.

* * *

> We have always covered our mouths in front of Cindy when we want her to listen and repeat various sounds. Our latest sound is panting. That is making the sound with our breath in and out and not using our voices, and Cindy repeats this.

Cindy likes to whisper. She whispers back to me when I whisper, repeating what I say and not looking at me.

Once a child can blow, he will be able to form the voiceless consonants. Speech, however, is not just a series of puffs of air; it requires a steady supply of air, and this can be encouraged once a child has learned how to blow. He can blow a twist of Kleenex® off his high chair, "cool" his hot food, blow a ping-pong ball across the table, blow a paper windmill round and round, and he can make a candle flame dance. He can blow a paper figure folded over a pencil back and forth. Speech books contain many ideas suitable for young children.

(When the child blows, the clinician or mother *says,* "Blow." Thus, understanding of a word develops with the muscular skill. As always, the child's vocabulary is "stretched" each day by using new phrases or sentences. So we add, "Blow the candle out." "Blow the bubble. Blow it up! Blow it to me!")

Mouth Smacking

This is sometimes used by children to indicate enjoyment of food or as a vocal game with mother. Then they call it "blowing raspberries." A child also enjoys saying *Brr* to represent the engine of a car.

Tongue Clicking

This is easily learned by playing with toy horses or clicking the tongue in time to a musical clock or metronome.

Sucking and Chewing

It must be remembered that the primary functions of the speech muscles are chewing and swallowing. The clinician may find several children who have not learned to chew well with the lips closed, and in view of Froeschel's findings in 1941, we should not overlook this important prespeech activity. Chewing with vocalization can be practiced with marshmallows in therapy time. Sucking does not have to be learned, but it should be repeated so that the sound of sucking is learned—sucking through straws at snack time and sucking up paper fish with straws as a game. Sucking vigorously should aid somewhat the movement of the soft palate. Unfortunately, many hearing-impaired children raise the back of the tongue as a closing mechanism instead of the soft palate. This results in a nasal voice quality.

Tongue Exercises

The tongue movements of severely deafened children are generally flaccid, and exercises for the older preschool child are included in speech pathology books and need not be described in detail (Ling, 1976).

A baby is always intrigued by the adult's tongue poking in and out, and wagging side to side like a dog's tail. He will try to sing *la-la-la* with an adult model when pretending to play a toy guitar or piano, or when turning the handle of a music box, or riding his rocking horse. He may enjoy trying to lick a lollipop that is held in front of his mouth. Then he can turn the tongue up to reach it when it is held beneath the nose, and down when it is held above the chin. A side-to-side movement is a good muscular exercise. Next, it is fun to lick honey off of the top lip and the bottom lip and then the top and bottom teeth. The older preschool child can push chewing gum onto the teeth ridge and roof of the mouth with his tongue tip. By this time he is ready to sing *la-la-la, da-da-da, na-na-na*. Additional tongue exercises such as trilling for *r,* and humping for *ng,* should be given only if the child fails to develop these sounds spontaneously by school age.

DEVELOPMENT OF AUDITORY SCHEMA

Stimulation for Vowels

It is easy to stimulate young children with vowels and some diphthongs as part of their play activities. They love to watch bubbles, and as the adult blows and the bubble floats to the ground, we say, "OO----!" When baby cuddles a soft toy or strokes a kitten, we say, "OH----" in a warm, appreciative tone. Toddlers who enjoy trying to string large, wooden beads hear the adults say, "OO----," as the blue bead is pulled down the string, "OH----" for the yellow, "AH----" for the orange, and "EE----" for the green. Hopefully the adult is also talking about the activity, too: "Here's a blue bead. Push it through. All the way down. OO----. More? or Another bead?" and so on.

Most infants love the color cone. Each ring can be held in front of the mouth and a vowel sound said through the ring before it is placed upon the cone. This encourages an open mouth position for vowels and prevents nasality.

The most popular game devised by a mother for infants was a variation of "This Little Pig." As she touched each toe, she said, "oo, oo, oo," and so on with all the vowel sounds. This game was repeated with the consonants and later with vowel and consonant syllables. The same game can be played on the child's fingers.

Other mothers report that their children practice vowel sounds through cookies, Cheerios, onion rings, or whatever is at hand. They become part of the diaper changing games, too. One child always imitated vowels during the time he was being dressed. While his mother put on his clothes, they echoed each other back and forth. The mother then used high and low pitches and different rhythm patterns such as *oo-oo-oo.* This led to naming parts of the body at the same time—*eye, ear,* and so forth.

Clay Activity

An activity which combines many skills and which is enjoyed by infants aged eighteen months and over is clay activity. Put clay on the table. Say, "Roll, roll, roll, roll." Roll the clay into a ball and say, "I roll it to you. Now roll it back to me." Roll the ball of clay back and forth. (Add names such as: "Roll it to Mommy," and so forth.) Now take the ball and pat it firmly with the palm of your hand and begin to say *rhythmically,* "Pat-a-cake, Pat-a-cake, baker's man," and so forth. The young child may imitate independently or may need help. Now say, "Look, we have made a cake." Take out a candle and put it into the cake. (Afterwards show a picture of a child blowing out a candle on a birthday cake, but at first do not confuse the child with too many associations.) Light the candle and if the child tries to touch it, say, "That's hot. Ow!" Next say, "Blow!" and demonstrate. Repeat, helping the child to blow out the candle. If the child tends to look at the speaker's face, cover your mouth casually when you say, *Blow,* or sit beside the child with your mouth close to his hearing aid. This activity will be enjoyed for a long time. Later it can be used for number work, counting the number of candles rhythmically, "One-two-three." It can be used on birthdays— "How old are you? One-two-three-four. I'm four."

Next, the clay is used to teach *vowel sounds.* Although the shapes made with the clay correspond to the shapes formed by the lips, no attention is drawn to this. It is simply a "gimmick" which has proved highly successful to help the child place his mouth in the correct position for the vowel sounds. The vowels are nevertheless learned auditorily. The clay is now rolled into a long piece. Run the child's finger along it and say, "That's long." Then form it into a round circle about two inches in diameter and let the child feel it. Say, "That's round." The child works with his own piece of clay or watches the clinician, who now holds the circle in front of her mouth and says, *Ah.* If the child does not want to participate, the clinician may hold it against the mother's mouth. Often when a child sees his mother participating he will imitate her.

Continue with the long vowels and diphthongs which are easier to imitate because of their duration. The clay is next broken and a very small circle made, about the size of the small finger tip. The clinician holds this against her mouth and says *oo* as in *shoe.* If the child imitates well, the same procedure is followed for the next series of vowels. If the child cannot imitate them, the first two should be practiced daily until he is ready to continue. All this is hearing-controlled; the clay actually conceals the mouth, but in trying to say the sound through the little clay hole the child is encouraged to shape his lips correctly.

Use a clay "doughnut" about the size of a thumbtip for the sound *Oh* as in *boat;* the size of three fingers for *Aw* as in *fall.* Now form a longer, narrowing ring for *Ee* as in *sea; I* as in *my; Ay* as in *day; Ow* as in *how.* The component elements of each diphthong must be elongated, since this is heard more clearly through the aids. The child will produce a natural and pretty sound. The vowels have been selected in order of their lowest frequency formants and in terms of their highest intensity.

In their studies of premeaningful vocalizations of infants, Smith and Oller (1981) found that front and central vowels of mid to low tongue height occurred most frequently.

The author usually begins with *AH, OO, OH,* and *EE,* although it may be months before some children are able to match an EE or any other phoneme.

The short vowels appear to be learned more easily if they are presented in a word. As an example, roll up the clay into a ball again, rolling it back and forth. Now say, "Let's throw it up. Up! Up! Up!" An infant will invariably say *Uh* when he does this. The same week, of course, the mother will be asked to use the word *up* whenever possible. The following week throw the ball down and use the word *down* in other activities. The child usually imitates *ow* spontaneously. The element *o* as in *hot* can also be learned at clay time, when the clinician lights the candle. The mother will find many ways to repeat this at home—hot food, hot water, hot stove. This is a very important concept! Most parents report that the word *hot* is whispered at first and is vocalized later on. Clay is a relatively quiet and satisfying activity for a young child which does not detract from receiving strong auditory impressions.

Technique for Encouraging Imitation

A clinician should establish good eye contact with the child. She then says, "LISTEN!" and covers her mouth with her hand. (An index card or piece of paper can be used with a schoolage child.) She makes the sound (vowel, consonant, or word), and then places her hand in front of the mother's mouth. The mother makes the same sound, and then *her* hand is placed in front of the child's mouth, indicating that the child is to imitate that sound. Frequently, the first attempt on the part of the child to imitate will be unlike the model, the second attempt will be closer, and the third attempt to match the model may be correct. No more than three attempts should be tried at one time, and in each case the child receives praise by being hugged, clapped, or reinforced by "Good try."

Young children are so naturally imitative that the hand technique should not be overused or it will be resented. Once a toddler understands that he is expected to imitate, he accepts this as part of the activity. Later, the hand technique is an effective way to encourage a more correct match when a child has reached the stage of self-monitoring.

Imitation will only occur, however, if the adult and child have a playful and loving relationship. Sometimes parents or clinicians are too anxious for results and this will inhibit the child's speech.

Babbling and Lalling

Although studies show that hearing-impaired infants tend to follow normal patterns of babbling (Smith, 1982), the development of consonants is influenced by the configuration of the audiogram, and the Laradon Chart given in this chapter may have to be modified for a child with a very severe hearing loss.

There are three main discriminations to be made by the child before he can produce consonants: the manner of production, that is, nasal or oral, a stop or a fricative; the place of production, that is, with the lips, tongue, etc.; and whether the sound is voiced or devoiced.

Most phonemes in English are paired:

| Place of production | Oral & Plosive | | Nasal & Prolonged |
	Voiced	Voiceless	Voiced
	w	h	
Lips	b	p	m
Tip of tongue on alveolar ridge	d	t	n
	l		
	(not plosive)		
Back of tongue against soft palate	g	k	ng (as in song)

Phonemes which develop later, usually after the third birthday, involve more complex movements but again follow the pattern of pairing.

Upper teeth & lower lip	v	f	
Teeth together; tongue either behind upper or lower teeth	z	s	
Teeth, tongue and lips	3 (as in measure)	sh	
	j	ch	

One phoneme, [r], is unusual in that it is the only one formed in English by curling the tongue backwards.

In learning to imitate, children have to become aware of the essential features of each phoneme: is it nasal or not, is it said with vibration of the vocal cords or not, is it a plosive sound or not? But none of this involves *conscious* effort when a child learns to listen and imitate what he hears.

If the infant is babbling *bbbbbbb* spontaneously, he is showing an ability to make a sound with his lips together and the nasal passage closed. It may then be appropriate to continue with labial sound stimulation at that time, that is, with [w] and [p]. If he is babbling *dddddd* spontaneously, it may be more effective to stimulate with other tongue tip sounds: [t], [n], and [l].

Many deaf children use spontaneously the labial sounds [b] or [m] which are highly visible, and it is surprising how many words in a young child's vocabulary begin with b: baby, bunny, bottle, bye-bye, bath, bed, ball, bear, and so on; but the normal hearing infant begins by making sounds toward the back of the mouth, often called cooing sounds, perhaps because he is lying on his back. As he sits up and later crawls, he produces sounds at the front of the oral cavity. The author prefers to begin babbling stimulation with *gggggg*, and an activity involving the word *go:* for example, letting a wind-up toy move when the adult says: "G-g-g-go." Other games enjoyed by toddlers are the following:

Father stands at one end of a hallway with mother and child at the opposite end. Father shouts, "GO!" and mother and child run to him. Father lifts the toddler up in the air with much laughter.

Father carries the child on his back. He says, "GO!" and gallops around the room. When he stops, the child may try to say *GO!* This game can also be used to encourage singing, when Father sings "Yankee Doodle" as he jogs around the house with baby on his back.

In view of the difficulty encountered by older deaf children in learning to say [g] and [k], it is interesting to note that very few infants fail to develop these sounds naturally when they are taught auditorily.

Normally, the voiceless component of each voiced consonant can be learned soon after the voiced consonant, providing the child can blow and imitate whispering. Thus, after *b*, *p* should be presented. However, for many profoundly deaf children, only the voiced consonants are acquired first: thus, one might present *m*, *b*, *n*, *d*, *g*, *l*, and the semi-vowels *w* and *y*. The author recommends babbling each phoneme for about two weeks to develop a clear auditory schema; thus, fourteen weeks will have passed, constituting several months of listening experience. When the clinician returns to work again with the *b* sound, she can present the voiceless *p* immediately afterwards; the *d* sound can then be followed by the *t* sound; the *g* by the *k* sound, and so on. For the two-year-old to three-year-old child it remains only to present *h* and *f* and he will have a repertoire of sounds appropriate for the vocabulary of his peer group. The phoneme *sh* can also be introduced on the first level. This is rarely articulated *correctly* by a normal hearing infant, but it is used by his parents frequently—*Shhh!*, *she*, *wash*, *show me*, *push*, and so on. It is a sound of relatively high intensity and accompanied by a characteristic gesture, so that the limited hearing child should be given the opportunity to add this to his listening repertoire.

Throughout the program of phoneme stimulation, the clinician has to make decisions based upon the progress and needs of each individual child. One immediately uses a phoneme in words, and then in phrases or sentences because no consonant is used alone in conversation and its production is influenced by the vowel which precedes or follows it. (Thus, at first a child may be able to say *cut* but not *key.*)

Suggestions for First Consonant Units:

    g activities which use: go, all gone, good girl, go get . . .
    k cut (with a plastic knife), cookie, or cracker.
   w say wow wow (dog barking), wash, wind wind using wind-up toy)
      oo
    h hhh (dog panting), hi! hot!
   m mmm (with an airplane), more, mama, meow (for the cat)
    b bbbb (with a toy motorbike), bye-bye, boo!
    p ppppp (to blow a toy sailboat), pop! push, pull, pop
    d dddd (down) dada
    t Ttttt (for a clock), turn (around), toe
    l lalala (singing)
    n night-night, say: n n n n NO! (shaking your head).

Special Techniques for Consonants in an Initial Position

Small children often repeat the vowel sound in a word and ignore the initial consonant sound. To "highlight" the initial sound, babble it several times and then say the whole word. For example, say, *g-g-g-g-g-go, p-p-p-p-push,* or *d-d-d-d-d-down!* This will not cause the infant to stutter!

"Highlighting" can also be used in speech correction. A child who says *goggie* will self-correct if the parent or clinician says, *"Listen! d-d-d-d-doggie."*

Special Techniques for Consonants in a Final Position

Consonants which occur at the ends of words are usually much quieter than the preceding vowels and are therefore often omitted. There is a simple solution. Young children enjoy the two-beat rhythm, as in *bye-bye,* and frequently change single syllable words into two syllable words: doggie for dog, horsey for horse, kitty for cat, and so on. When the final consonant becomes a *medial* consonant, it is much louder. Thus, a "g" which is omitted in *dog,* is heard and imitated in *doggie.* Later, the diminutive *ie* will be dropped.

Special Techniques for High Frequency Phonemes

Special techniques are needed for high-frequency phonemes which may present problems for children with high frequency loss. Huizing and Kruizinga (1962) demonstrated that the *whispered* voice remains clear with a clear grade of intelligibility, and that a child with a sloping audiogram acquires better discrimination ability and improved speech, and adapts auditory control function to his handicap when the clinician uses an amplified whispered voice. Part of the difficulty for a limited-hearing child has been vocal inversion: the strong, low components mask out the high, weaker components, as in the word *hot.*

Amplified whispering of the whole word is one technique used to stimulate the child. A second technique is to use adjustments within the hearing aid and receiver so that the high frequencies are amplified. In general, it is better to fit a receiver with a wide frequency response than a limited response which appears to give more power. It was noted that one child was saying the *t* phoneme within a few days after being fitted with a wide-range receiver, and as her discrimination improved, she needed less amplification for average conversation. This is also true when two hearing aids are worn rather than one.

A third technique is the occasional use of an amplifier which amplifies a wider range of frequencies than a wearable hearing aid.

Kinesthetic Cues

If no feedforward occurs after a reasonable period of time, a decision may have to be made by the clinician to add kinesthetic or tactile cues. For example, a child who has poor lip closure can feel his lips together as the clinician presses upon his upper lip, or if he cannot produce S or TH, she may let the child feel her breath upon his finger. She should not say: "Look in the mirror," or "Look at my tongue and lips," until it becomes obvious that no success will be obtained auditorily or kinesthetically. This is very rare. Shaping the muscle movements for speech with the hands or fingers has been described in books on motor kinesthetic speech facilitation (Vaughn and Clark, 1979). Note that if the clinician uses her hands and then withdraws them, the child is left without a feedback mechanism; therefore, the child should use his own hands, too.

One very helpful technique for children who experience difficulty with [k] and [g] but can articulate [t] and [d] is the following:

The clinician asks the child to imitate *dddddd*. Then she presses her finger down upon the tip of the child's tongue and again directs the child to say *dddddd*. The tongue tip will be unable to rise, and the child will raise the back of the tongue instead, saying *ggggg*. The same technique is used with t in order to obtain k.

It is also useful to know that *K* and *EE* usually develop at the same time because of a similarity in tongue position. Practicing words like *monkey, donkey,* and so on, with a firm plosion on the k sound will produce a much clearer *EE* sound.

These techniques are seldom necessary with young children, with the exception of those who have severe motor defects, such as dysarthria. For these cases, the clinician needs to work in association with a physical or occupational therapist (Crickmay, 1966).

Examples of a Clinic Session

First Level

1. ***Babble.*** We need to plan an activity in which *m* can be hummed over and over and then spoken on varying pitches or notes. One family used a jar of bubbles. When they stirred the plastic ring round in the bubble jar, they said, *mmmmmm,* with a variety of inflections. A harmonica is useful if the child cannot yet blow it. Hum *mmmmmm* on the harmonica on a low note and then on a higher note. Hum *mmmmmm* while "flying" a toy airplane.

2. ***Highly Motivating Word.*** Next, an activity should be planned to introduce the sound in a highly motivating word which begins with the phoneme. Eat cookies or drink milk and say, *mm-mmm, good!* Then ask the child, "Mmmmm-ore?" (Prolong the *m* sound,) We give him a little more, and again ask, "Mmm-ore?" and so on. Most infants imitate the word *more* quickly, irrespective of degree of hearing loss.

3. ***Calling Game.*** Then we need a highly motivating calling game. Call, "Mama," and she appears around the door saying, "Here's Mama." Or she looks out of the window. "Mama," we call, and she turns around and says, "What?"

4. ***Use of Scrapbook.*** Cut out a house, cut out the door so that it opens, and partially paste it into the scrapbook so that mother's

photo can be slid behind the door. Knock on the door, pretend to ring the bell (*Ding-dong*), open the door and say, "Hi Mama!" . . .

5. ***Home Assignment.*** The home assignment for this lesson is frequent repetition of the sound in babbling, frequent use of a few highly motivated words beginning with *m,* and the calling game. Single-syllable words should not be the only words selected — two-syllable words are just as easy. If the child can imitate *m,* encourage attempts to use this phoneme, as for example when he wants *milk* and *more.* If he wants his mother's attention, do not let him scream or pull on her arm. Help him imitate *mama.* Parents are reminded to talk in appropriate sentences, as for example: "Do you want some more?" "What do you want, more milk?"

SUMMARY

Guidance of a young child toward development of auditory-verbal communication involves reaching the following stages:

1. Communication with Crying.
2. Cooing, Laughing.
3. Vocal Play (which includes vowel play).
4. Babbling and Lalling.
5. Echolalia.
6. Blowing and Whispering.
7. First Words.
8. Jargon (communication by strings of inflected vocalization).

Chapter 10

THE DEVELOPMENT OF
SPOKEN LANGUAGE 2:
COGNITION, SEMANTICS, SYNTAX
AND PRAGMATICS

When an infant begins to use amplification his attention is drawn to environmental sounds and the human voice. Within the first year, he must change from vocal to verbal behavior. His attention is now directed to listening to spoken language which he will imitate spontaneously when motivated within an enjoyable activity.

COGNITION

In recent years, researchers have investigated the relationship between cognition and language, with some linguists asserting that cognition occurs before language, while others feel that they occur simultaneously. Probably both theories are true at different stages of a child's development. Certainly an infant must recognize the "shoeness" of an object regardless of its size, shape, color, and style, before he can label it a shoe. But if an adult waves an infant's hand and says "bye-bye" when another person leaves, cognition and language occur at the same time.

LANGUAGE AND THOUGHT

Some writers hold the view that language is identical to thought while others say that language and thought are independent because the ability to think is innate while language is acquired and the product of thought (Wepman, 1976). Piaget (1952) stressed that a child's thought stems from information derived from his sensorimotor activity. Sensorimotor information gives him an inner frame of reference which can be verbalized by the adults who provide appropriate language. Vigotsky (1962) thought that the way a child perceives and responds to the world is largely determined by the language forms surrounding him because the adults direct his attention to certain aspects of his experience.

Luria (1973) describes an unpublished investigation by Homiskaya in which a child who had just started school was evaluating colors. If the child was instructed to evaluate the shades in words (by saying pale or dark) and to give the appropriate response at the same time, the accuracy of discrimination between the shades was considerably increased. The inclusion of the child's speech enabled the differential features to be distinguished, made sensitivity more selective, and the responses much more stable.

A Colorado study of ninety-six children under the age of three years (Day, unpublished) used symbolic play to study the relationship between cognition and language development. Day used the MacArthur Communicative Inventory and the Calhoun Play Assessment Questionnaire. This study found the following:

1. There is a high correlation between symbolic play and language.
2. The ability to represent a concept symbolically is highly related to talking.
3. The play item analysis indicated a linear development of symbolic play. Children with hearing loss and under the age of three follow the same developmental progression of play skills as normal-hearing children.
4. Degree of hearing loss does not predict language success or failure.
5. Females score higher than males.

The Auditory-Verbal Approach takes all these points of view into account. The child is given enriched and stimulating play experiences in a one-to-one situation so that the adult can provide the appropriate language to fit the experience and to increase the child's exposure to useful input (Gatty, 1992). Then the child is encouraged to verbalize his own experience, as for example, saying *up, up, up, all fall down* while he is building blocks, or to say *wind, wind, wind it up,* if he is winding up a toy.

In this chapter, the term language will include receptive and expressive language, that is, semantics, syntax, and pragmatics, but not speech or motor skills which were described in the last chapter. An auditory approach must keep a balance between emphasis on the mechanics of speech and the dynamics of language. Parroting without understanding is not language, although it is an observable step in learning to communicate (Lenneberg, 1962).

Since educational audiology follows normal sequential stages, it is important to study the development of language for communication in normal-hearing children because this can apply to the hearing-impaired child who has no significant multiple handicaps. A child who wears hearing aids or a cochlear implant during the first three years of life is able to acquire natural language during the normal psychological and physiological period, although it is not impossible to start at a later age.

NORMAL DEVELOPMENT OF LANGUAGE

1. Sound Is Used for Communication

From the time of birth, a normal-hearing baby begins to understand that sound is used for communication: he cries, and someone attends to his needs; he coos and gurgles, and everyone in his environment responds and makes delightful sounds back to him.

2. Sound Has Meaning

As the months go by, a normal-hearing baby learns that sound has meaning: this sound means his food is on the way; that sound means the family dog is barking; yet another sound means Dad is home and will soon be bouncing him up and down, and so on (Levine, 1956).

3. The Beginning of Word Understanding: Functional Words

A long period of listening to conversation leads to a "passive" understanding of each routine situation. Thus, inner language is developing for a long time before it becomes spoken language (Johnson, 1973).

From the sixth to the twelfth month is a period when nonverbal or gestural communication also develops: shaking the head, waving, extending the arms to indicate a wish to be picked up, and so on. It can be easily observed that early or functional words are accompanied or replaced by gestures: *bye-bye, no, up, sh, hi, so big, more,* and *all gone* (the last one expressed by open palms and raised shoulders). It is interesting to note that a baby learns *no* before *yes* and that this has been interpreted as part of the rejection gesture when he turns his head away from food.

At the same time, an infant is beginning to understand and use vocal intonational patterns: as, for example, he shouts to get attention and can interpret angry versus happy voices.

By the ninth to the twelfth month, he should respond when his own name is called and should use one word clearly and meaningfully, as for example, *hi, no,* or *dada.* He is moving toward the *symbolic* level (Huizing, 1959), when passive word understanding comes into being, and the *oral* level, when he uses more less articulate speech for symbolic use.

One of the most important warning signals that language processing problems may occur is the failure of an infant between nine and twelve months to understand that an extended hand means *Give that to me.* Normal-hearing babies will automatically respond appropriately and place some thing, after a brief hesitation, into the extended palm. Children with severe language learning problems will only mirror the gesture.

4. Symbolic Language

a. Vocabulary Development. Words have Meaning

It is a major milestone when a child understands that a word, that is, a pattern of sounds, is the symbol for a person, object, or feeling.

Early symbolic language is learned by gesture, intonation, and action. It arises out of a process of using all available clues within the total situation.

For example, when a child touches the stove or iron, this makes a very vivid impression. Simultaneously Mother shouts "Hot!" The next day the child is playing outdoors in the sunshine. He climbs onto a metal wagon or upon a metal slide which has been standing in the sun. He yells, "Hot!" The feedback cycle of hearing, understanding, and *using* the word has been completed, without the same visual clues or further repetition of verbal stimulus. The initial impact upon the child was so impressive that language learning immediately took place.

In contrast, a child who depends upon lipreading or manual communication loses the *simultaneous* association of word and experience, for he has to look up and away from his activity to the speaker's face or hands.

Understanding of nouns or labels develops more slowly. For example, Mother points to the toys on the floor or indicates them by looking at them, and says: "Pick up your toys." At this point in time, her infant does not understand *toys* outside this context. Another example might be *slippers.* Every night, Dad comes home, takes off his shoes and says: "Get my slippers," and points to them. As these daily routines are repeated a number of times, the child's brain perceives a variety of sounds which become organized into a pattern. Patterns which are labels begin to stand out, and thus acquire a meaning. This presupposes that the infant, usually around his first birthday, has observed the similarities in spite of the differences. He will not learn *shoe* until he perceives the "shoeness" of an object: that, in spite of the differences in color, shape, size, and texture of all the shoes in the family, these objects are only placed on the feet. At that point, an infant can learn to label these objects *shoes* and can understand when someone else uses the label *shoes.* This normally occurs around 1.6 months of age.

Most parents of normal-hearing children do not think about these basic experiences or steps and assume that their child understands or will understand what he hears. In the case of a child with a hearing loss or a language learning disorder, it has to be explained to the parents that their child is relying upon many other clues in the situation.

"Does your baby understand the word *shoes?*" asks the clinician.

"Oh, yes!" replies the mother.

"Tell me about that. . . . How do you know?"

"Well, when I am dressing him, I put on his socks and then I say, *Get your shoes,* and he does."

"Do you point or look at the shoes?"

"Yes, I guess I do."

"Do you think he would get his shoes if you were not dressing him, but standing in the kitchen?"

"Mmmm, I don't think so."

As concepts form in a child's mind, he learns symbols for the whole concept or for each of its parts and qualities, and these new concepts become part of the concept also (Woodruff, 1961). As new symbols are acquired, the potential for new thoughts or ideas is increased. For example, a small child plays with toy cars, which differ in size, shape, and color. He rides in a real car, and observes that it makes a noise, goes beep-beep, that it needs gas, that it goes slowly and quickly, in and out of a garage, that it can be washed and so on. He then learns that some wheeled vehicles are not *cars.* They are *trucks.*

The Abstraction Ladder of Learning. Another aspect of vocabulary development is the tendency of young children to label what they perceive as most important; that is, the action, not name, associated with an object. Thus, they do not say *cup* but *drink;* a chair is a *sitdown;* a bed is a *go night-night;* a table is *eat,* and so on.

In general, children learn first to label and answer the agent, as in: *Who's that? (Daddy.)* or *What's that? (Car).*

This stage is followed by recognition of contrast: *That's not a car,* and later still, by a finer discrimination: *That's truck.* Thus a child begins with a very narrow meaning and broadens it gradually.

If we listen with a child's ear, we find that learning labels is a difficult process. In his home, he sees a four-legged animal with a tail, and his mother says: "That's a doggie." At the neighbor's house he sees another four-legged animal with a tail, and he says, "Doggie!" "No," says Mother, "That's a kitty cat." The family goes for a drive. He sees a larger animal with four legs and a tail. "Look. Doggie." "No, that's a cow (or horsey)."

In this case, the child is observing a category, *animals,* which he labels *doggie,* and gradually learns specific labels, followed by such general terms as *livestock, farm animals, pets,* and so on. This has been called the abstraction ladder of learning (Korcybski, in Hayakawa, 1939).

In the same way, a child's first family label may be *Dada,* which pleases his father very much, until he shouts, "Dada," when the milkman comes to the door! Many children call their teacher *Mama* when they first go to school.

Thus, children seem to like large category words and the most common name used is probably determined by the naming practices of adults in that family (Brown, 1973).

Meanings of words for a young child both expand and contract. One child used *ticktock* not only for a watch, but for the elevator bell, the bathroom scale, the gasometer, and so on. On the other hand, in dealing with opposite pairs, one word of a pair is learned first and may also be used for its opposite. An example of this is the word pair, *up and down.* *Up* may be learned first and used for both up and down. Later, the child will deal with opposites by using a negative: *outside-not outside, hot-not hot,* before he eventually learns both a word and its opposite.

The semantic component of language development cannot be separated from cognitive and pragmatic development. Not only does the infant see similarities which he labels, but he must perceive object permanence; that is, he understands that a ball which is out of sight under a chair still exists, and he can ask for it. In addition, he has to learn how to *use* words: that *HI!* will contact someone, or that *hot!* will express feeling, and that *Daddy — ball!* will mean *Get my ball. I have thrown it out of the playpen,* and will bring help.

Multiple Meanings. After the child has learned the primary meaning of a word, he then learns multiple meanings. A few amusing anecdotes are all that are needed for the parents to be alert to the need for explanation, since many children will not verbalize their confusions. For example, one small boy overheard his mother say, "I must run now, or I will never catch the bus." He cupped his little hands in front of his body and asked in a very puzzled voice: "Catch . . . a *bus?*"

There is another difficulty for a child who is learning the meaning of English words, and that is, many words which *sound* the same have different meanings, as for example: *fly, nails, trunk, pair (pear), two (to, too).* At thirty-nine months, one child understood two meanings of fly: the name of an insect and the word for a bird's activity (McNeill, 1970).

Abstract Expressions. Abstract expressions such as, "Wait a minute," "I need that," and "I don't know," are also acquired as a part of the total experience and are picked up auditorily by the child and used spontaneously.

A child with a severe unaided hearing loss heard a lady use the expression, "I'm cuckoo," when she did something silly. Several weeks later his mother also did something silly, and he said, "Cuckoo," spontaneously to another adult in the room. So the limited-hearing child can learn abstract language auditorily.

Growth of Vocabulary. The second year of life is the year of a great increase in *naming* activity and the beginning of continuous speech for the normal hearing child. This is also true of the limited-hearing child, except that the second year means the second year of wearing a hearing aid.

The clinician must be aware of the enormous number of words which the limited-hearing child must acquire. Fitzgerald (1949) quotes several studies which estimate the rate of increase in the size of a normal-hearing child's vocabulary. One study estimated the rate between the ages of three and six as from five hundred to six hundred words a year. Watts (1944) says that the average child enters school at age five with a vocabulary of at least two thousand words. With an increase of about seven hundred words a year, a child of fourteen should be in possession of from eight thousand to ten thousand words. It has been said that deaf children must be taught on the average five new words a day from the beginning of first grade work at six-and-a-half years of age, in order to prepare them for high school.

It will sometimes be observed that a child can *hear* a word and be unable to understand it readily. Once he has *repeated* it, the association between the auditory pattern and its meaning is made more quickly.

b. The Development of Structure

(1) Vertical Construction. The One-Word Stage. Lois Bloom (1973) has observed that virtually all normal-hearing children go through a fairly long period between nine and eighteen months during which they only utter one word at a time. However, she feels that this is not only a stage in which the meaning of words is learned but also special relationships between words and their experiences.

Only when children begin to combine two words together can there be an emergence of grammar, but neither Bloom nor Crystal (1976) think that normal-hearing children know as much about sentences in this early period as has so often been assumed. However, it seems clear that an infant is engaged in some syntactic analysis during the one-word stage which is reflected in his accurate perception of sentences spoken to him and in his own utterances later on. Linguists have pointed out that examination of larger segments of parent-child interactions show important pattern in word choice during the one-word stage and the beginning of sequencing when one event follows another.

Scollon (1976) described how a nineteen-month-old named Brenda used a series of one word utterances; that is, a vertical construction, to express what an adult would say with a horizontal construction of sentences.

> Brenda: "Car" (pronounced Ka). "Car, Car, Car."
> Scollon: "What?"
> Brenda: "Go, go. Bus" (pronounced baish). "Bus, bus, bus."
> Scollon: "What? Oh, bicycle? Is that what you said?"
> Brenda: "Not" (na).
> Scollon: "No?"
> Brenda: "Not."
> Scollon: "No, I got it wrong."

Brenda was perhaps trying to say: "Hearing a car reminds me that we went on the bus yesterday. No, not on a bicycle."

Thus, the one-word stage is not just a time for learning the meanings of words, but a period in which the child is developing hypotheses about combining words together and is already putting expressions together in meaningful groups. In this case, new functions are expressed by old forms. Van Uden (1977) has much to offer about developing the combinability of words in his Maternal Reflexive Method.

The parents of a hearing-impaired or language-delayed child need to be reminded that a normal-hearing child does not begin speaking in grammatically correct sentences, but is certainly hearing them. Therefore, although they have to spend time on "labeling drills" in order for new words to be learned, those words should be used in short sentences or phrases immediately.

The average, normal infant is able to label some family members and some parts of the body, such as eye, nose, etc., by one year, six months. The actual choice of additional words depends on the environment: a child growing up on a ranch will learn a different set of early words from the one who is growing up in a city.

(2) The Two-Word or Telegraphic Stage. Although adults are using complete sentences to the average eighteen month to two-year-old with normal hearing, the child himself responds with a two-word utterance.

> "Did you see the truck?" asks Mother.
> "See truck," says her child.

Here the child is preserving the word order but selecting the most important or high information and stressed content words, and omitting functors, auxiliary verb, and so on, in order to stay within the range of two to four phonemes (Brown and Bellugi, 1964). This is not just related to his auditory memory span, but to neuro muscular growth, because a child may remember a large number of words at this stage. It is also related to cognitive or conceptual development. Young infants, for example, do not use pronouns for a long time unless they are part of a sentence which has been learned as a unit: *Put it back, Stop it,* etc.

In this telegraphic stage, which persists onto a three-word level at three years of age, words are not always in the right order. Linguistic encoding is not necessarily imitative, nor is it a shortened form of adult language. Indeed, linguists feel that it is not "telegraphic:" If the child is leaving out items he could have put in, perhaps he does not know these items. Rather, he often combines words and word groups already learned to express his own thoughts: *Train go bye-bye. Where man gone? No more big, bad wolf. All gone big, bad wolf.*

With the omission of functors, *of, to, with,* etc., the meaning of normal children's utterances is usually guessed from the context or from stress and intonation patterns. Bellugi and Brown (1964) give the example of *Eve lunch*. This can be interpreted by the mother to mean: *Want my lunch*, or *Finished lunch*, or *Is it time for lunch?* according to the circumstances.

Menyuk (1969) feels that there is tremendous importance to the intonation of contours or "markers" in the development of sentence and meaning. The sentence melody and stress is an integral part of the structure. For example, a rising inflection usually indicates a question, but with a different stress and pitch, the meaning changes.

The two-word stage includes many different types of expressions (Bloom, 1973, 1975). Among the most frequently used are the following:

Topic Comment:	That car. Here ball.
Noun plus modifier:	Big boat.
Possession:	My shoe. My turn. Daddy car.
Negation:	Not tired. No down. Don't bite.
Verbing (Pres. Progressive):	No biting. He hitting. I'm painting.
Questions:	What that?
Recurrence:	More Cars. Another cookie.
Attributes:	Light hot. Other cookie.
Commands (or imperatives):	Help me. Open door. See car. Turn around.
Demands:	Want more. Come here.
Locative:	Sit down. Up there. Right there!
Declarative:	Broken! All done!
Adverbs:	Too late! All wet. That's enough.
	(These adverbs are only used at an early age when they are part of a phrase learned as a unit.)

The two to three-year-old also perceives that words can be used in different positions:

In isolation:	Ice cream!
As a subject of a sentence:	Ice cream is melting.
As the object of a sentence	I want ice cream.
As a predicate nominative:	That's ice cream.

Some of the best known examples of a child practicing two and three word combinations are given in Weir's *Language in the Crib* (1962). The child uses a number of words in different combinations. Parents report that children with a hearing loss also practice new words at night when they are in bed, or they may use jargon.

Kernel Sentences

Hearing-impaired children can also become aware of "Kernel patterns" and enjoy combining words as is described in excerpts from mothers' diaries:

> *Luann:* (C.A.—4-6; Hearing Age—14 months; Av. loss) 100 dB, ISO level, better ear)

I should not have neglected to write for so long because this last month Luann has really blossomed. It first began with: "Where?" "Where's Tammy? Where's the purse, bathroom,"—and everything else that comes to her mind. Everything is: "Where is the—?" Luann tries to talk about everything now and really tries to say the words she knows, and even pops out with words I didn't think she knew but certainly does! Her understanding has improved so much—I can almost see the change daily. Things like: "No, you can't do that *now*—but *tomorrow.*" She accepts this and even remembers it the next day. This all amazes me and, needless to say, thrills me to no end.

Her hearing range is very much improved; I can call her from quite a distance outside and she snaps around immediately. She hears the doorbell almost any place in the house and races to the door, even when she is totally absorbed in something else.

What amazes me is the discrimination of words—she seems to fairly whiz along on these with very little trouble on very few words. She has also gotten the 'sh' sound pretty good.

She loves to say "No," and delights in teasing and saying "No." For instance, she points to a pair of women's shoes and says, "Daddy shoes," then laughs and says, "No," shaking her head and giggling and going down the hall like that.

All in all, I am so very pleased with her progress. I really didn't expect it, this soon, or this good. I keep asking myself where she would be if we were still plodding through lipreading.

I often think of the E.N.T. doctor in . . . who told me Luann would never talk and to plan on placing her in a residential school as soon as she was old enough. No help, no instruction, no encouragement—no nothing. I suppose I am a little bit too bitter, but I will never forget the hopeless black feeling I had that whole day—every time I looked at Luann after that I felt like bursting into tears.

> *Cindy:* (C.A.—3.6 years; Hearing age—2 years; Av. loss—103 dB ISO)

Cindy says, "Open the door." "Pick it up." "Hi, Mamma." "Bye-bye, Daddy." Etc.

When an airplane flies overhead, she says, "I hear that airplane." When we turn on the radio, she says, "I hear that radio." When the telephone rings, she says, "I hear that telephone."

When we go for a ride Cindy talks about the various sights. "*That's* a very pretty house. That's a pooie house. That's a blue car. That's a purple car. That's a bus. I hear that bus, Errrr. That's a little bitty truck." Etc.

Cindy has learned to answer questions. "*What's* your name?" "My name is Cindy." Then she asks me, "What's your name?" Etc. We also ask *where* members of the family have gone, and *who,* concerning things that certain individuals have done. Example: "Who fell down?" or "Whose car got broken?" We also ask, "*What's* that?" "*That's* my dress." When we ask, "Where is Daddy?" she replies, "Daddy bye-bye car." When she wants something taken off she says, "*Watch* off, coat off," etc.

Cindy loves to tease by giving obvious wrong answers. I say, "What's my name?" She replies, "Daddy." And she laughs. I'll ask, "What's your name?" She might say, "Mona."

We have used a lot of identifying games, both puzzles and lotto types. Cindy enjoys these. My requests are made from across a table with my mouth covered. Some things she identifies are names of animals and objects, and she describes pictures such as, "Mamma sweeps the floor, the baby is crying, the little boy fell down, the little girl takes a drink of water," etc. Lately Cindy likes to be the requestor and she uses only language and no pointing when she wants me to hand her a particular picture. If I make a mistake and hand her the wrong picture, which I sometimes do purposely, she says, "No," and will not accept anything except the picture she mentions.

(3) Syntactic Stage. Between three and four years of age the normal hearing preschooler enters the true syntactic stage of language. This is accomplished in three different ways: by continual expansion of comprehension, by imitation of particular instances, and by building of analogies and rules.

This is the time when plural endings are added, and verb tenses, prepositions, and conjunctions are used. As the normal-hearing child sorts out the regularities and irregularities of the language, he makes many errors.

The development of rules seems to follow the same pattern as in semantics and phonology: the child breaks down the system into its smallest combinable parts and then develops rules for combining the parts. In other words, the most general rules are hypothesized first and then are narrowed down.

Plural S. Examples given by linguists include the observation that in learning plural *S,* the child observes that *S* can be added so he uses it in *foots* as well as in *cats.* Later he hears *houses,* and may add this ending to all plural nouns to make *footses* and *manses.* The use of this ending is quickly narrowed down and finally, the irregular plurals are learned: feet, mice, and so on.

Later, the use of final *S* has to be learned to express possession, as in *Mary's book* and verb tense, as in *he puts* (Moskowitz, 1978).

Negatives. Bellugi (1967) found three stages in the acquisition of negatives. At first, a child attaches no or not to the beginning of a sentence to make it negative, as in *no play that*, although the author's daughter always used *none*, as in *none more, none milk*. In the second stage, *no, not, can't,* and *don't* appear after the subject and before the verb: *I don't like it. Don't leave me. He no bite you.* In the third stage, children include forms of "to be" and correct use of the auxiliary *do*, as in: *I am not . . . , I don't have. . . .*

Some linguists feel that there is a developmental sequence to the *use* of negatives and the auxiliary negative verbs; first to express non-existence, as in *all gone puzzle*, or *no puzzle*, and then to express rejection, as in *no*, and *not*, and finally for denial, as in *don't* or *no dirty* (Bloom and Lahey, 1978).

Verb Tenses. Young children seem to develop verb tenses in a similar manner. At first, they are exposed to many imperatives: *go get* your shoes; *chew* it well; *wash* your hands; *open* the door. Next, they learn to use the present progressive in answer to the question: "What are you *doing?*" "Cutting my hair!" "Going outside." This leads to a form of the future tense: *I'm going to* (eat lunch now).

The development of the past tense has also been observed to involve several stages, with the first stage consisting of adding *ed* or the *t* sound to the stem. Unfortunately, there are many irregular verbs, but children tend to use the regular past tense for all their verbs; for example, "I doed it," "I drinkt it," "I seed it," and so on. The author observed that her normal-hearing daughter continued to make up her own past tense according to the regular rules almost through third grade, although she possessed a mature vocabulary otherwise.

The third person singular of the present tense is always a problem, and *He eats it* is generalized to *He brokes it* in the past tense. Similarly, there is confusion which arises because *he* is not plural, so *He eat it* may be used, with the idea that only nouns which are plural are associated with *S* endings.

Eventually, the development of predication involves the action agent: *Who swims? What cuts?* and later, the ability to process questions such as as, What do you *do* with (a knife)? and What do you cut with? See with? etc.

(4) Expansion Phase. The last stage of structural development involves using various structures for the same thought, and much expansion, including the use of auxiliary verbs. Examples of this stage are:

> What does it look like? or What looks like . . . ?
> What do you do with scissors? What do you cut with?
> Middle means inbetween.
> This phase was described by Susan's mother in her diary:

Susan: (C.A.—3.6; Hearing Age—2 years; Av. loss—103 dB ISO level)

Susan's vocabulary has begun to "snowball." It is gathering in momentum and growing in size. Her ability in attaining the words, comprehending them, and using them is quite wonderful to see. Her comprehension in the abstract part of language is slower. It's amazing, however, when she does understand a certain abstract expression, how each bit of this knowledge seems to open a door to so much more for Susan. And, when she learns more ways in which to express herself, we learn even more about our Susan, her personality and abilities. For example, it was suggested we work on the concept of 'looks like.' When Susan learned to use and understand this expression she let us know that she can distinguish every car that she has ever had occasion to notice. Susan is aware of each car that is possessed by all our relatives and friends. She indicates that she recognizes them by style and make, and although she doesn't know the automobiles by their brand names, as we ride along the street she watches out of the window and says, "That looks like Helen's car," or, "That looks like Debbie's Daddy's car." Susan recognizes cars from the back, sides, or front and from great distances. She hasn't yet made a mistake. If someone gets a new car she remembers both the old and the new ones, and when she sees one like them she says, "That looks like Bubie's old car," or, "That looks like Bubie's new car."

Auxiliaries. Auxiliaries are learned in a very restricted fashion at first and with many errors of placement and ommission: *Kitty no bite; Why the kitty can't stand up? What Daddy do?*

The Development of Questions. Between two-and-a-half and four years of age, normal-hearing children use a large number of WH questions. They begin with the forms which give only one piece of information:

> What's that?
> Where's that?
> What's he doing?

Who, which, and *how* questions follow later, and finally *when* and *why* because time and cause and effect require a lot of information and more mature thought processes (see Table 10-I).

It has been said that 50 percent of parent-child conversation consists of questions and only 30 percent for labeling and giving directions. Parents, however, use questions for a great variety of functions, as for example:

- to request information: *Would you like . . . ?*
- to control behavior: *Would you do . . . ?*
- to express sympathy: *Are you O.K.?*
- to threaten: *Did you hear me?*
- to maintain contact: *Where are you? What are you doing there?*

PRAGMATICS

It has been said that language is caught, not taught. It arises out of a social need and as part of the development of social skills, not in front of a blackboard.

Pragmatics, or the purpose of language, has its own developmental sequence which has only recently been studied in detail (Caz den, 1972; Gallagher and Prutting, 1983).

It begins with the prelinguistic period from zero to nine months, with perlocutionary acts, such as crying, sucking, laughing, and with illocutionary acts such as pointing and showing.

Turn-taking appears very early when the infant struggles to vocalize in response to the adult's pleasant tones.

The next stage, which is really stage one, from nine to eighteen months, involves using language for a variety of functions and intentions, such as labeling, greeting, and protesting.

Stage two, from eighteen to twenty-four months, involves true conversation, both mathetic, to inform, and pragmatic, to get things done.

Stage three, from two to three years, includes rapid topic change and lots of questions.

In stage four, from three years and up, the normal-hearing child begins to sustain a topic, role play, and maintain a conversation.

The last stage develops into adult competence, anticipating what kind of a response is required, together with the knowledge of who can say what, where, and when.

The one-to-one conversational therapy during daily routines and play in partnership with the parents, which is the strategy used in the Auditory-Verbal Approach, produces a normal pragmatic development.

TABLE 10-I
THE DEVELOPMENT OF WH QUESTIONS

Related to Persons		Related to Details	Related to Objects
Who's that?			What's that?
		That's not _____.	
	or	That's hot, cold, big, more, all wet, all gone, etc.	
		That's my _____.	Which one?
What's he doing?..............		Present participle....................	What's it for?
What happened?................		Past Tense	
What's the matter?			
		Begin numbers.......................	How many?
		1 2 3 (4 5)	
Where's _____?.............		Begin Prepositional Phrases.....	Where's _____?
		Begin Colors..........................	What color?
		Begin Plural s.	
How do you feel?..............		Begin Adjectives	How does it feel?
		Sad, happy, tired.	
		Rough, sharp, etc.	
Why?			What is it made of?
Action Agent			Action Agent.
Who swims?			What grows?
What do you _____ with?			What do yo do with a (e.g. knife)?
When?..............................		Introduce time	When?
		Introduce future tense:	
		I'm going to:	
		Concept: not now, later.	
How do you do that?..........		More verbs	How does it work?
		Detailed parts; e.g. of..............	What's missing?
		a car.	
			What belongs to?
		Add names of shapes...............	What does it look like?
			Is it the same?
			Is it different?
			What is the opposite of?
			What kind?

In summary, one must stress that there is now a large body of literature devoted to all aspects of the development of language in normal-hearing children, the study of which is crucial for successful guidance of language development in the limited-hearing child.

TEACHING STRATEGIES

The auditory approach diverges from the traditional approach in teaching language to hearing-impaired children in two main ways: first, in the choice of vocabulary taught, and second, in dealing with correctness of word order.

Teaching at the Vocabulary or One Word Level

Choice of Vocabulary

It has long been the custom to first teach those items which are easiest to say or lipread (Gallaudet, 1950). When speech is taught with an emphasis upon lipreading, such words as *shoe, bow, tie, boot,* and so on are selected first. But a child who has been trained through auditory stimulation is much more likely to say *button* first, and not *bow,* because of the inflectional pattern. No limits are placed upon the vocabulary used in an auditory approach, although a plan is necessary in the teaching situation.

Functional Words

An auditory approach frees the clinician and parent from a vocabulary which is easiest to say or lipread and makes an early vocabulary of functional words possible. These are the words a child needs to communicate in his everyday experiences and they bear little resemblance to vocabulary lists devised to teach language to deaf children.

It has often been stated, as by Watts (1944), that proper names and nouns are the first parts of speech acquired. Experience has shown that the words first understood and used by infants are *No, Bye-bye, All gone,* and so on. An example of these can be given from the case whose audiogram is given in Figures 3 and 4. There are only five nouns although some words may be *used* as nouns:

First Words: *Bye-bye, All gone, More, Oh, Off, Nice, Rough, Hi, Up, Down, Yummy, Ow, Hot, Cold, Light, No, Yah, Pooie, Peeoo, Uh-Huh, Stop, Cut, and Knock-knock.*

First Phrases: *Open the door. I heard that. Pick it up. Bad girl. Bye-bye in the car. Daddy shop. I love you. Come here. Thank you. Peek-a-boo.*

After the infant sits up and begins to take a more active part in the communication process, certain words should be selected every week and used as frequently as possible. These, of course, are the functional words already described. Each parent will select his or her own words when recognizing the need for them, but a few examples should be demonstrated by the clinician. (There are always some parents, of course, who need very specific instructions, but the author has found that eventually they become alert to the child's needs.) One example might be "Up." The clinician demonstrates that this word can be spoken over and over again during the daily routine. "Up," when the parent lifts the child out of the crib, the high chair, the stroller, or baby carriage; "Up," as the parent carries or walks him up steps and stairs; "Up," when he begins to climb on boxes and chairs; "Up, look up," when an airplane or bird flies overhead; "Up," when they throw a ball; "Up, Up, Up," when he runs to Daddy at night and is lifted up in the air; "Up," when he sits on Daddy's feet and is raised up and down.

After "Up" has been emphasized, the word "Down" should follow, because many concepts are learned more readily in contrasting pairs—not that this procedure should be used to an extreme.[1]

Another example to give to the parent might be "Where?" Once an infant sits up and throws his toys "overboard," he needs the word "Where?" As he throws and then looks, the parent says, "Where is it? Here it is." About the same age, that is, six to ten months, "Peek-a-Boo" becomes a favorite activity. "Where is Mother? Where is baby? Here's Mommy. Peek-a-Boo!"

These functional words are gradually associated with more difficult concepts or abstractions. The one-year-old child loves to crawl round and round an arm chair, chasing after the elusive parent who says, "Where am I?" The toddler of two years enjoys a more sophisticated version, when an adult or sibling calls out from various parts of the room, and parent and child look for him. Gradually, this game, like so many children's games, has prepared the way for everyday activity. At dressing time, the parent may say, "Here's your shoe. Where's the other shoe? Go get it." On another occasion, they may say, "I lost. . . . Where can it be? Let's find it."

Developing the First Nouns

As soon as an infant recognizes from five to ten sounds associated with toys (that is, meow for the cat, mmmm for the airplane, and so on, as

---

[1]It has been a frequent criticism of deaf education that the deaf child receives so much of the matching-nonmatching, or contrast black-white type of teaching, that he tends to see the world in this way and loses the concept of gradation and subtlety.

described in Chapter 9) and as soon as he uses a few functional words, such as up, or bye-bye, it is time to plan a program to accelerate the development of symbolic language.

For the more severely impaired child, it is usually necessary to teach the first nouns in the following ways:

Select a word which is motivating to an infant. For example, *eye*. Point to the eye on a toy animal or baby doll and say, "What's that? That's an *eye.*" Point to your own eye; "Here's my *eye*. That's Daddy's *eye.*" Look in the mirror and say, "There's your *eye*. Say, *eye.*"

We try to teach one word for each routine of the day so that there is a word which the child understands and uses in each daily situation. Gradually, another word is added for that situation, and then another. For example, if a child likes to play with toy cars, we point to each one, saying: "What's that? That's a CAR. That's another CAR." We drive the car into a cardboard garage; we pretend to fill it with gas; we make it go up and down a ramp; we make it go fast and slowly, and so on, stressing the name *car* many times.

For the two-year-old child, pictures can be added: parent and child look through magazines and find a picture of a car which they paste upon a sheet of paper and hang on the wall. Each day they paste another picture on the paper, until the child names the car spontaneously. The pictures can also be pasted into a scrapbook. (This can be made out of newspapers folded into a book.) The parent gets the glue and spreads around all the pictures they have cut out of the magazine. "Get a car," says the parent, and guides the child's hand to the correct picture and pastes it into the book. The parent can use this opportunity to say, "Press it; put some glue in this corner, in the middle. That's enough. That's *too much.*"

Family members continue to point out cars when they are outdoors. It is best to take about one week for each new word at first, until the child understands that everything has a name. Then it is no longer necessary to repeat one word many times; indeed, several new words have to be learned every day.

The development of vocabulary is shown in Figure 10.1. The first level of the circle around the "core activities" includes the following vocabulary:

1. A few names, including the child's own name, *Mommy, Daddy, baby, doggie,* and names of siblings.

2. A few verbs, such as *listen* and *push.*
3. A few adjectives, such as *loud, hot* and *more.*
4. A few nouns, such as *hat, cookie,* and so forth.

As we look out along the radii of Figure 10.1, we see the vocabulary increasing in depth. For example:

Names: The second circle will include names of friends and other relatives. The third circle will include names of community helpers who are most interesting to a child: the mailman, the milkman, the fireman, and the doctor. The fourth circle includes special people associated with holidays or new experiences to which a preschooler is beginning to be exposed: the circus clown, Santa Claus, a snowman, Easter bunny, and so on.

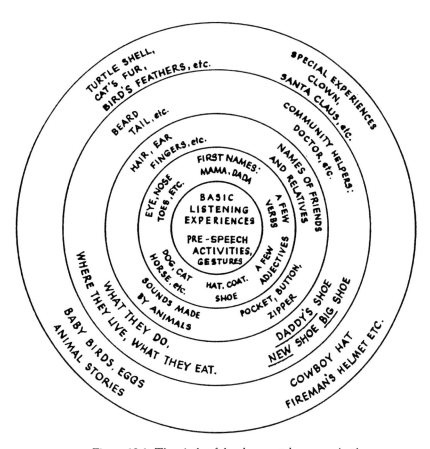

Figure 10.1. The circle of developmental communication.

Another radius is concerned with parts of the body. This begins with the infant's interest in the eye, the nose, and the fingers and toes. Later on, it will include a beard for Santa Clause, and at Easter time the rabbit's tail and long ears. At Halloween we have an opportunity to review the parts of the face. On Pet Day in nursery school, we learn about the turtle's shell, the cat's fur, the bird's feathers, and so on.

Another radius will include clothing. Clothing begins with those items most interesting to a young child: his hat and coat, maybe his shoes or boots, depending upon the season. He learns to take them *off* and put them *on*. He learns button, zipper, pocket, and sleeves. He learns possession: *Daddy's* shoe is too big. Put *brother's* socks in his bedroom. He likes to wash clothing and hang it up. He learns the colors of his clothing and what it is made of. When he is interested in community workers, he enjoys dressing up with cowboy hat and boots, a policeman's cap and whistle, a fireman's helmet, and so on.

The clinician must plan carefully around each circle to ensure that she is developing all the language concepts to fit the needs of each activity.

Developing Language Units

Planning language units is easiest when one thinks in terms of a child's interests and activities and the toys or materials available. Some examples of these are the following?

Parts of Body:	Eye, nose, toes, hair (wash, comb)
Family Names:	Mama, Dada, baby
Food:	Names of foods and dishes, together with verbs such as stir, cook, eat, drink. Lead up to preparation of foods, shopping, and ordering food from a menu. Also needed are more, enough, no more, another.
Clothing:	Names of clothes; possession (Mummy's shoes, my boots); on-off (put on, take off). Parts of clothes (button); colors. Washing and drying clothes (dirty, clean). Kinds of fabrics (fur, wool), plaid, polka-dots. Special clothing (cowboy boots, fireman's hat).
Weather:	Cold, hot, snowing (to be associated with kind of clothing as in Willie the Weatherman flannel board).
Animals:	Pets. Sounds associated with animals. Parts of animals (tails, whiskers). Verbs associated with them (barking, hopping). Their homes; what they eat. Baby animals; farm and zoo animals.
Vehicles:	Names; sounds associated with them; verbs (dump, go, fix, stop, take off); adverbs (fast, slowly); also: accident, flat, gas. Later, parts of vehicles.
House:	Names of furniture; rooms; upstairs-downstairs. Parts of house (roof, back door). Activities in a house (watching TV, cooking, etc.). Prepositions (in a closet).
Shapes:	Playskool materials; puzzles; Montessori materials. Shaping clay. Later, learning names of shapes. Making valentines.

Colors:	Playskool materials, beads, finger painting. Traffic lights.
People:	Fireman, policeman, doctor, mailman. What they ride in; what they do; what they wear; what equipment they use. Friends. Indians. Astronaut.
How they feel:	tired, mad, happy, surprised, disappointed.
Objects:	Their names and what we do *with* them.
Woodwork and tools:	*Hammer, nails. Make a tunnel. Long, short, thin, thick wood; measure.*
Trains:	Train goes round and round. Fast. Stop. Go. Through the tunnel. Over the river. Across the bridge. Depot. Signal.
Buildings; places:	Store, church, mountains, school.
Money:	Dime. Penny.
Games:	My turn, your turn, jump, swing, spin it, kick, catch.
Sports:	Swimming, skating, ball games.
What things are made of:	Paper, glass, wood. How things feel, such as sticky, rough, soft, taste.
Seasons:	Winter (making a snowman). Spring (planting a bean seed).
Holidays:	Easter eggs, summer picnics, fishing, Christmas tree, making decorations, opening presents, making cards and cookies, painting pine cones.
Calendar:	Most important words: Tomorrow, today, last night.
Clock; time:	Time to eat. Not now, later.
In the water:	Duck, fish, boat, frog. Fishing, swimming.
In the sky:	Sun, moon, rainbow, star, cloud, airplane, kite, rocket.
On the tree:	Birds, nest, bee, leaf, ladder, tree house.
Nursery tales:	Three Pigs, Goldilocks, Three Little Kittens.
Nursery Rhymes:	Hickory Dickory Dock, Humpty Dumpty, etc.
School:	Teacher, children's names, routines, following directions.

Input Versus Output

Part of the problem at this stage of vocabulary development is the incompleteness or paucity of input for the child with a severe hearing loss, in comparison with his normal-hearing peer who hears words spoken many times over, on the television, radio, across the room, and so on. The normal-hearing child hears, as it were, on the run, but the hearing-impaired must hear at close range. Another road block arises from the inhibition of normal conversation observed in parents who know that their child is "deaf." Parent guidance must overcome this barrier to encourage parents to talk more, not less, and not *assume* that words will be "picked up."

Although there is a time and place for vocabulary drill, it is usually difficult to learn words apart from experiences. To facilitate learning words, labels must be supplied at the appropriate time experientially as an integral part of the child's cognitive development. After the enriched association has taken place, drill has its place.

The art of a clinician or teacher lies in contriving situations, by dramatizing real-life situations, or by actual experiences such as field trips, demonstration home activities, etc., in order to show families how to give the extra input needed by the child with a hearing loss.

Unfortunately, the very words which parents and teachers may have worked so hard to teach are not necessarily the first words which a child uses! Sometimes a word like *candy* will be said one time only and because of motivation or interest level, the child learns it immediately. But then he may not use that word again for a long time, and the parent feels that it is lost.

The author's one-year-old son was taken to a picnic and placed in his stroller in the shade under some trees. The adults were sitting at a table some distance away. When Mother brought out a cookie tin, he stood up in his stroller and yelled, "Cookie!" That was the first time he had used the word and he did not say it again for about six months because he did not feel the urgency again. At the picnic, he apparently thought he was not going to get one.

This also happens to children with a hearing loss as described in the following diary excerpts:

Ricky: (C.A.—2 years; Hearing Age—9 months; Av. loss—103 dB, ISO)

> While Ricky gets dressed in the morning, I try to make these few minutes worthwhile by talking to him and trying to put a few things across to him. This morning we were working on parts of the body. Without my having initiated it, Ricky pointed to my eye and very clearly said, 'eye.' He hadn't said "eye" for about four months. It is interesting to note Ricky's speech is developing very much the same way as his sister's did. He kept this word locked in his memory until he was good and ready to use it again.

David: (C.A.—4.8 years; Hearing Age—2 years; Av. loss—90 dB, ANSI, 1969)

> A year ago, David was playing 'Doctor' with Mrs. Pollack. She said to the doll, "Don't cry, baby," and pretended to give her a shot. David has not had occasion to use this vocabulary since. But last week we took the cat to the vet's and when the vet gave a shot to the cat, David said, "Don't cry, Kitty." He sounded just like Mrs. Pollack.

TEACHING AT THE SYNTACTIC LEVEL

Menyuk says that most normal-hearing children possess the majority of transformations for communication by first grade, but Chomsky (1965) says there are still others to be learned between six and ten years.

Hearing-impaired children follow the same developmental sequences, but at a later age, and in therapy we have to start where they are and move on from that point. As soon as a number of single words are used spontaneously, we encourage the child to combine two and then three words together.

Unfortunately, many educators have taken the position that the hearing-impaired child cannot learn syntactical structure without visual clues and have tried to teach complete, grammatically correct sentences, either by charts on a blackboard, as in the Fitzgerald Key (1949) or by using colored blocks, and so on, the result of which has been that a deaf child uses correctly what he has been taught, but spontaneous conversation is meager or rigid.

Gantenbein et al. (1965) took the following structures and found that with 169 words they could make 22,380 sentences.

Subject-Verb-Direct Object—"I want a cookie."
Subject-Verb-Predicate Nominative—"I am a cowboy."
Predicate-Adjective Pattern—"My shoes are new."
Intransitive Verb Pattern—"The boy cried."

The choice of words, of course, was rather crucial in terms of their usefulness in conversation.

One of the main criticisms of such a teaching approach *with young children* would be that children do not usually converse in complete sentences. The teacher asks, "What do you have there?" The child says, "A new ball," or "Lookie, a ball." He does not say, "I have a new ball." Furthermore, a preschooler does not arrange his sentences in adult form. He turns words around to fit his limited thought processes and vocabulary and still gets his meaning across. He will be heard to say, "Measure me. How tall me?" On other occasions, the child selects key words from the speaker's sentence patterns and fills in other words as he matures. An example of this would be, "I want to go to the park." A two-year-old will say, "Go park." The three-year-old will say, "I want to go park." The four-year-old will say, "I want to go to the park." (Lee, 1966)

A child who is taught through visual language programs loses the real subtleties of language and communication which are acquired so easily through hearing. Thus, blackboard teaching has serious disadvantages, a fact discussed many years ago by Miss Sullivan, the teacher of Helen Keller (1961):

> We visited a little school for the deaf. Two of the teachers knew the manual alphabet and talked to her without an interpreter. They were astonished at her command of language. Not a child in the school, they said, had anything like Helen's facility of expression, and some of them had been under instruction for two or three years. I was incredulous at first; but after I had watched the children at work for a couple of hours, I knew that what I had been told was true, and I wasn't surprised. In one room some little tots were standing before the blackboard, painfully constructing "simple sentences." A little girl had written: "I have a new dress. I love mamma." A curly-headed little boy was writing: "I have a large ball. I like to kick my large ball." When we entered the room, the children's attention was riveted on Helen. One of them pulled me by the sleeve and said, "Girl is blind." The teacher was writing on the blackboard: "The girl's name is Helen. She is deaf. She cannot see. We are very sorry." I said: "Why do you write those sentences on the board? Wouldn't the children understand if you talked to them about Helen?" The teacher said something about getting the correct construction, and continued to construct an exercise out of Helen. I asked her if the little girl who had written about the new dress was particularly pleased with the dress. "No," she replied, "I think not; but children learn better if they write about things that concern them personally."
>
> There was the same difficulty throughout the school. In every classroom I saw sentences on the blackboard, which evidently had been written to illustrate some grammatical rule, or for the purpose of using words that had previously been taught in the same, or in some other connection. This sort of thing may be necessary in some stages of education; but it isn't the way to acquire language. Nothing, I think, crushes the child's impulse to talk naturally more effectually than these blackboard exercises. The schoolroom is not the place to teach any young child language, least of all the deaf child. He must be kept as unconscious as the hearing child of the fact that he is learning words, and he should be allowed to prattle in monosyllables if he chooses, until such time as his growing intelligence demands the sentence. Language should not be associated in his mind with endless hours in school, with puzzling questions in grammar, or with anything that is an enemy to joy.

There is a time for a structured language program and insistence upon correctness, but it is only after the hearing-impaired child has been given time to develop language naturally.

The Role of Echolalia

In an auditory approach, on the infant and preschool level, sentences develop as we converse with the young child about his activities, feelings, and needs and encourage him to echo back what we say. We usually tailor sentence length and complexity to fit his present auditory memory span and cognitive level. If the child is able to imitate two or three words at a time, it is easy to act out a story or talk about an activity in two or three word "chunks" and the child can imitate those sentences. For example, we put a toy kitten in a "tree" (a branch which is in a vase):

Adult:		Where's kitty?
Child:		Where's kitty?
	Adult:	Up in the tree.
Child:		Up in tree.
Adult:		Get down (kitty). (Child imitates each statement.)
		Don't fall!
		Be careful!
		Come down (kitty).
		Pour, pour, pour.
		Here's your milk. Etc., etc.

As the child's auditory memory span lengthens and his motor speech skills mature, we can encourage imitation of longer sentences, and especially the use of "kernel sentences."

A doll's house and doll family are excellent materials. We can say: "Daddy's home. Sit down Daddy. Time to eat. Come here baby. Sit down baby," (names of other family members). If the child has a dog or cat, we make the animal jump on the chair. "Oh no! Get down. . . . " We talk about watching TV; we tell the children to "go pottie"; go night night; take a bath, and so on. The hearing-impaired child echoes back each phrase or sentence as he manipulates the toys.

Play Dough is fun. We take turns to make something and say, "I made a. . . . " We dress up and practice saying, "I'm a cowboy. I am a fireman," etc. We look into a View Master or out of the window and say, "I see. . . . "

The child enjoys the clinician's activity and imitates everything she does. Soon he is also imitating the sounds or words she makes. But the child should not continue indefinitely to echo everything we say. We must teach him to listen and then reply *without echoing what we have said.* This can be achieved best in question and answer activities, and in general conversation. "What color do you want?" "How many cookies?"

"Where's Daddy?" However, a limited-hearing child does tend to repeat back some of the things which have been said to him, probably to reassure himself that he has heard correctly.

Use of Books

The enjoyment of books is very important for the following reasons: (1) Books provide the opportunity to teach many concepts which one cannot present in a clinic or even in the home; (2) they foster development of imagination; (3) books offer another opportunity to repeat and reinforce new concepts and experiences. Libraries today are full of delightful ones which duplicate a small child's activities. For example, a three-and-a-half-year-old will enjoy *The Lock-Out Book* after his mother has accidentally locked herself out. This happens to every family, and creates rather too much excitement at the time for language learning. So the experience can be repeated through the story book: "I'm locked out. I can't open the door. I forgot my key. Help me!"

A small child whose hearing is severely impaired may not enjoy books as soon as a normal-hearing child. One has to prepare for them in the following way. After an activity has been used in a natural way, a picture symbolizing it can be shown (for example, blowing out the candle). The first story book should have one picture on each page and the clinician should have a matching toy for some part of the picture. She should act out the picture; for example, ride the horse, build the blocks, and so on.

The first books for limited-hearing youngsters are very successful if they contain more than one dimension (for example *Pat the Bunny* and *The Touch Book*) or have pages which are opened or turned back to reveal something. Later on, books such as *The Boogle House* are used with some toys so that the story can be acted out. As soon as possible, however, the book should be read without objects so that the child attends only to the conversation.

Nursery Rhymes and Stories

Watts (1944) points out that nursery rhymes and stories play a valuable part in the linguistic education of infants between three and five years of age. In any forty nursery rhymes there will usually be found at least four hundred different words which will suffice to introduce the child to a world of great interest and to a wealth of knowledge about it.

The nursery stories also contain many repetitive sentences such as, " 'Who will help me?' said the Little Red Hen. 'I won't,' said the pig. 'I'm tired.' 'I won't,' said the dog. 'I'm *very* tired.' 'I won't,' said the cat, 'I'm *so* tired,' or I'm *too* tired,' " and so on. There are commercial materials for flannel board nursery stories or one can cut out picture and glue on a felt backing. Nursery rhymes can be learned while playing with the excellent jigsaw puzzles available which depict the main event, as for example, Jack and Jill falling down the hill.

This phase of language training continues for a long time, and requires ingenuity to encompass the enormous subtlety of the English language. If one meaning of a word is learned, we must race on to experience other meanings of the same word. Ahead of us lie the idioms, expressions and riddles enjoyed by eight or nine-year-olds; for example, "You're trying to butter me up," "I have a green thumb," and so on. Other examples of language activities are given in Chapter 11.

Experiential Stories and Scrapbooks

At this point, many of the teaching devices used in programs for the deaf can be adapted for an auditory program, such as stories made up about the child's experiences (Groht, 1958). These can be learned auditorially at first.

> Cindy enjoys talking about a series of events that have happened to members of the family. We echo each other back and forth. Sometimes she leads and sometimes I lead. We say, "What happened to Do-Do? Do-Do fell down and hurt her back. Poor Do-Do. Do-Do went to the Doctor's office. Doctor gave Do-Do medicine. Do-Do's all better now."
>
> We have noticed that lately Cindy's memory for discussing past events has become more developed. Last week I mentioned that a friend of ours has a new little baby. This morning I mentioned this person's name again and Cindy told me that "Mary has a little baby."

Most children, however, learn first by participating in an activity and talking about it with some clues. For example, take a box containing a hammer, nails (both long and short), and some wood. Begin by saying, "What's that? That's a hammer. What's that? That's a nail. That's another nail. That's a long nail." The child hammers the wood and nails together and makes an airplane. Ask, "What did you make?" The child is taught to answer, "I made an airplane." Then he can have great fun running around, pretending to fly it and making a great deal of noise.

When he sees other people he says, "Look, I made an airplane," or "Lookie, my airplane—I made it." One may have to put a little pressure on him to repeat the whole sentence.

After such an experience one can draw simple pictures to illustrate it, and the child will derive great pleasure from bringing out his picture story and talking about it when relatives or friends visit his home. "I had a hammer. I had a big nail. I had two little nails. I got some wood. I went bang, bang, bang." Mother said, "Careful! Don't hit your thumb." "Ow! I hit my thumb. Look! I made an airplane." The number of details will be varied according to the age, auditory memory span, and conversational ability of the child. These conversations can soon be practiced *without pictures.*

This is a project a mother can continue by herself for a long time, but she must understand that a young child needs a great deal of repetition. In the three-year-old activity just described the same sentence patterns can be used when they make a tunnel, bridge, a boat, or just a hole.

Limited-hearing children also need to act with toys and picture events which are going to happen—"Here's Ricky's old house. Here's a big truck. It's a moving truck. The man is coming into the house. He is carrying the table. He's putting it into the truck. It's heavy. Now he's driving the truck. Here's the new house. Now the man is carrying the furniture into the new house. He is carrying the bed. . . . " Experiences such as these help to teach *sequencing* of events. One can use commercial sequencing picture cards later on.

Children love to act out their experiences over and over again.

It is also important for the clinician to watch the child at play, and provide opportunities to learn the sentences she observes to be needed. It is necessary to reenact everyday experiences for several reasons:

1. Real-life situations are complex and confusing and complete sentences may not be heard. Therefore the situation is re-created in the clinic or in the home and simplified, so that attention can be paid to the conversation.

2. One mother commented that each time her daughter advanced language-wise, she seemed to deteriorate speech-wise, just as she had seemed to become confused at an earlier age when she acquired a new speech element. Any type of change and progress acts as a kind of disorganizing element until the new skill is integrated. In this case, the new language unit or new grammatical construction has not been used orally before. With repetition the articulation will

improve and the situation stabilizes for a time until the next advance.

3. We are also faced with the problem that articulation and voice quality are excellent when a child is directly imitating an adult, or is using phrases which have been spoken many times, but it may be difficult to understand him when *he* is trying to describe something which has happened. However, normal-hearing children pass through this phase also, and it is quite a common experience in all homes for only the mother to understand because she knows what the child has experienced and is trying to communicate. The author's own children at kindergarten age still talked about playing in the "bacon lot" (vacant lot) and the "tangerine" in band (tambourine).

SPEECH CORRECTION

If the child is nearing school age, it may be time to begin speech correction. Drills may now be valuable. As Ling (1976) has documented, the normal-hearing child says 134 to 210 words per minute, but deaf children may say only 28 to 145 words per minute. Depending upon the nature of the hearing loss and functional use of amplification, speech errors may consist of distorted vowels, omission or distortion of consonants, particularly in blends or in a final position, nasalization, devoicing, restricted pitch range, and so on. Only systematic drills will lead to automaticity and normal rate.

Distorted vowels can often be corrected auditorially by using the Resonator Scale (Aikin, in Fogerty, 1923). This is contained in Standard English in the following sentence:

Wh*o wo*uld kn*ow au*ght *o*f *a*rt m*us*t l*ea*rn *a*nd th*e*n t*a*ke h*i*s *ea*se . . .

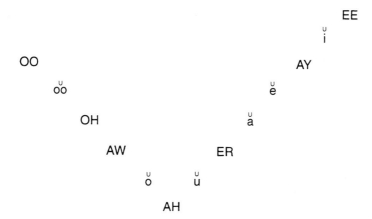

If we ask a four or five-year-old to imitate auditorially he will usually have little difficulty with the first part of the scale, OO to AH, because it involves primarily a change in lip shapes. The vowels AY, i, and EE present the most difficulty, but as the child begins with u and moves upwards to EE, the tongue gradually makes the correct adjustments in position. Of course, these sounds must then be practiced in combination with all the consonants.

For the older child who has the motor control and motivation, the LING evaluation and target practices are recommended (Ling, 1976).

Kinesthetic Cues

If no feedforward occurs after a reasonable period of time, a decision may have to be made by the clinician to add kinesthetic or tactile cues. For example, a child who has poor lip closure can feel his lips together as the clinician presses upon his upper lip, or if he cannot produce S or TH, she may let the child feel her breath upon his finger. She should not say: "Look in the mirror," or "Look at my tongue and lips," until it becomes obvious that no success will be obtained auditorially or kinesthetically. This is very rare. Shaping the muscle movements for speech with the hands or fingers has been described in books on motor kinesthetic speech facilitation (Vaughn and Clark, 1979). Note that if the clinician uses her hands and then withdraws them, the child is left without a feedback mechanism; therefore, the child should use his own hands, too.

THE ROLE OF THE PARENT
IN LANGUAGE DEVELOPMENT

Parents do, in fact, "teach" language to their children, but some parents are much better teachers than others! The clinician's role is to model and guide parents to provide the most productive stimulation at home.

In studies of good parent-child interaction, the parent has been observed to do the following:

1. Attach meaning to the child's vocalizations, that is, to talk to the child as if the child is conversing.
2. Use rising inflections and a sing-song voice. This seems to be feedback productive: a child listens more to pleasant inflections and tries to respond.
3. Reduce complexity: this is sometimes called "baby talk" when the vocabulary and grammatic complexity are simplified, but good parents seem to know instinctively about short memory span and many of their sentences are very short: *Come here. Don't touch. Put it back! Are you tired? Be right back.*
4. Model a sentence and encourage imitation: "Jimmy, say thank you."
5. Repeat a sentence several times: good parents frequently say everything twice to draw attention, but repetition also occurs naturally because of repetitive daily routines and behaviors: *Drink your milk. Where's your shoe?*
6. Ask questions and model the answer: *What are you doing? Washing your hands?*
7. Expand and correct: *Yes, that's a doggie and not a goggie. That's a very big doggie.* (We are not sure that expansion, or taking the child beyond his own response is necessary.) Ling and Ling (1974) observe that most parents do not correct or model a child's utterances, but continue talking about the subject at hand. However, parents of the child with a hearing loss do have to provide clear models and correct errors. In this case, the expansion should be one of the child's own sentences or should be a verbalization about his own activity. If used appropriately, it helps the child view his world through adult eyes.
8. Accelerate learning: *That's round . . . that's a circle. Yes, that's a boy like Jason. Jason is a boy; Melissa is a girl.*

In recording examples of conversation between children and adults, Tough (1974) demonstrated the extent to which a child is dependent upon adult communication to build up the widest possible range of resources of language and strategies for learning. However, some parents talk a great deal but not about the subject in which the child is showing interest, or with much scolding and complaining, and some talk too much without giving the child a chance to respond. Both Tough and Ferguson (1977) give very helpful studies of interaction.

Ewing (1963) states that linguistic development seems to be more especially related to the personalities of the parents, to the family structure and home conditions, rather than to economic or mental capacities. It behooves the clinician, therefore, to pay considerable attention to these, and go occasionally into the homes and devise a program best fitted to the conditions she finds there (Proctor, 1983).

A number of clinics and schools have set up demonstration homes, where the clinician can model and guide adult-child interactions during everyday activities, such as cooking, cleaning, bedmaking, and so on.

Many programs video parent-child interactions to help parents observe and analyze both their conversations and the child's responses. Parent guidance can, however, occur satisfactorily without expensive equipment. If there are siblings in the family, they, too, should be included in the guidance program.

There are several difficulties encountered in guiding parents of hearing-impaired children: if the young child does not respond to conversation, the family members become more silent or use too many gestures. It is obvious in watching interactions between normal-hearing babies and their parents that it is a delightful turn taking game, with babies responding to parents' vocalizations and vice versa. This reciprocal vocalization may not occur for a long time with a profoundly deaf child and his family simply stops talking to him often without realizing it. But turn-taking has been called the essential initiation of communication.

Then there are parents who know that the child is "deaf" and assume that he will not understand if they talk to him. A very good example of this was related by a mother. She was walking across the parking lot with her two children, one on either side of her. She took out a candy bar, broke it in half, and gave one piece to her normal-hearing son, saying: "You have to share it with Debra. Here's your half." She then turned, and, *without saying a word,* gave the other piece to her "deaf" child and was surprised when Debra had a tantrum.

Related to this is the tendency for parents to stay on a simple level and fail to use more mature language: "Do you have an owie?" instead of "Did you hurt your knee?"

Other parents talk to the hearing-impaired child, but not enough to make up for the lack of input before the hearing aids were fitted or for the incompleteness of the input after the aids were fitted because a hearing-impaired child may only hear clearly at close range. Parents rarely consider that normal-hearing children have thousands of hours of input in order to learn one language ... perhaps as many as 25,000 hours from ages zero to six. Therefore, they have to talk about everything over and over again to make up for "lost time" with a hearing-impaired youngster.

Some parents do talk a great deal but fail to encourage or expect their children to respond. This problem, however, is more typical of the special classroom, where the teacher does most of the talking.

HOME TRAINING FOR LANGUAGE DEVELOPMENT

There are two main ways in which a parent can carry out home training. He or she can join the child in his play, supplying the language and sounds he needs, and then guide him into expanding his play in order to teach new concepts, or she or he may set up a situation in which all this seems to occur spontaneously but is actually planned and the parent is really the leader. This should never be rigid—there should always be time to follow up a child's spontaneous ideas, even in a structured situation. Too much parent education for the deaf has stressed control of the situation by the parent, with loss of spontaneity and imagination.

Some parents are quite shocked by the idea that they will have so much to do, and feel that the training is the responsibility of the clinician. The clinician must decide if this arises from the insecurity in his or her role, or rejection of the child. Insecurity can be overcome by discussing the fact that a child normally learns his basic language and speech patterns from his parents, and that we are not asking them to do something for which parents normally receive special training. We are simply asking them to do a little more than the parents of a normal-hearing child would do. We may walk a rather slender line at first between giving just a few simple instructions which a parent can carry out confidently within the normal schedule, and giving them enough to effect the progress which the family expects to see.

Most parents grow into their role and think of many original ways to provide the necessary stimulation, and their children's response is gratifying. This can best be illustrated by the case of a deaf and blind girl whose hearing loss was not suspected until she was four years old. It had been assumed that she was mentally retarded and the expectation level of her home training had been geared to that diagnosis. After being fitted with hearing aids, marked changes in her behavior, evidences of real mental growth, learning, exploring, and so on, were observed. She had not been expected to learn, and she did not do so. When the expectation level and the family attitude were changed, she surprised everyone by her ability. The family became excited and eager to provide new experiences—a picnic by the river to hear and feel the water on the rocks, playing with gravel, throwing it and hearing it hit something, a picnic fire to learn heat, how to walk around the fire, and so on. Within a few months, they were talking about possible nursery school attendance.

> When the baby cries, I rock the crib and I have showed her how to do this, too. I show her things to play with, and we encourage her to climb and swing. She used to sit on the back porch all the time; now she is climbing over the fence and visiting around the neighborhood. She has learned that if she stacks up two pillows and pushes them to the door, she can climb up and reach the chain and get outside. She climbs on a chair and plays with the door knocker. Now when someone knocks, she recognizes the source of the sound and goes to the door. She listens to the voice, and if it is not her playmate she walks away. If the TV is too loud, she walks across the room and turns it off.

Within a few months her progress report covered pages. She began to babble, click her tongue, blow, drink from a cup, laugh, cough, dance to music, play "train," and bang on her plate with her fork to get attention. Yet for four years this child had shown minimal behavioral development; she had shown no response to sound, no speech development, no particular interest in people, and very little exploration of her environment.

Unfortunately, the increasing number of mothers who have to work outside their homes during the infant and preschool years has introduced another problem in terms of language input. Rarely does a babysitter or preschool teacher give the same one-to-one input that a good mother gives in her home. The input for early language development for the child with a hearing loss should be normal conversation about highly motivating activities and daily routines, and no child with a significant hearing loss will succeed without daily, enriched stimulation and conversational interaction within his home.

Many mothers try to work part-time and devote as many hours as possible to carrying out an Auditory-Verbal Approach. If the father and siblings are also actively involved, the results are, of course, even better. The alternative offered currently is a sign language program, and it is definitely more difficult for working parents to become fluent signers.

Chapter 11

A CURRICULUM OUTLINE FOR
AUDITORY–VERBAL COMMUNICATION

The Auditory-Verbal Approach is a developmental approach, based upon the sequential stages of learning communication skills observed in normal-hearing infants. Listening skills cannot be isolated from the entire communication process: listening, language, speech, and cognitive and sensorimotor development are interacting, inseparable components.

But development is not a simple progression from less to more, nor is it simply an unfolding of built-in structures. An individual does not operate at a fixed developmental level: he has a *range* of operations. Thus, any skill that is acquired on a simple level stays with the child and becomes more sophisticated. It is a process that grows and flows like a stream, which begins as a spring and becomes a river, always subject to influences from environmental change. Therefore, it is important to leave no gaps.

A curriculum can include many different aspects of learning: objectives, content, methods or procedures, and evaluation. It is subject to many outside influences, such as the teaching environment, teacher attitudes, economic pressures, and so on.

In the curriculum guidelines given here, the author has tried to separate the basic auditory, speech and language skills (which are normally acquired during the first year or two of life), and place them in a hierarchy which can be used to evaluate the level of development reached by the child and decide what he has to learn next. Too many details are not given because it is intended to be a child-centered curriculum, and children with hearing losses enter the program with different degrees of loss, at different ages, and with different basic skills. The important principle is to begin at the beginning and move forward as rapidly as possible, but moving, as it were, with the flow of the child.

In describing developmental sequence, we do encounter the problem of a time frame. What is a reasonable amount of time to reach each level?

If we set up our objectives in a stimulus-response framework, we will expect to elicit a certain response to each activity, but the time frame will depend on the individual child: is he a quick learner overall or a slow one? If there is *no* response, is he ready for this level, or are we encountering learning problems? Therein lies the art of the teacher-clinician and her evaluative skill.

We do know that progress is not achieved smoothly. After stimulation, change occurs, but the child must then "take in" new information before moving forward, and there will be a "plateau." After new kinds of stimulation, change and progress occur again before another plateau is reached. Sometimes, before a step forward occurs, the child seems to regress, as if the new information is causing temporary disorganization until it is incorporated with the old information, and is then reorganized so that progress can take place.

Sometimes, a small amount of new information opens many new doors, as it were, but at other times a large amount of time and information is needed to produce a small change. During the plateau periods, both parents and teachers may become discouraged, but just when everyone "gives up," the child moves forward again. One cannot, however, wait indefinitely. If several different approaches to the problem have been tried, reevaluation must then take place.

At the beginning of the program, the adult "feeds" in large amounts of information and the child gives back very small amounts. All kinds of toys and activities appropriate to the child's age must be used, many of which have been described in previous chapters. They have also been demonstrated in videotapes available for rent or purchase from the Alexander Graham Bell Association.[1]

LEVEL ONE

Objectives:
- To change the learning environment.
- To develop auditory awareness, vocalization, and the use of sound for contact.
- To conduct Baseline Evaluation.

---

[1] Pollack, Doreen: Five Videotapes: "Teaching Strategies for the Development of Auditory-Verbal Communication." A.G. Bell Assn., 1981.

TABLE 11-I
INTERRELATIONSHIP OF THE DEVELOPMENT
OF AUDITION, SPEECH, AND LANGUAGE

AUDITORY	*SPEECH*	*LANGUAGE* *"MILESTONES"*
Understanding	Spontaneous Speech	Receptive and Expressive Language
Processing Patterns	Jargon	Development of Syntax
Sequencing	First Words	Symbolic Language: Concrete and Abstract
Auditory Memory Span	Blowing and Whispering	Functional Words, Often Associated with Gestures
Auditory Feedback	Echolalia	
Discrimination	Babbling and Lalling	
Localization	Vocal Play	Sounds Have Meaning
Distance Hearing	Cooing and Smiling	
Attention or Listening		
Awareness	Crying	Sound is Used for Communication

Materials:

- Individual hearing aids or cochlear implants.
- Music: radio, tapes, CDs, musical instruments, music box, songs.
- Toys that make a sound: rattles, marimbas, squeaky toys. Begin with loud sounds and later use quiet sounds.
- Human voices: male and female, adults and children.

Activities:

1. Child is learning to wear appropriate amplification throughout the waking hours.
2. Natural conversation to accompany every parent-child contact.
3. Play with toys that make a sound, and listen to music. During this time, the child's attention is drawn, by gesture and words, to the fact that other people are aware of the sound, too, and that sound is *on* or *off, loud,* or *quiet, musical* or *noisy,* and so on.

Parent Guidance:

- Reminds parents that infant can now hear through his aids and should be spoken to as if he is a hearing child and not a deaf child. Parents should speak clearly, close to the aids, and with a lively

inflection. Every experience should be verbalized in short, natural sentences, and with much repetition.
- This guidance is given in a demonstration home or in a child's own home, as Mother changes diapers, feeds and plays with the infant, or in the case of an older child, as she makes the beds, dusts the furniture, sorts the laundry, and fixes a meal.

Evaluation:

As soon as a child is comfortable wearing aids all day long, and shows some awareness of sound, move on to Level Two.

Suggested Early Developmental Tests

Communication Evaluation Chart from Infancy to Five Years, Ruth M. Anderson, Madeline Miles, Patricia Matheny, Educators Publishing Services, Inc., Cambridge, Massachusetts. 1963.
Denver Developmental Screening Test, W. M. J. Frankenburg, M.D., and Josiah B. Dodds, Ph.D., University of Colorado Medical Center, Denver, Colorado. 1966.
Play Assessment Scale, R. Fewell, University of Washington. 1984.
Receptive-Expressive Emergent Language Scale, Anhinga Press Assoc. Publications, Inc., Gainesville, Florida.
Vineland Social Maturity Scale, E. A. Doll, American Guidance Service, Inc., Publishers Building, Circle Pines, Minnesota, 55014.

LEVEL TWO

Objectives:
- To develop auditory attention or listening and more vocalization.

Materials:
- Toys which make a sound, such as a drum, horn, rattle, snapper, a saucepan and wooden spoon, etc.
- Environmental sounds.

Activities:
- Focus child's attention upon sound by saying two or three times: "Listen, I hear something. What is that?" Pat your ears, but do not show the source of the sound until child is listening.
- Reward attention by showing the source of sound.
- Encourage feedback from child; that is, encourage imitation. Change

roles and let him make the sound and you show a big reaction (see Ch. 8).
- Create situations for spontaneous behavior of this type.

Parent Guidance:

- Continue to talk about every activity as to a *hearing* child.
- Continue to use music and singing.
- Take "listening walks."
- Parents should imitate sounds made by the baby and make this into a game.
- Child's own vocalizations are accepted and responded to as if he is talking.
- Parent begins to keep a diary of child's reactions.

Evaluation:

- Baby looks up, or turns around, or reaches out, or pats his ear, or has a "listening" facial expression whenever a sound occurs. Baby grabs toy and repeatedly makes a sound with it.

LEVEL THREE

Objectives:

- To develop auditory localization and distance hearing.
- To teach appropriate response to a sound.
- To make sounds meaningful.
- In speech development, there is laughter and increased vocalization.

Materials:

- Noisemakers
- Music
- Blocks
- Rocking horse
- Bubbles
- Musical clock, box, or radio

Activities:

- For auditory localization and distance hearing, see Chapter 8.
- Responses: Play games with sounds: open door when someone knocks; dance to music; ride a rocking horse to music and stop

when the music stops; clap to music; wind up musical clock or music box if it stops, and wave arms and rock body in time to music; build with blocks when a sound is heard; march to a drum; pick up phone when it rings, etc.
- In speech, laugh a lot while blowing bubbles. Laugh back and forth reciprocally. Hum and sing to music. Encourage "Hi!" Child may begin to imitate coughing, sneezing, crying, as well as greetings.

Parent Guidance:

- Parent to continue all previous activities.
- Parent to teach child to turn in the direction of sound, both to noisemakers and to voice.
- Parent to make a list of all the sounds baby responds to, remembering that awareness of new sounds continues throughout one's life.

Evaluation:

- Child is now attentive to certain sounds and looks for the source of them. He is aware when a sound stops. Child is beginning to turn when his name is called.
- As soon as orienting reaction is observed, move toward to the next step.

LEVEL FOUR

Objectives:

- To develop vocal play.

Materials:

- Stuffed toys
- Large vehicles
- Clay or Play Doh
- Large beads for stringing
- A plastic cone and rings

Activities:

- For vocal play, see Chapter 8.
- Make lots of sounds when playing with toys, especially animal and

vehicle noises: growl for the teddy bear, meow for the cat, click tongue for the horse, etc.

- Play pat-a-cake, peekaboo, ride-a-cockhorse, and other games. Blow kisses. For other games, see: *How to Play with Your Child and When Not To* (Sutton Smith, 1974). For older infants, play Ring-a-Round-a-Rosy, do fingerplays, play with puppet.
- Begin vowel games described in Chapter 9, using clay, large beads, plastic cone rings, etc.

Parent Guidance:

- Parents are shown how to set aside short but frequent time periods to play these games, and also how to introduce them into everyday routines.
- Parent begins to cover his/her mouth to encourage listening.

Evaluation:

- Child may attempt to imitate pitch, rhythm, and volume of the adult vocal model.
- Child tries to imitate one or more of the vowel sounds, either spontaneously or when parent uses the "hand strategy" (see Ch. 9).

LEVEL FIVE

Objectives:

- To begin to develop auditory discrimination.
- To develop Auditory Feedback and Feedforward through babbling.
- To learn that we live in a world full of sounds and that sounds are meaningful; that is, symbolic of an object or person.

Materials:

- Small toys, cars, boat, airplane, train, bike, cat, dog, bird, etc.
- Baby doll
- Cardboard box
- Picture books with large pictures, or books representing sounds, such as the *Ear Book*
- Building blocks

Activities:

- Review vowel sounds and vary pitch, loudness, and rhythm: *oo---* versus *oo-oo-*. For example, build a "train" with blocks and say, *oo-oo* or *oo----*, as you push it on the table.
- Play with lots of toys which can be represented by babbling: *mmmmm* for the airplane, *bbbbb* for the bike, *lalala* for a baby crying, etc. Encourage imitation of these sounds, varying the rate, rhythm, and loudness.
- Use the cardboard box for a house, as described in Chapter 9.
- For the older infant, look at books, making similar sounds for the pictures: "See, there's birdie." (Whistle.) "Listen, I hear that birdie." Match a toy to the picture.

Parent Guidance:

- Parent continues to keep a diary.
- Parent is shown how to listen for child's imitation and how to give lots of praise when the child tries to imitate.
- Parent should not talk all the time, but stimulate, and then wait to give child a chance to talk, too.

Evaluation:

- Child begins to babble some sounds. He may be more vocal when he plays by himself, but is quiet, because he is listening, when the adult talks. Child is responding to more environmental sounds.

LEVEL SIX

Objectives:

- To develop auditory discrimination and short term memory.
- In speech, to practice pre-linguistic skills (chewing, blowing, etc.) and to encourage echolalia.
- In language, to use those sounds which can be babbled in child's first words, which are usually functional words. Gestures should be used meaningfully.

Materials:

- Toys
- Inlay puzzles

- Noisemakers
- Recordings and percussion band instruments
- Book of Sounds, or a "listening book"
- Wooden board and stairs

Activities:

- Discrimination activities include teaching discrimination of noise-makers. With older infants, one may use recordings of sounds.
- Percussion band instruments are enjoyed.
- As described in Chapters 8 and 9, place toys upon the table with an edible reward in front of each toy. Cover your mouth or sit behind the child. Make a sound for each toy, and teach the child to select the correct toy and pick up the reward. Inlay puzzles with pieces which portray animals or vehicles can be used, too.
- *Speech:* Incorporate prelinguistic skills into games: Tongue clicking while riding the rocking horse; lipsmacking while feeding the toy baby or dog; licking a sucker; singing *lala* while riding the horse or riding on parent's back; blowing food which is hot; blowing bubbles, candles, kleenex; chewing with the lips together; sucking through a straw; whispering games.
- *Language:* When child can imitate a phoneme, that phoneme is incorporated into words. For example, if he can hum *mmmmm* for the airplane, he is encouraged to say *mama* or *more*. If he can imitate *bbb*, he is taught to say *bye-bye*.
- A young child enjoys a wooden board which is placed upon a box. He finds many ways to go up and down: sitting, standing, prone or supine. He makes his toy vehicles roll down. Parent says, "Ddddd Down!" or "UpUpUp," (while helping child to walk up the board).
- Child enjoys making the doll family walk up the stairs, or making toy animals walk up a ramp into a wagon.

Parent Guidance:

- Parents continue to introduce all previous activities into the daily routine, but also set aside time to "test" the child's discrimination as demonstrated in the clinic. Parent either makes a Book of Sounds or uses a clinic-made book (see Chapter 8).
- Parent now encourages the use of functional words and gestures: *up! bye-bye, no, more, hot!* and so on (see Chapter 10).

Evaluation:

- Child can identify and recognize the meaning of some environmental sounds: he may run to open the door or answer the phone. He may hear the dog barking outside and open the door for him. He can recognize the sounds made by the parent for about five to ten toys, pick up the correct reward, and imitate the sound for each toy. He may also be able to change roles, and make the appropriate sound for the toy so that the parent or sibling can pick up the toy. Child may take out his Book of Sounds and spontaneously "read" it by making the sound appropriate for each picture.
- He should be using a few functional words, such as *bye-bye* and *all gone,* although they will not be perfect reproductions of the adult model.
- In these ways, child is showing that auditory memory is present and that he is beginning to self-monitor auditory feedforward.
- In evaluation on this level, check the following behaviors:
    1. Can child recall word associated with a situation? Example: bye-bye.
    2. Can child recall sound associated with an object? Whistle means the bird, meow means the cat. He selects the correct toy.
    3. Can child imitate the sound? (Good motor skills)
    4. Can child recall the sound? Example: he picks up the toy flute and makes a high pitched sound with his voice, or picks up the horn and makes a low pitched noise.
    5. Can child remember which sound is associated with a toy and make that sound spontaneously? Picks up the toy and says *mmmmm* for the airplane, or says *ppppp* for the sail boat.
- This sixth level should be attained from six months to one year after hearing aids are fitted unless the infant has a very profound, left corner audiogram. This level must be reached after two years of wearing aids at the latest. The next level may be attained spontaneously or only as the result of many hours of formal teaching.

LEVEL SEVEN

Objectives:

- To develop auditory processing.
- To develop echolalia to the extent that the child will rarely need to be reminded to imitate.
- To develop symbolic language: the first nouns and verbs.

Materials:

- Toys
- Objects around the house
- Pictures and photographs
- Doll family
- Inlay puzzles
- "Sticker Books"

Activities:

- A great deal of auditory input is usually required before the child realizes that everything he sees, does, and feels can be labeled. For some children, especially those with more residual hearing, this symbolic labeling happens spontaneously, just as it does for the normal hearing infant. For others, structured teaching of pointing and labeling, etc. may be necessary, to accelerate the birth of symbolic language, as described in Chapter 10.
- The activity may be very simple and structured, as in pointing to eyes and saying, "What's that? That's an *eye.*" It is easy to say *eye,* and infants like to poke the toy cat's eye, Mother's eye, etc.
- The activity may be part of a game: we throw *the ball* to Dada; we catch *the ball,* we kick *the ball,* etc.
- We play with the doll family, calling them by name first. We look at the family photo album and name the family members.
- Predication is equally important. We line up chairs and pretend we are in a bus or car, and we *drive, stop,* and *go.* We play with the doll family and make them *eat, sleep, walk, sit down, wash,* and so on. As described in Chapter 10, the development of predication includes the present participle in answer to the question: "What's ...*doing?*" or to the question, "What's it for?"
- Children like to act out a few nursery rhymes such as Humpty Dumpty *falling,* Jack Be Nimble *jumping,* and so on.

- In speech, the child is encouraged to imitate within moderation, and to use those words he knows, as for example, saying *milk* when he wants some, or *pour,pour,pour,* when he pours the milk. As soon as he is using a few single words spontaneously, he should be encouraged to say two words together, as in *bye-bye Daddy.*

Parent Guidance:

- On a one-word level, parents are given the "vocabulary" of the weeks, as it were, and are shown many different ways to incorporate it into their daily life, and are also asked to practice in rather more formal ways: hanging pictures on the wall, making a scrapbook or pasting pictures on a table mat so that the new words can be pointed out during mealtimes, and so on. It is helpful to begin a vocabulary listing and watch the number of words grow (see the Circle of Communication in Chapter 10).
- At the same time, parents are reminded to continue with natural conversation about every experience, or some of them will get into the habit of talking in single words. Even the practice of single words must be part of a conversation, for example, as answers to the questions: "Who's that?" or "What's that?" or "What did Grandma bring?" or "What do you want?"

Evaluation:

- Child's vocabulary increases steadily, showing evidence of long term memory span, sequencing ability, and auditory recall. Parents usually report that it is much easier to communicate: the child seems to be understanding the gist of a conversation, and uses the words he knows.
- *Commercial Tests:*

Vocabulary and Language Tests:

Peabody Picture Vocabulary Test-forms L & M, Leota Dunn, American Guidance Service, Inc., Circle Pines, Minnesota. 1981.

Pre-School Language Scale. I. L. Zimmerman, Steiner and Evatt, Charles E. Merrill Publishing Co., Columbus, Ohio. (Ages 2–8). 1979.

Reynell Developmental Language Scales, Western Psychological Services, Los Angeles, 1990.

SICD, Hendrick, Prather, & Tobin, 1984.

One can repeat the early developmental tests also.

LEVEL EIGHT

Objectives:

- To develop auditory processing of patterns.
- To increase the auditory memory span.
- To increase the vocabulary.
- To promote good articulation.
- To develop syntax.

Materials:

- Everything and anything enjoyed by infants and preschoolers:
- Toys, especially preschool toys
- Doll family and doll house
- Dishes
- Dressing-up box
- Clay (Play Doh)
- Scissors and paste
- Tupperware blocks
- Inlay puzzles
- Lotto games
- Fisher-Price Village
- Tools
- Flannel board
- Books
- Montessori materials
- Picture cards
- A Buzz Box
- Experience Book
- Paints
- Puppets

Activities:

Auditory

Once a child has learned a few nouns, the Buzz Box can be used for auditory discrimination.

One parent designed an ingenious device to test a child's recognition of words. He made a box containing a large battery, a buzzer, and wiring. The top of the box slopes down to a ledge upon which are placed objects or pictures. Underneath the ledge, along the edge of the box, are six knobs to press. At the back of the box, not visible to the child, are six interruptor switches. When the clinician or parent says, for example, *doggie,* the child has to press the correct button. The appropriate switch has been turned on. The child's discrimination skill is thus rewarded by a loud buzzing sound. If the child touches an incorrect button, no sound is heard because the matching interruptor switch is in an "off" position.

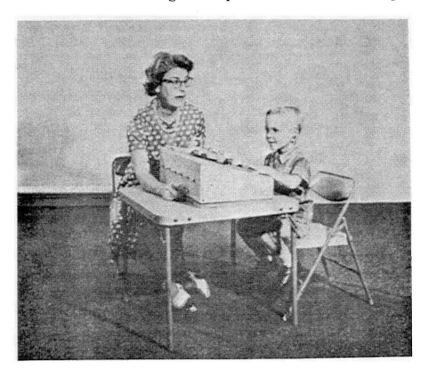

Figure 11.1. The buzz box.

More Listening Activities for Words

Use pre-primer cards or homemade cards, with one picture upon each card. Ask the child: "What's that?" or "Who's that?" as each card is placed upon the table. Then, call out the name of each card as you move to different parts of the room. The child listens and picks up the card named. Turn your back upon the child at times. This activity should only be used when the child can say the words, usually after two years of training.

Discrimination is also exercised in all other language activities. In using inlay puzzles (such as enjoyed by the two or three-year-old), we ask the child to pick up the various pieces which represent animals, vehicles, and so forth, and place them in the puzzles. "Get the boat, please. Get the fire engine, please." When we are setting the table, he is asked to select the cups, forks, and so on, in response to the directions: "I need a cup. Get me two forks." When we play restaurant, we order different foods (which are on pictures) and the child has to bring them to us.

The next stage is to construct similar games in which the child listens and identifies sentences. "The mother is sweeping the floor." "The boy fell down," and so forth. There are several inexpensive commercial lotto games for this purpose. Flannel board games are also enjoyed.

Auditory Memory Span Activities

These are appropriate for children about three to four years of age, providing that they can say the words.

1. Repeat the activity of naming and putting the flash cards upon the table, as used in the listening exercises. Use only a few cards at a time, and place them in a column. Ask the child to listen for, and pick up one card at a time, then two, then three, and so on. (Five is usually the limit.) At first, the child does not pick them up in the correct sequence.

2. When the preschooler can remember three at a time, place three of the cards in a row. Tell the child to hide his eyes. Remove one card and ask, "What's missing?" The child looks up and names the missing card.

3. The number of cards in a row can be increased.

4. Play a game of giving commands to each other, as for example: *turn around, clap hands, open the door,* etc. These must be given without visual clues.

5. As soon as a child can say two to three word units, he can begin to learn rhymes, such as:

   • One, two, buckle my shoe, etc.
   • Teddy bear, Teddy bear, turn around. Teddy bear, Teddy bear, touch the ground.

   These are more fun if they are acted out.

Speech

In speech, refinement and correction have *not* begun, although the child is encouraged to monitor himself and do his best; that is, if he imitates spontaneously, he may be encouraged to imitate more closely by listening to the adult model two or three times and trying again. This correction should not be overdone, nor should it be allowed to interrupt an enjoyable experience.

As soon as a few words are known, we encourage two-word combinations: *more pop, my shoes, bye-bye Daddy, another cookie, want juice, two candies, yellow paint, right there,* and so on.

Language: (a) to increase vocabulary
(see the Circle of Communication in Ch. 10)

This is the time to begin "units": for example, washing the baby to learn parts of the body; setting the table and learning spoon, cup, cookie; planting seeds, and learning dig, water, bigger.

Units can become complex: parents look *up in the sky* and talk about what goes up in the sky or what we hear up in the sky: birdies, airplane, kites, the sun that is so hot and so bright that you have to put your fingers over your eyes. In the clinic we have a flannel board which represents the sky, and the child has to learn and discriminate the vocabulary which has been used outside: "Where's the helicopter? Make it fly. Put it up in the sky." "Where's the bee? Zzzz. Oh, go away! Don't sting me! Put it up in the sky."

We use whatever is appropriate to the season: we plant seeds; paint pine cones to hang on the Christmas tree and learn the names of colors; make hot chocolate; cut out a pumpkin and review the parts of the face, and so on.

Words can also be learned in categories as we play with farm animals, or zoo animals, or different vehicles.

Example of a Language Unit: Parts of the Body

Infant: Baby is first interested in eyes, nose, toes, hair, fingers and mouth. Name these parts of the body during daily routine and vocal play: "I'll wash your hair. I've got your toes." In using the word *nose,* say, "That's Mummy's nose. That's Daddy's nose. That's doggie's nose." (Begin with *eye* which is easiest to say.)

Look in a mirror together and say, "There's baby. There's his nose. There's my nose." Gradually add the following: *ears, hands, feet, legs, face,* and so on. For example, when a child crawls, you have to scrub his knees!

Children Over One Year But Under Three: Begin as above, and continue as follows:

Take a large washable doll, a bowl of water, and a cloth or paper towel. Say, "Oh, dirty doll! Let's wash him. Let's wash his face. Wash his nose. Wash his eyes," and so on. Then say, "Let's dry his face," etc. "Now he is clean!" Put on some article of clothing and put him into a toy bed (which can be a shoe box). "Night-night, baby! Sh, Sh! Baby's asleep." (Note: when washing doll's body, teach *tummy* or whatever word family uses.)

The child may now wish to participate. Name each part as he washes the doll. With some children, one can control the activity and guide the child's hand to the part named; with others one has to name the parts *they* choose to wash! Next, some parts of his stuffed animals can be named.

For children approximately two and one-half years and over, use the following equipment: large blackboard, large paintbrush, chalk, and container for water.

Child is seated in front of the board. Say, "*Look!* Here's a face." Draw round shape. Say, "Now, here's the eye," drawing eye. "I drew the eye," and so on. Next draw a body. (I have always drawn a very simple figure, stick arms, fingers and legs, and a round body, like a child's drawing.) Of course, the young child does not draw a neck, or even a body. Omit the neck, but include a body or tummy. With older children, the neck should be included. (Small children like to have buttons, hat, etc., but these should *not* be included until after the clothing unit has been taught.)

Now say, "Let's paint the boy or girl. Here's some water. Here's the brush. Paint the face. Paint the hair." When the child wishes to participate, try to control the activity if possible; otherwise, name parts the child chooses to paint.

Remember, you are presenting lots of visual clues, but the names of the parts of body should be presented aurally.

Language: (b) To Develop Syntax

The teacher-parent can use many different approaches:

1. Create a situation in which a specific sentence pattern is practiced as a natural part of the activity: as for example, walking outside and saying, "I hear a car. I hear a bird. I hear an airplane. I hear the wind. I hear my shoes," or, playing a picture lotto game and saying, "I want the.... I want a.... "

2. Use the nursery stories which include repetition of sentence patterns, as for example, the "Little Red Hen" in which occur the sentences:

   > Who will help me?
   > I won't. I'm tired. (Which can be changed to: I'm *too* tired. I'm *very* tired.)
   > Then I'll do it myself.

   In this story, there are wonderful opportunities for role playing, and for varying the pitch and rate of the voice for each animal, as well as for changing the adverb.

3. Acting out stories. Children especially enjoy using toys to reproduce the action in books about animals, children, and so on. Lois Lenski books are excellent and so are many of the Golden Books.

4. Create an Experience Book. Every day or so, parent or teacher draws, uses photographs, or pastes pictures into a sturdy scrapbook to represent an interesting experience: the birthday party, the visit to Grandma's house, a walk in the park, buying an ice cream cone, being sick in bed, building a snowman, flying a kite, the first day at preschool, and so on. At first, the child may be able only to point out and name something or someone, but as the adult models simple sentences, he learns how to talk about his experiences. Later, he can relate these experiences to the days of the week, or months of the year.

5. Play table games which include repetition of certain phrases, as for example: in *Go Fish*, we say, "I want a yellow fish," and "I don't have one." "Go fish." Other games are: Hickety Pickety; Candyland; Hi Ho, Cherry Ho; and Picture Dominoes.

6. Three-word sentences become six- or seven-word sentences once prepositional phrases have been learned and added to the basic sentence patterns.

   In this kind of activity, it is advisable to practice one prepositional phrase until it is understood before adding another one, as for example, hiding easter eggs, and saying, "Look *under the chair, under the pillow,* " etc., or putting toys *in a* bowl of water, saying, "Put the fish *in the water;* put the turtle *in the water;* the frog hops *in the water,* " etc. Eventually, the phrases can be used together, as in building a zoo, and putting some animals "in a cage," others "in the water," or "on the rock," and others "behind a fence."

Other patterns to be practiced include the use of words such as *of:* a bottle of pop, a box of chocolates, a piece of pie; and also the particles, as in look *over,* look *back,* etc.

At this level, children enjoy learning *adjectives:* the concepts of color and number are introduced. They like to feel in a sack and pull out objects which are rough, hard, rubbery, and so on. They will sort out objects into big and little categories.

Parent Guidance:

- It is extremely important to work with the parent-child conversation on this level. Van Uden (1977) calls this the "seizing method" —parent and teachers "seize" the child's attempt to converse, and model correct sentences. Too many parents do not talk enough, and accept single words from the child, instead of using each situation to teach sentence patterns. This does not mean *interrupting* the child, nor correcting *everything* the child says. On this level, children often attempt to converse by using jargon, and the parent has to guess at the meaning.
- Sometimes the child's auditory span is short, so parents have to break the sentence into shorter chunks, as for example: "Billie say: I want to go/to the swimming pool."
- It is very helpful if parents encourage regular visits to the library, and enjoy reading to their children.

Evaluation:

- In addition to reviewing previous lessons, and testing the use of new concepts and language in different situations, there are many formal test materials on the market today. These include the tests already mentioned and the following:

The Language Tests

The Houston Test for Language Development, Margaret Crabtree, Ed., 10133 Bassoon, Houston, Texas. 1963.

Utah Test of Language Development, M. J. Meacham, J. L. Lex, and J. D. Jones, Communication Research Association, Salt Lake City, Utah. 1967.

Verbal Language Development Scale, (Ages 1–16), Mecham, American Guidance Service, Inc., Circle Pines, Minnesota. 1958, 1971.

The MacArthur Communicative Development Inventory: Words and Sentences, San Diego, California, Center for Research in Language, University of San Diego, California. 1993.

Auditory-Verbal Therapy, Warren Estabrooks, Alexander Graham Bell Association, Washington, D.C. 1994.

Speech Tests

Arizona Articulation Proficiency Scale: Revised, Western Psychological Services, 12031 Wilshire Boulevard, Los Angeles, California, 90025.

Goldman-Fristoe Test of Articulation (Ages 2 and over), American Guidance Service, Inc., Circle Pines, Minnesota.

TABLE 11-II
PREPARATION FOR MAINSTREAMING

Auditory processing: following directions, answering questions, etc.
Auditory tracking
Auditory closure
Increased memory span and sentence structure
Categorization
Similarities, rearrangement, inferences, etc.
Kindergarten concepts: calendar, Boehm's basic concepts, etc.
Integration of speech and phonics
Language of math, etc., etc., etc.
Use of local school curriculum guides

LEVEL NINE

Objectives:

- To prepare the child for formal education.
- Auditorily, to continue to expand the auditory memory span.
- To discriminate against a background of noise.
- In speech, to begin formal speech correction, and to associate speech sounds with written symbols.
- In language: to hold conversations to describe and to select on the basis of descriptions, to tell a story and answer questions about it,

to learn school readiness concepts, and the rules of games, to work in a workbook.

Materials:

- Tape recorder
- Toy xylophone
- A question and answer book
- Blackboard
- Workbooks
- Materials for shapes, colors, numbers, textures, especially Montessori materials
- Materials for phonics (such as Houghton Mifflin boxes and toys[2])
- Calendar
- Toys, objects, pictures
- Basic Concept Materials

Activities:

Auditory

- Child may learn to clap or dance to different rhythms; he may learn to tap out a tune on a toy xylophone or imitate a number of drum beats. As he matures, he learns the words of fingerplays.
- He has to learn to count to ten, say the alphabet, days of the week, his address and telephone number, nursery rhymes, holiday songs, and prayers.
- He must remember two or three directions at a time.

Speech

- Formal speech correction is begun, and may be associated with the written letters.

Language

1. **Question and Answer Book.** (For the questions, see Chapter 10, Table 10-I).

   The scrap book begins with the question, "Who's that?" On

---

[2]Obtainable from: Houghton Mifflin Co. 1900 S. Batavia Ave. Geneva, Ill. 60134. Sets I–III 1-26073 (plastic objects). Set 1-26066 (22 boxes).

each page following, are photos of family members, neighbors, and community people, such as the mailman, the fireman, policeman, and doctor.

The next question, "What's that?" may be followed by pictures of new vocabulary, words like *dial* on the telephone, stadium, circus, and light bulb; that is, words which are not learned spontaneously.

The next section is, "What is . . . doing?" Pictures are used to teach the pattern:

Daddy is painting.

Baby is crying.

Mummy's cooking.

Later, the same pictures can be used to teach pronouns:

He's painting.

She's crying.

The book continues to illustrate the answers to such questions as:

What color is that?

How many . . . ?

How does he/she *feel?*

Where is that? (Use photos of familiar places.)

The child must learn to answer *and* to ask the questions.

2. **Descriptions and Riddles:** Place three similar objects on a table. Describe one of them: It is white, it is round, and it bounces. One of the clues is definitive. In this case, all objects are round and white.

3. **Directions:** Older preschoolers love to give directions. Begin by giving one direction to each other, such as *turn around.* Then give two directions at a time, then three, and so on. *Simon Says* is a good game, too. Following directions in a workbook is important, too: the child learns to circle, underline, put a cross on, check, and draw a line from . . . to . . . There are many books available in the dime stores and one entitled *The Book of Directions* (Rush, 1977), can be purchased from A. G. Bell Association.

4. **Blackboard Activities:** this is an excellent time to have fun on the blackboard. Children like to draw together with parent or teacher. "Here's the house. What's in front of the house? Draw Daddy's car. What's above the house? Draw an airplane," etc., etc.

Many of the Basic Concepts can be illustrated on the board.

For example: *every.* Teacher and child draw a number of cars, cats, balls, and cups. The child is told to "circle *every* cat or erase *every* ball."

Other blackboard activities include: drawing shapes, such as a circle, and asking the child, "What does it look like?" The child completes the drawing to look like a cookie, a balloon, a sun, and so on. He has to say, "It looks like a . . . ;" or, drawing objects and asking, "What goes with what, or what do you do with it?"

This is a good time to introduce the action-agent concept, and after drawing many objects upon the board, ask, "What flies? What grows? What swims?" and so on. The child erases the correct one or circles it.

5. **Opposites:** Children at this level have to know *opposites:* hot — cold, friend — enemy, young — old, etc. There are commercial pictures of opposites for a flannel board.

6. **Phonics:** The blackboard can be used again. Write a large "b" for example, several times on the board. Let the child trace this letter with his finger saying "b" each time. Let him erase a "b" each time he hears the adult say "b" or he can write the letter himself. Change roles, and have him say "b" while you, the adult, erase the letter. After he has learned several letters, he can begin to collect pictures of words beginning with "b" and also sort out the Houghton Mifflin toys into appropriate boxes.

The number of activities at this level is limited only by the teacher's expectation and the child's progress in learning new concepts and the language which accompanies them. It is important to re-emphasize that the child is expected to process *auditorily.* The adult stands behind the child, at increasing distances, or covers her mouth, for all these activities.

Parent Guidance:

• It is, hopefully, routine for parents to review and use new vocabulary at home, and to converse about everything and anything! Many parents are also able to sit down for daily lessons just as parents help their normal-hearing children learn the alphabet, practice music, and so on. Some parents are able to demand good articulation but this must be handled carefully.

Evaluation:

The Peabody Pre-School Language and Utah tests can be repeated. In addition, the following tests are recommended:

Auditory Tests

Test of Auditory Comprehension of Language, Elizabeth Carrow, Educational Concepts, Austin, Texas.

Goldman-Fristoe and Woodcock Test of Auditory Discrimination, American Guidance Services, Inc., Circle Pines, Minnesota.

Auditory-Visual Test

Illinois Test of Psycholinguistic Abilities, Samuel A. Kirk, James J. McCarthy, and Winifred D. Kirk, University of Illinois Press, Urbana, Illinois. 1968.

Syntax Tests

Northwestern Syntax Screening Tests, Laura Lee, Northwestern University Press, Evanston, Illinois. 1969.

Grammatical Analysis of Elicited Language, J. Moog and A. Greers, C.I.D., St. Louis, Miss. 1980.

Language Test

Language Sample Analysis. See *Language Development and Language Disorders.* Bloom and Lahey, Wiley and Sons. 1978.

Speech Test

Phonetic Speech Evaluation Sheets, Planbook and Guide to the Development of Speech Skills, Ling, Alexander Graham Bell Assn., Washington, D.C. 1978.

Concept Tests

The Basic Concept Inventory. Siegfried Engelman, Follett Educational Corp., Chicago, Illinois. 1967.

Boehm Test of Basic Concepts, Boehm, A. E., The Psychological Corporation, New York. 1967, 1969.

Bracken Basic Concept Scale, Bruce Bracken, Chas. E. Merrill Publ. Co., Columbus, Ohio. 1983.

Visual Tests

Frostig Developmental Tests of Visual Perception, Pre-Kindergarten—Grade 3, Consulting Psychologist Press, Inc., Palo Alto, California. 1963.
Goodenough-Harris Drawing Test, Dale Harris, Harcourt, Brace, and Jovanovich, Inc., Atlanta, Georgia. 1963.

School Readiness Tests

First Grade Screening Test, John E. Pate, Ph.D. and Warren W. Webb, Ph.D., American Guidance Service, Circle Pines, Minnesota. 1966.
Metropolitan Readiness Tests, Gertrude H. Hildreth, Nellie L. Griffiths, Mary McGaurian, Harcourt, Brace, and World, Inc., New York. 1964.

LEVEL TEN
AND ON, AND ON, AND ON!

At this point, the Auditory-Verbal Approach has opened the door to formal education, and future activities will be coordinated with academic subjects. Auditory skills must always be practiced because they regress very quickly, especially since so many visual materials are used in schools.

Objectives:

- Auditory tracking.
- To receive and process information without visual clues.
- To use inner auditory feedback to remember and self-monitor.
- In speech: to continue speech correction.
- In language: to use a language arts program, to learn new vocabulary as it is relevant to daily experiences and formal academic subjects.

Materials:

- Tape recorder and other self-monitoring equipment.
- Practice telephones from the Telephone Company.
- A Speech Therapy Program, such as the LING Program 1976).
- A Language Arts Program.

Activities:

A. **Auditory:** to track on a tape recorder

The adult uses a book with many illustrations. She records the story, using one sentence for each picture (or each page). The child is present during the recording, and then replays it, turning the pages appropriately.

The "Muffin stories" are enjoyable for this purpose, because they also involve recognition of environmental and animal sounds.

B. **When a Child Is Beginning to Read, the Tape Recorder Can Be Used in the Following Ways:**
1. Adult records a list of reading words which are also written on index cards.
2. Child listens to the recording and selects the correct cards as he hears the words.
3. Adult records sentences using those words, and writes the sentences on cards. It is best if the child can formulate his own sentences.
4. Child selects the sentence cards as he hears them.
5. Child records the words and sentences, and finds that he has to speak very clearly!
6. When he begins to write little stories, he can record them.

C. **Reading Aloud:** Adult reads aloud from a sentence in a book. Child has to follow in his own book and has to be prepared to read as soon as the adult stops. Later, play reading is an excellent activity.

D. **Telephone Usage:** It is advisable to begin with a special program to instill confidence in the hearing-impaired child; that is, by using single words at first, such as *names, hello, goodbye,* and then routine sentences as: *How are you? Is your mother home?* Some profoundly deaf children handle the phone very well with the aid of a special speaker or amplifier; others require a special "code" when they call home (Castle, 1982). Every child should be encouraged to practice using the telephone because progress can be made. If, however, the residual hearing is not functional for telephones, a TTY should be purchased.

E. **At This Level,** the child needs a great deal of practice in listening for information. The author usually begins by reading one sentence, and asking a simple question, as for example: "What sort of weather did they have?" She may use the sentences for auditory closure, in which the child has to supply the last word.

Later, she reads short paragraphs and asks for many different kinds of information, such as: "Name the three main facts you learned about bears," or "What was the main idea in this paragraph?" There are many good commercial programs for this type of activity.

F. **Using Internal Repetition.** Children from a visual program frequently ask, "What?" and expect repetition of questions and directions because they cannot "hear inside their heads." The auditory child learns how to repeat aloud the question or direction before giving an answer. Then he learns to do this silently to himself. Auditory feedback used in this way greatly expands the memory span.

Similarly, too many deaf children speak correctly, but write down something which is quite different from what they have just said. Internal repetition helps them to write down what they hear themselves say, or to correct their written mistakes.

Parent Guidance:

- Some children enjoy having a special "lesson time" with their parents. New concepts and language must be reviewed.
- Parents need to keep in constant touch with the classroom teachers so that they or a tutor can prepare the child for new vocabulary which will be used in school.

Evaluation:

Auditory Tests

Detroit Test of Learning Aptitude, Baker and Leland, 1935. 3 Years to Adult. Bobbs-Merrill Company, Inc., 4300 West 62nd Street, Indianapolis, Indiana, 46268.

Lindamood Auditory Conceptualization Test. P. Lindamood. Preschool to Adult. Teaching Resources Corporation, 100 Boylston Street, Boston, Massachusetts, 02116.

Roswal-Chall Test of Auditory Blending, 1st to 5th grade. Essay Press, P.O. Box 5, Planetarium Station, New York, New York, 10024.

Wepman Test of Auditory Discrimination, Auditory Memory Span Test, and *Auditory Sequential Memory Test,* Wepman, Morency, 5 through 13 years. Language Research Associates, 175 East Delaware Place, Chicago, Illinois, 60611.

Test of Auditory Comprehension, L. A. County Southwest School. N. Hollywood, Foreworks. 1979.

Written Language Test

Picture Story Language Test, Helmer R. Myklebust, Grune and Stratton, New York. 1965

Screening for Language Disability Tests

Screening Tests for Identifying Children with Specific Language Disability, Beth Slingerland, Educators Publishing Service, Cambridge, Massachusetts. 1967.

Academic Achievement Tests

Brigance Diagnostic Inventory of Basic Skills, Brigance, Curriculum Associates, Woburn, Massachusetts. 1977.

Peabody Individual Achievement Test-R, American Guidance Service, Inc., Circle Pines, Minnesota. 1989.

Wide Range Achievement Test, J. J. Jastak and S. R. Jastak, Guidance Associates, Wilmington, Delaware. 1965.

Additional Lesson Plans are Given in the Following Books:

Courtman-Davies, M.: *Your Deaf Child's Speech and Language,* London, Bodley-Head. 1979.

Estabrooks, W. and Birkenshaw, Fleming L.: *Hear and Listen, Talk and Sing.* Arisa, Toronto. 1994.

Fowler, William: *Curriculum and Assessment Guides for Infant and Child Care,* Boston, Massachusetts, Allyn and Bacon. 1980.

Mavilya, M., and Mignone, B.: *Educational Strategies for the Youngest Hearing-Impaired Child* (0–5). New York, Lexington School, 1977.

Simser, Judy: *Auditory-Verbal Philosophy: A Tutorial.* Washington, D. C., The Volta Review, Summer, Vol. 95, No. 3. 1993.

Sitnick, V., Rushmer, N., Arpan, R.: *Parent-Infant Communication.* Beaverton, Oregon. Dormac, Ind. 1977.

Stovall, Dene: *Teaching Speech to Hearing-Impaired Infants and Adults* (ages 0–36 months). Springfield, Illinois. Charles C Thomas, 1982.

Vaughan, Pat: *Learning to Listen.* Washington, D.C., A. G. Bell Assn. 1981.

Estabrooks, W. and Birkenshaw, Fleming L.: *Hear and Listen, Talk and Sing.* Arisa, Toronto. 1994.

Chapter 12

PARENTS AS PARTNERS

THE DEVELOPMENT OF
HOME TRAINING PROGRAMS

For many years, education of the deaf child was not begun until the child was six or seven years of age. During the 1940s, many programs for the preschool child, aged three to six, were started in the public schools. These were patterned after the curriculum for older deaf children, rather than nursery schools for normal-hearing preschoolers. The children began their day seated in front of the blackboard, and followed a highly structured program. When hearing aids were used, they were usually kept at school and sent home only during the vacations.

During the same decade, audiologists were learning how to test the hearing of children too young to attend public schools, and in 1946 the Ewings published a book, *Opportunity and the Deaf Child*, which described how parents could begin the training at home under the guidance of a clinician or teacher of the deaf. The Wright Oral School and the Tracy Clinic correspondence courses, the *Volta Review*, and other publications in the United States of America recognized the importance of strong parental support, and the value of home training before a child entered special school. The suggestions they gave to the parents were, however, still reminiscent of classroom procedure. It now seems as if the true nature of the parents' role in relation to normal patterns of child growth and development was not wholly understood at that time. It has been particularly unfortunate that teachers of the deaf have regarded their role as the developer of a child's communication, with parents feeling somewhat on the periphery of their child's education.

THE PARENT–CHILD RELATIONSHIP

The author personally began to realize the significance of the parent-child relationship during World War II. In England, all women from ages eighteen to forty-five had to work in essential war work unless they had a baby under one year of age. The children were cared for in government nurseries. As the war dragged on, it became apparent that the group as a whole showed adequate language understanding, but were delayed in speech development. We surmised that this was caused by the lack of a one-to-one relationship with a loving mother who normally talked to her child all day as he played on, under, and around her feet.

In the literature of psychology and speech pathology there are many references to the role played by mothers in speech and language development, and to the communication problems of children who are raised in institutions. Wyatt (1959) describes how the young child learns to talk through continuous close association with a particular adult, usually his mother, who, with endless patience and constant interest, teaches him the patterns of his mother tongue through unending repetition of sounds or words. Margaret Mead (1930) reports hearing an adult and child repeat back and forth for sixty times the word, *me*.

The author observed a young father and his son enjoying a similar game across a restaurant table. "Nanny, Nanny, no!" said the little boy. "Nanny, Nanny, yes!" said his father. The child continued this game many times using different inflections, stress patterns, and laughter.

Unfortunately, parents of a hearing-impaired child may be unable to fill their natural roles when they realize that their child is "different." It has long been customary to think that counseling should be directed toward helping the family "accept" the handicap or impairment. But one mother complained, "Acceptance means resignation," and this will not encourage the best efforts to work with and *overcome* a handicap.

If, by lectures, books, and counseling, the deafness or "difference" is emphasized, a barrier between parent and infant is almost inevitable. To the lay mind, the term "deaf" has the connotation of a *total* impairment, and in spite of advice to "talk, talk, talk," the parents can be observed to gesture more than they talk. Unconsciously parents change their mode of communication. Amusing vocal play ceases, and they no longer draw the child's attention to environmental sounds.

Since a hearing infant perceives nurturing by hearing voices and the sound of approach, the deaf infant may find it more difficult to perceive the relationship between his behavior and an adult response.

This lack of playful interaction may impede facilitation of an attachment of the mother to her baby and cause feelings of frustration and a feeling of incompetence because of the infant's unresponsiveness. In this regard, deaf babies of deaf parents have been reported to fare better (Meadow, 1980). However, at least 90 percent of hearing-impaired infants have two normal-hearing parents to whom deafness is a traumatic diagnosis. In an auditory program, the parents have to see the child as a child, first and foremost, not as a handicapped child. Even if he is profoundly deaf, he can have a lively, happy, outgoing personality, as the Vassar experiment demonstrated (Fiedler, 1952).

PARENTS AS COMPANION "THERAPISTS"

Since home training is a radical departure from the traditional approach in which children are sent to a residential institute, or to a special day school, the question arises if all parents can undertake such a difficult task as communication training for the deaf. Overlooking at the moment that no professionally trained person claims equal results in all cases, it is undeniable that some parents are more successful than others, or perhaps it would be truer to say that clinics have more success with some parents than others. (Obviously, since there are large numbers of speech-defective, *normal-hearing* children, speech and language development is not a simple process, and a great deal of guidance is needed.) However, in Sweden, where home visitors help the family, some of the best results have occurred in the northern part of the country where it is very primitive, because the mother and father live close together with the child. On the other hand, cases in Stockholm are seen where the results are very poor, because the parents cannot understand their function and try to pay their way out of the difficulty. Bentzen, of Denmark, has found that a mother may come with ideas and observations which are better than a professional person can have in a short time with the child.

Wyatt (1959) stated that a mother's capacity for cooperation frequently cannot be assessed during the initial interview, but only after a period of working with her. Some mothers who appear rigid or overanxious during the initial stage are amazingly capable of following guidance and of cooperating effectively, often in spite of difficult home situations.

Parents naturally differ in their readiness to become cotherapists. In general, they fall into two groups: (1) those who show readiness to become co-therapists, and (2) those who do not. Those in the first group are reasonably concerned, even bewildered, but willing to help only if they know how to proceed. Once these parents understand the principle of therapeutic communication, they are able to use their own imagination. Parents in the other group seem highly irritated by children's peculiarities. Their relationship to the child, as well as to the clinician, is ambivalent and inconsistent. Particularly striking is their behavior when they are asked to observe the clinician at work with their child. They seem to rival the child for her attention.

Questionnaires and commercial tests can be used to confirm the clinician's observations and to determine parental attitudes and abilities as co-therapists. One example of these tests is the Mother-Child Relationship Evaluation (Roth, 1961) in which the mother completes a questionnaire which gives scores along a continuum for *acceptance, non-acceptance* (overprotection, overindulgence, and rejection), and *confusion-dominance.*

One new parent complained bitterly about her only child's behavior to the point of saying she did not like to be in the same room with her little girl. The child was indeed out of control and exhibited very bizarre behavior. The mother scored at the highest point of the range on *rejection* and *permissiveness,* thus giving obvious reasons for the child's impossible behavior. Her answers to many items on this questionnaire indicated that she had no concept of parenting. The mother later revealed that she had had a mentally ill mother and had left home at an early age. A great deal of individual counseling for the mother and play therapy for the child resulted in positive changes. In this case, the father refused to see the counselor. The child did learn to talk but required special education.

Another parent who had two hearing-impaired sons scored at the 75th percentile for acceptance, at the one percentile for overprotection, below the scale for overindulgence, and at the 20th percentile for rejection. She had a strong dominance score. In this very strict, high achieving family, both sons were mainstreamed in their neighborhood schools, with the older boy (who had a profound hearing loss) developing into a high achieving personality, but the younger son, who had more residual hearing, a very shy, average student. The mother elected to stay home and devote most of her energies to helping the boys succeed in a number of extracurricular activities as well as in their school work and therapy.

Although the role of a mother has been emphasized throughout this book, it is recognized that many mothers are working outside the home or are divorced, and the clinician may also be working with another caretaker or the father. However, national studies have reported that the mother of normal-hearing children are usually the primary caretakers.

When the fathers participate actively in the program, rather than as a supportive family member, the results are even better.

Factors for Success with Parents

There are several factors in the success of parents in an Auditory-Verbal Program.

A major factor is the goal the parents have in mind for the child. Do they feel all their problems should be solved and will be solved when they send him to a special school? If the attitude is held that it is someone else's problem, a family cannot be helped by an Auditory-Verbal Program. In this case, the clinician can advise that whatever path is chosen, the parents must follow it with their whole heart. A child should not be caught between two opposing points of view, for he will become so confused that he is likely to withdraw. Do they wish for him to speak and to live as normal a life as possible? The parents who hold this attitude are asked to follow the Auditory Approach until their child is at least five or six years old unless the clinician's regular evaluations show a need to change. The years of work ahead are not minimized, for educational audiology has no miracle cure to offer.

The second factor is the image parents have of their hearing-impaired child. Do they see him first and foremost as a *child* who has a hearing loss, or do they gain satisfaction from seeing him as a *handicapped* child?

The third factor is the success of the clinician working with the family to establish rapport with them and give them long-term guidance and support.

An important factor is the type of program given to the parents. It must be individualized so that they can meet with immediate success. If the parents are overly concerned with long-range goals, the best advice to them is as follows: "This is a long-range program and many years of work are involved, as with all children. Take one day at a time and step by step you will get there. However, remember progress sometimes seems two steps forward and one step backward."

Another major factor is the type of counseling available. Among the recommendations of an international conference on early management of hearing loss (Mencher, 1981) was one which stated that guidance and counseling should be initiated immediately upon informing parents of suspected hearing impairment, and that such counseling should be aimed at fostering the development and use of both new and existing networks, that is, the extended family, parent groups, parent organizations, and the habilitative team.

Luterman (1979) prefers group counseling for a number of reasons: he feels that the group meets fundamental personal needs, such as inclusion or having feelings of worth within a group; control, or the desire to make decisions regarding one's welfare; and affection. The group is wiser than any individual member and will aid other members in a sensitive and spontaneous fashion. Luterman describes other ways in which group counseling lies at the heart of the parent education program: the group is an important vehicle for building self-confidence and for sharing feelings, and it is an efficient vehicle for processing information. Professionally handled, the group can be a very powerful resource for promoting the growth of its individual members. Luterman, however, admits that some parents never reach the point at which they can accept the group. Unfortunately, with so many mothers working outside the home, few of them have time for regular groups. In a group of 50 families in one area, only 10 are actively involved.

The Grief Process and Its Effect Upon the Parent-Child Relationship

In recent years, it has been recognized that a good relationship between parent and a handicapped child will not develop unless the parents work through the natural grieving process which follows a diagnosis of deafness.

All parents dream of having a perfect child, and a disability has been called "a spoiler of dreams and hopes." The grief process which occurs in separating from someone or something significant that has been lost involves certain affective states which should be viewed as positive stages of growth toward the emergence of "coping." These states should be facilitated, not denied, by the professionals (Clark, 1982).

The most common affective states are as follows:

1. **Denial.** This appears in a number of different ways; by not following through on suggestions, by arguments over diagnosis, and so on. During this time, the parent cannot effectively engage in habilitation but will begin to acquire information and build some inner strength.

2. **Guilt.** This arises from a feeling that the world is just, so "bad things happen to bad people." They, the parents, caused this handicap in some

way . . . by genetics, drug usage, alcohol usage, and so on. This attitude is often related to the religious beliefs of the parents.

3. **Depression and Anger.** Depression is anger turned inward. The parents feel impotent because they could not prevent the handicap. On the other hand, some parents feel angry at this child who has disrupted their lives, and this anger may be displaced upon other people, such as the doctors or the professional who is trying to help them.

4. **Anxiety.** This is a generalized feeling of responsibility, conflicting with a temptation to run away from it all. The professional has to be careful of the amount of responsibility she places upon some parents or they will feel overwhelmed and end up doing very little.

The counselor or clinician has to allow time for parents to work through these feelings and then guide them toward appreciation of their child *as he is* and for whom they can build new dreams. Sometimes this takes place in group counseling, sometimes in individual counseling (Moses and Wulatin, 1981).

One of the ways we have tried to bring out these feelings for discussion is through a questionnaire. For example, when asked: "When it appeared that my child was hearing-impaired, I . . . ", the parents' responses revealed their true feelings:

- I cried.
- I thought it would only be a temporary condition. I was sure an operation would cure it.
- I didn't really believe it at first, and then was very depressed.
- I was very upset and hurt, wondering how her life would be, if she would talk, etc.
- I knew I had to learn a great deal about it. I tried to get the best medical help for her.

To the next question asked: "When I think of my child, I . . . ", parents answered:

- I am filled with love sometimes and frustration other times.
- I feel sad sometimes.
- I smile and thank God for them. (She had two hearing-impaired children.)
- I feel fortunate that her handicap is not worse.
- I think of all the future problems.
- I usually think of what I have to do next, where I have to take him, etc.

PROBLEM FAMILIES:
WHEN PROGRAMS DO NOT WORK

There will always be problem families and sometimes it seems almost impossible to elicit consistent cooperation or follow-through with them. One clinician who had struggled to impress upon a mother the importance of wearing the hearing aid continuously, was delighted to see the little boy arriving at the clinic finally wearing his hearing aids. But later she became suspicious of his lack of response and found there were no batteries in the aids! Some parents seem quite incapable of setting limits upon their child's behavior. It is very difficult to teach a child who is permitted to do whatever he pleases at the drop of a temper tantrum. These parents need a great deal of guidance and support in child management.

Among the parents who experience difficulty in a parent-infant program are the parents who have many children, the parents who speak another language, the clinic-hopper who is always seeking a cure, and the single or divorced parent who has to work full time and leaves the young child with a busy sitter who has several other children in her care. It is very difficult to carry out consistent and sufficient stimulation under these circumstances. On the other hand, one young mother of triplets was able to employ some household help, and the two normal-hearing siblings (talkative little girls) gave their severely hearing-impaired brother so much stimulation that he developed above average language skills!

It is often thought, mistakenly, that only mothers from the higher income groups can successfully undertake home training. Other clinicians have reported that families from a higher income level are more likely to feel they must send the child to a private school or provide a tutor, rather than undertake the home training program themselves.

One of the most challenging homes in which to carry out an auditory approach is that in which both parents are deaf. This has occasionally been solved by seeking the help of normal-hearing relatives who take the child into their home during the week, or by placing the child into a normal-hearing environment on a daily basis, such as a Head Start preschool. But it is not always possible to find two deaf parents who equally share the goal of oralism. In a sense, this would be a negation of their own successful adaptation to their hearing loss. If they have never worn hearing aids successfully, they do not understand what we are trying to accomplish and why. Furthermore, since a child identifies with his parents and uses only manual communication, it will be difficult to help this child auditorially.

TYPES OF PROGRAMS FOR PARENT GUIDANCE

There are two main types of parent-infant programs: those which are primarily parent-centered and those which are primarily child-centered. An Auditory-Verbal Program, however, is for both a child *and* his family.

Soderkvist (1963) has described a system of ambulating teachers in his country. (In England they are called *peripatetic.*) These teachers visit the homes and give the parents an idea of the preparatory activity at the age in question, observe the child, and give him appropriate educational training. As a parallel to home guidance, special courses are arranged every year in different parts of the country in order to give the parents a deeper knowledge and understanding of the problems which the treatment of a deaf child involves. Soderkvist feels that homes normally have an atmosphere which, to a much greater extent than the school, stimulate a child to learn to speak. When the child becomes four or five, the period of training only at home has passed, but the continuation of parents' work should be stimulated in all other possible ways.

In England, health visitors visit the homes and believe that it is very important (by conversation with the parent and observation of the child) to find out the immediate needs and then work by demonstration with whatever is at hand.

In some American cities, families receive their training in a home owned by a clinic, as in the "Home Demonstration Program" of Nashville, Tennessee (McConnell, 1974).

Luterman (1979) describes the program which has been in existence for a number of years at Emerson College, Boston, in which the children are placed in a special nursery which can be observed by parents, but the main focus of the program is the parent counseling group. Each family has to contract to spend from one to two years at Emerson. They seek additional and continuing help in other facilities.

The John Tracy Clinic in Los Angeles, California, has long been noted for its correspondence course which reaches out countrywide. It can be particularly helpful to parents in rural areas but has the disadvantage of relying upon written communication skills without any personal contact.

Morag Clark, an English consultant to many third world countries, has found that an Auditory-Verbal approach is very successful for families that have limited resources. Since they do not have access to professional clinics, they are receptive to assuming the responsibility for developing communication for their hearing-impaired children.

Programs which are child-centered can be found in private agencies and in schools. Public school programs often suffer from a number of disadvantages: they are frequently dependent upon special funding which can be discontinued at any time, they are usually suspended during the school vacations which are lengthy, and they rarely foster true parent participation and guidance. Most school programs group the child in groups of four or more, sometimes with wide age variations, or with different handicaps. These are called noncategorical groups. A model school existed in Minnesota for a number of years and has been described by Northcott (1978).

The Acoupedic Program was in two settings: one in a university (Stewart, 1965), and the other in a hospital clinic setting (Pollack, 1974). The parents, and siblings on occasion, participated in the clinical session for a year or two, depending upon the age and behavior of the child, after which time the child received individual clinical teaching while parents observed and carried out home assignments. During the clinic visit, parents received a great deal of individual counseling and guidance. If it was felt that there were significant problems within the family, parents were referred, or could self-refer, to the family counselor. Parents were expected to attend group meetings.

Parent Organizations

Experienced parent volunteers have been very helpful in making home visits to give support to new families and were instrumental in forming a fund-raising and support organization for the Acoupedic Program named the LISTEN FOUNDATION.[1] This group also purchased a house where out-of-town or out-of-state families stayed for short-term clinical help. Later, LISTEN operated its own center. The Beebe Center in Pennsylvania also has a similar house. A similar group, Voice for the Hearing Impaired, in Toronto, Canada, has promoted publications, conferences, and support for parents from a number of different programs.

---

[1] For their publications, write to LISTEN, 3535 So. Sherman, Englewood, CO 80110.

Chapter 13

PARENT EDUCATION PROGRAM

Every child is a promise
of something that will happen;
of something that will be;
of someone becoming fulfilled.
Every child is a promise
for each of us to nurture,
to support, to cherish, to encounter.
Every child is a promise
of dreams undreamed,
of hopes unspoken,
of fantasies not yet imagined,
of life yet to be lived.
Every child is a promise
for each of us to keep intact,
by allowing the child, as promise,
to emerge, free—to BE.

by Pat Greene

In the last chapter, the parent counseling program was described in terms of facilitating parental affect rather than in terms of providing content, but parents also need information before they can be expected to participate meaningfully in the habilitation of their child. A major factor in the success of any program is the participation of well-informed, enthusiastic, and committed parents.

Information can be given in group or individual counseling sessions. It is, of course, more cost-effective and less time-consuming to impart information to large groups of parents. The reality is, so many mothers are working outside the home (in all countries) that they do not have time to attend many meetings. This is unfortunate because it was in the regular group meetings of the Acoupedic Program that parents received not only information, but group support and reinforcement for their commitment.

The topics to be discussed are the following:

1. *Audiology:* Normal and abnormal hearing mechanisms; amplification technologies.
2. *Spoken language:* The development of a listening function, phonology, and the development of speech and language.

3. *Sociology:* Education and vocation, including legal implications.
4. *Psychology:* Psychological effects of a hearing impairment upon child, family and community.

The more personal questions about home training, parental attitudes, and family problems should be discussed in individual counseling sessions, or as part of the training sessions. The clinician has a responsibility to be aware of those parents who need psychotherapeutic counseling and should either refer them personally to a clinical psychologist or family counselor (usually a MSW) or send them back to their physician with a letter explaining to him that it is felt they should be referred to a psychiatrist or mental health clinic.

Participation in parent education sessions by other professional personnel (such as a psychologist, social worker, and otologist) is excellent providing that a clinician is present who is working with the child and knows the family, home situation, and so on.

For a long time parents will be mainly interested in such information only as it pertains to their own child and to themselves, and will often ask questions which will be answered more effectively by someone who knows the family and child personally.

In time, parents do extend their interest further and work toward helping others. For example, one mother, the wife of a minister, said they had never before considered the needs of deaf people in their church, and they were planning to initiate services especially for them.

A major problem often arises when the parents are challenged and made insecure outside the clinic by conflicting opinions, well-meaning advice (much of which consists of "old wives' tales"), prejudice, and even disbelief, which they encounter frequently within their own families as well as in the neighborhood. Therefore the author has always invited parents to bring relatives and friends to group meetings. The benefits may be far-reaching.

The foundation for participation may well be laid in the initial diagnostic testing situation. For the majority of parents, the appointment for audiological tests represents a difficult emotional experience — the culmination, perhaps, of months of doubt and anxiety, of medical examinations, and so on. This day they are asked to accept the observations and advice of an impartial observer and adjust to the undeniable fact that their child has not responded normally to the test sounds. The audiologist will observe that the parents hope there is a cure available, or that the hearing impairment can be explained by "slowness," allergies, tonsils, and so on. Occasionally they will appear relieved that the impairment is one of hearing rather than mental retardation or whatever they have feared. But it should not be forgotten that all of them are hopeful for, and desirous of, normalcy. Since this is not possible, the audiologist must send them away with a positive and hopeful attitude toward habilitation.

As soon as possible after the test, parents and child should begin a training program because anxiety fades with the realization that much can be done.

FIRST ORIENTATION SESSION

Before parents acquire the information which is needed for full participation in the program, it is wise to hold a group orientation meeting in which new parents introduce themselves and are encouraged to describe their feelings and experiences. A clinician leader who knows their case histories can ask such leading questions as:

> How did you suspect or find out that your child has a hearing loss?
> How did your relatives react to the news?
> Why did you choose this program?

Parents are reassured when they discover not only that their anxieties, hostilities, and so on are accepted by the group but are shared by the other parents. This session can then end with specific orientation to the philosophy of the Auditory-Verbal Approach.

Because of all the publicity in American newspapers and movies, parents may have many questions about "Total Communication."

Two books discuss this topic very well. Gray, in her book *Yes You Can, Heather!* (which recounts the life of Heather Whitestone, Miss America of 1995), describes her visits to various programs so that she could make an informed decision.

> When I observed a classroom in which all instruction was done totally in sign, I experienced one overwhelming reaction. I felt completely left out—as if I'd walked into a silent and alien world. If I felt left out, what would those kids feel when they walked out of their classroom into the hearing world? That one visit convinced me that I could never be comfortable choosing a communication method for Heather that did not include some oral aspect.
> When I observed a TC classroom I could understand more of what was

happening. But the speech being used seemed to be very sporadic: much of the communication relied totally on sign . . .

After visiting a classroom where the children relied on lip-reading, and where Gray felt that the speech wasn't very clear, there was only one other option to visit: the auditory-verbal method. Gray had already ruled out "CUED SPEECH" as the result of her reading and research. She writes:

> The visit to Porter Memorial Hospital in Denver turned out to be the most exciting and encouraging development yet . . . What impressed us the most were the kids themselves. We met and talked with several — all different ages. And what seemed to be even more amazing to me was that we actually did talk to them. They understood us. What seemed even more remarkable — we understood them. Some spoke more clearly than others. But we communicated easily with them all, without signs or special instruction . . .

Bonnie Tucker (1995), in her book *The Feel of Silence,* explains why TC does not result in a child who both speaks clearly and signs simultaneously.

> When they sign and speak at the same time, their speech becomes distorted. Many English words have no corresponding sign. Those words, therefore, must be fingerspelled . . . which means that the signer has to make a separate sign for each letter of that word . . . the spoken word must be dragged out to correspond with the lengthy sign. Further, people who sign and speak simultaneously sometimes do not speak all the words they sign.

For reasons described in Chapter 3, it is a difficult task for a young child who does not yet know language to pay attention to so many different facets: listening, looking, speaking and signing simultaneously. Signing is a manual and visual language, speaking is auditory. Nevertheless, parents must have the right to choose the option with which they feel most comfortable.

SECOND ORIENTATION SESSION

When parents set as a goal for their hearing-impaired child an independent life in the hearing world, they must realize that they are charting a long-term program for the whole family. One might say to them: "You are laying the foundation now. Sometimes it will seem to be years of work. Understanding and speaking will develop more slowly than for a normal-hearing child and it will take more energy and persistence for a long time."

Some of the responsibilities of parents in an Auditory-Verbal Program can be printed in a brochure or discussed personally. They include the following:

1. To learn all they can about hearing loss, amplification and child development, and so on. They can attend parent meetings, borrow books and pamphlets from the clinic library, and go to local or national conferences.
2. To determine what goals they want and look for a program which shares their goals so that they are not caught in the middle of professional controversies.
3. To keep all medical, audiologic, and therapy appointments. Helping a child become independent means being part of a team.
4. To keep the hearing aids in good working order and worn comfortably during the waking hours.
5. To talk as if their child can hear, and expect him to listen and show him how to respond appropriately.
6. To follow through on assignments, and maintain active communication with the clinic or school personnel.
7. To prepare the child socially. He needs to accept the same rules and responsibilities as the other members of the family. Of course, it may take more time and ingenuity and patience at first to demonstrate what is required of him, but his potential to understand should not be underestimated. The public already feels a barrier when they see a hearing aid, and the barrier will be increased if the hearing-impaired child is allowed to misbehave.
8. To teach self-discipline. For example, a child should remain reasonably quiet while others are speaking and try to remain part of the group conversation. (The author has seen many mothers of deaf children, and particularly those who use sign language, allow constant interruptions when their normal-hearing child would be told to be quiet and wait.) The child should also greet and thank people, and be taught to say *please* and not grab at something. In most ways he will develop normally if he is given a normal environment; that is, if he is not "spoiled" or overprotected. Unfortunately, children who are not raised in this manner use all their time, energy, and thoughts in manipulating the situation so that they do what they think *they* want to do. They are very difficult to teach!

9. To allot time to themselves. Living with any handicapped child imposes more strain upon a family. Parents need relaxation and interests away from their hearing-impaired child, whose hearing loss should never be allowed to dominate "pillow-talk" or the dinner table conversation.

The parents are now at a "crossroads"—behind them lies, without a doubt, a time of much anxiety and guilt, even despair. They need to establish a rapport with their counselor and express such feelings. But most of all they need to be shown the road ahead, along which their child will go, not as a "handicapped" child but as a child with a specific problem for which help is now available.

PARENT EDUCATION SESSIONS

Hearing Loss and Hearing Tests

The author begins each education program with general orientation, then talks in lay terms about normal hearing, causation, and effect of hearing loss, and about audiometric and other hearing tests. An otologist may be invited to discuss the medical aspects. The group may request a talk by a geneticist too.

A pictorial representation or model of the ear is shown and a brief discussion of each main part of the mechanism and its function is given. In order to hear normally, the parents are told there should be the following:

A conductive mechanism—
      an outer ear,
      a canal,
      an eardrum,
      a middle ear,
      with three ossicles, and
      a eustachian tube,

A sensorineural mechanism—
      an inner ear,
      the cochlea,
      nerve endings,
      hearing nerves,
      "hearing center" of the brain.

The ear can be compared to a telephone; the sounds which pass into the ear canal are changed by the eardrum into different forms of vibrations, which are eventually transmitted along the "wires" or hearing nerves to the brain where they are received and recognized as "sounds." If there is a breakdown between the canal and the cochlea, *CONDUCTIVE DEAFNESS* results; if there is a defect in the cochlea or hearing nerves, the result is *NERVE DEAFNESS;* and if the brain is unable to interpret the sound, the term *CENTRAL DEAFNESS* is often used.

Parents are interested in learning about the most common defects of this mechanism, for example:

> congenital malformations, such as atresia,
>
> impacted wax,
>
> perforations of the eardrum,
>
> "glue" ear,
>
> infection and blockage of the eustachian tube and middle ear,
>
> otosclerosis,
>
> high frequency deafness, and so on.

Some of the causes of hearing loss can be mentioned as follows:

> heredity, such as Waardenburg's Syndrome and Usher's Syndrome,
>
> meningitis,
>
> allergies,
>
> RH factor,
>
> prenatal virus damage such as rubella, influenza, cytomegalus virus, and so forth,
>
> high fevers,
>
> childhood diseases,
>
> anoxia at birth,
>
> skull fracture, and
>
> ototoxic drugs (Black et al., 1971) (Northern and Downs, 1990).

Otosclerosis should be clearly defined because surgery for this condition is given much publicity in newspaper and magazine articles. Parents are apt to pin their faith upon surgery to cure deafness without understanding that it is restricted to a very specific type of impairment and may not be performed upon a young child. Some other types of hearing impairment are, however, improved by surgery.

The clinician should emphasize protection of the hearing that remains, by regular visits to an otologist and by following instruction *to the letter,* because of the following reasons:

1. Hearing is so important that a child deserves the knowledge and skill of the specialist.
2. Prompt medical treatment can usually prevent permanent damage and may effect improvement.
3. A child's hearing can change and should be rechecked annually.

Next can be described the important part played by audiometric testing in the diagnosis of hearing impairment. The parents can take turns listening to the audiometer while the figures on the audiometric chart are explained. Each parent should have a blank test form, and there should be a large diagram or pegboard on the wall upon which each child's audiogram can later be represented. It is explained that speech and environmental sounds are not pure tones but a complex pattern with certain frequencies predominating. The most important frequencies for speech are as follows: 250, 500, 1000, 2000, and 3000 Hz. Some parents find it helpful to compare these with the piano. One can describe the nerve endings in the cochlea in this way: "If we unroll the cochlea it will be something like a keyboard: one end responds to low notes, and the other to high notes." Sometimes it can be described like a carpet full of cut loops, some of which are missing or thinned out. By such analogies, parents can understand why their child hears some sounds better than others.

Next, the figures on the chart should be explained: 0 decibels, 5 decibels, 10 decibels, and so on. They represent a measurement, expressed in decibels, of the loudness of the tone sent into the child's ear. The quietest sounds heard by the average normal ear may be said to be 0 decibels loud (although young people hear sounds quieter than 0). The loudness of the tone is gradually increased until the child shows awareness of it. It should be mentioned that responses to pure tones vary from test to test because of changes in a patient's emotional and physical well-being, and also because hearing, like vision, may become progressively worse over the years.

Audiograms can then be plotted upon the large chart to demonstrate that the child is able to hear much more, and in part, the distortion will be corrected. The child can be trained to listen and interpret what he can hear. He is no longer a deaf child, but a child who *can hear.*"

In conclusion, pamphlets and books can be given to supplement the session. Many are obtainable from The Volta Bureau, 1537 35th St., N.W., Washington, D.C. 20007.

PARENT EDUCATION SESSIONS

Amplification

This parent education session should be scheduled as soon as the therapist is ready to use hearing aids.

An audiogram and sound intensity chart is again plotted upon the board and reviewed to emphasize that although tones are from 0 decibels to 110 decibels, the human ear can detect louder sounds, up to 130 decibels (ANSI). The level of pain and its importance in hearing aid fitting is now explained. This represents the first limit we encounter. Some children will never hear sounds as we hear them, because sounds can be amplified so much and no more. Parents and relatives often believe mistakenly that a hearing aid gives normal hearing and they expect miraculous results! It must be emphasized that the aid is constructed to produce a specific output. It will amplify up to a certain intensity and is then, as it were, "clipped off" before the level of pain is reached.

A practical example can be given as follows: A child is fitted with an aid which will give him 45 decibels "gain." A conversational voice of approximately 65 decibels will be amplified so that 110 decibels are actually entering the child's ear: $65 + 45 = 110$ dB. If the child has a 60 decibels loss for speech, he will "hear" it as 50 decibels ($110 - 60 = 50$ dB) which is reasonably loud, although not as loud as the sound heard by the normal ear. If he has an 80 decibels loss, it will be heard only as a quiet voice (110 dB $- 80 = 30$ dB). The most important change is that the child wearing his hearing aid is no longer a *deaf* child—he *is* hearing the sound, even if he is not able to hear it at the same intensity as the normal ear. But if the sound stimuli is a loud noise, say 90 decibels, the aid would amplify this to 135 decibels ($90 + 45 = 135$ dB) which may actually cause pain sensations within an ear. This does not happen because the hearing aid will not amplify beyond a certain intensity level called *maximum output*. (The limit varies with different models; generally it is 110–140 dB.) It is helpful to demonstrate this with an aid which has automatic gain control. One can hear a loud sound being amplified up to a certain intensity. The noise appears to be "dampened" when the object making the noise passes by and then returns to a normal intensity when the object is further away. (A radio, or even a loud hand clap demonstrates this effectively.)

This explanation is, of course, greatly simplified for parents, but it is extremely important for them to understand the limits of amplification for two reasons:

FIRST, so that they do not misinterpret hearing aid "fitting" to mean something as precise as optometric fitting.

SECOND, so that they understand the need for intensive Auditory-Verbal training to enable the child to interpret through an incomplete channel.

Hearing Aids

The part played by amplification in an Auditory-Verbal Program is so crucial that parents must learn as much as possible about it. An auditory approach will not be successful unless the amplifiers are in good working order and are worn correctly. (For information about cochlear implants, see Chapter 7.) An engineer from a hearing aid company was an excellent resource speaker in Denver because he was familiar with the breakdowns which occur.

The following points should be discussed:

1. The parts of a hearing aid; and the ways in which adjustments are made.
2. The procedures followed in the clinic for hearing aid selection and evaluation (see Chapter 5).
3. The types of hearing aids currently used with infants and preschoolers. There are many developments in the hearing aid industry, including in-the-ear aids, transonic aids (which transpose the higher frequencies into the lower frequencies) and so on, but the usual aids used with small children are the ear-level aids. The body aids which were worn in early childhood by the graduates described in Chapter 15 are rarely used today.

   One of the problems with in-the-ear hearing aids is the fit of the earmold, because the receiver and microphone are so close. Earmolds must fit very tightly or feedback will occur and the volume may be turned down by wearer or parent. It is especially difficult to fit a baby's ear with its soft cartilage.

4. Maintenance and repair:
   a) How to wear an aid: in the case of ear-level aids which may slip off during active play, or may be removed by the infant, it is helpful to connect the two aids with an elastic band which runs at the back of the head under the hair. If an infant pulls out the earmolds, a ski-band over the ears or a bonnet can be worn. In the case of bone-conduction aids, worn by infants with atresia (a deformed or absent outer ear) the headband should be covered with ribbon or foam rubber.

   A child should be shown from the beginning how to handle his aids very carefully as a special possession. Parents need to accompany their young children to the bathroom to be sure that the aid or any of its parts is not being given a bath or flushed down the toilet! A preschooler should be taught to insert his own earmolds and to adjust the volume of the aids.

   Earmolds can be cleaned with a pipe cleaner or a toothpick wrapped in cotton.

   Unfortunately, earmolds, like shoes, are outgrown, sometimes within a few weeks, sometimes annually. The best indication that it is time for a new earmold is an intermittent whistling sound even when the insert has been correctly placed. It is tempting for the parent to turn down the volume but it is useless to provide a powerful aid and wear it at half volume.

5. Batteries:
   Batteries must be tested with a small battery tester at the end of the day. If they are checked in the morning, parents may find that some batteries have recovered during the night, but within half an hour of wearing the aid, they may be useless.

6. Hearing Aids:
   Although a parent can check an aid by listening to it, an aid should be regularly rechecked on a clinic analyzer designed for the purpose of charting its performance. When an aid has to be sent back to the factory for repairs, a loaner aid should be made available for the child unless the parents have purchased an extra aid. All new aids have to be checked too, as well as those returned from the factory for repair, because they do not always arrive with

the correct specifications for that child. The humidity of the climate causes problems, and the aid has to be stored in a special container. An aid which has become wet should never be placed in the oven! Nor should it be left in a car in the sunshine.

Parents will raise questions concerning the *cost* of maintenance, life of batteries, obtaining of service, insurance, and so on. They should understand that an aid is a device which, like any other appliance under constant usage, will break down and eventually deteriorate beyond satisfactory repair—very quickly if it is misused.

Such details in counseling are very important. The author has found that parents, after detailed instructions, handle the aids with confidence. Without them, they do not anticipate the mishaps and problems. It is discouraging to find children going happily on their way wearing hearing aids that are not working, and earmolds which are full of wax. Fortunately, a child who has come to value amplification is quick to indicate when he is not hearing anything. During the early months of training, however, we depend upon the alertness of the parents and their realization that the aid is now the child's "ear." If it is not working satisfactorily, the child has reverted to "deafness."

7. FM Units:

The main function of an FM unit is to bring the speaker's voice directly to the child's ear, thus eliminating the problem of distance hearing. Before the advent of cochlear implants, they were sometimes used instead of hearing aids for the most profoundly deaf children.

There are different opinions about the daily use of the FM units. Although it is generally agreed that they have made inclusion in the normal-hearing classroom much easier, the author does not believe that they should be used continuously. Limited-hearing children have to develop coping skills for distance hearing because they cannot use an FM unit in many situations. It may be tempting for parents to communicate from other parts of the house or outside the house, but they do not do much of this with the normal-hearing except to call the name. Limited-hearing children can learn to respond to their names, too.

Sometimes a bright child with a severe hearing loss becomes

not only an excellent listener but also an expert lip-reader (without special instruction) and will refuse to look different from his classmates by wearing an FM unit. The older child's feelings have to be considered.

8. Reevaluation:

Finally, parents should be urged to return to an audiology clinic at least once a year for a recheck of their child's hearing and hearing aid performance. Hearing, like vision, may change. Furthermore, progress in the hearing aid industry makes available newer and better prostheses. Certainly a parent should return immediately to the center if he or she observes a marked change or deterioration in the child's responses with an aid which has been ascertained to be in good working order.

PARENT EDUCATION SESSIONS

The Development of a Listening Function

It is very important to explain how a listening function develops. Emphasis is placed on the fact that the normal-hearing child hears something all the time, asleep or awake. Thus, he builds up a memory of sound patterns. He hears the same sounds many times over in similar situations so that they become meaningful to him. Then he recognizes them and pays attention to them. The limited-hearing child must have the same basic listening experiences as the normal-hearing baby in order to develop a listening function, but his rate of progress will depend to some extent upon the degree of his hearing loss, his personality, and the auditory environment which his parents create at home.

The Griffiths chart can be displayed and discussed. It is most helpful to read excerpts from diaries written by other parents to demonstrate that listening develops gradually. Parents should be encouraged to start their own diaries. Sometimes progress seems very slow at first, and the problems and defeats in raising a limited-hearing child may seem overwhelming. When parents read over the account of previous months they see what has been gained, not day-by-day but month-by-month. They realize that problems which loomed so large six months before are now solved, and they are preoccupied with entirely different ones. Thus they develop a long-range view.

OTHER EDUCATIONAL TOPICS

The following information should be scheduled to meet the needs expressed by each individual group or family. Some groups seem to be more concerned with education, some with personal problems, and some with community attitudes.

Speech and Language Development

Speech must be compared and defined in relation to language development. The normal stages of speech development are discussed, preferably with recordings of normal-hearing children. Books can be recommended. Few parents have consciously recorded the steps a normal-hearing child takes in learning to talk. In particular, the importance of vocal play must be emphasized. The amount of detail given by the clinician from preceding chapters of this book must be chosen on the basis of the interest level of each parent group. Most groups are very interested in the Laradon chart which shows the average development of speech sounds; some are also interested in the frequency components of phonemes and understand how limited hearing affects the perception of speech sounds.

One should emphasize that with the use of hearing aids or cochlear implants and intensive stimulation in the home, a hearing-impaired child can follow normal patterns of speech development. Ways to motivate speech should be described.

Fluent speech for the limited-hearing older child may require the skillful therapy of a speech pathologist, but parents' speech is the model for an infant and their voices need to be lively and more inflected. Many adults speak to infants in this way naturally, but it is helpful to make a recording or videotape so that parents can hear themselves.

When talking about language development, it is important to describe receptive and expressive language, and to stress that language is a natural outcome of listening within meaningful situations. The various levels of spoken language development should be described. Parents enjoy looking at the interrelationship chart in Chapter 11 and deciding which level their child has reached. Tape recordings and excerpts from parents' diaries are most effective in giving an overview of language development.

One needs to point out that what occurs naturally for the normal-hearing child will be the result of a more conscious, structured effort for the limited-hearing child who has not been fitted with hearing aids soon after birth. Parents often have to be shown how to use the home environment so that conversation includes repetition, reinforcement, turn-taking, and so on. For example, if a child uses one word, parents should use another way of saying this so that vocabulary will grow, thus lessening frustration and increasing self-confidence.

Many parents complain that they do not know what to say; that is, they "run out" of things to say. The author usually asks them to hand around a familiar object, such as a ball, and say something about it. The ball goes around the group several times before the parents can find no other word to describe it. They find they can talk about its shape, color, size, texture, decorations, weight, that it can be bounced, kicked, thrown, bowled, and so on. To increase and emphasize language development: if a child has one way of saying something, use another word or expand on the first word so vocabulary will grow. More vocabulary leads to less frustration for the parent and child, which leads to success and greater self-confidence.

The importance of motivation for the child in understanding and using language should be discussed. Learning to talk results from identifying with the parents from being praised, from getting results, from "need reducing" (i.e., reducing frustration), and so on. But anxiety on the part of the parents will inhibit this motivation.

Social and Emotional Development

This section is best handled by resource personnel. A psychologist or family counselor can be most helpful to the group. He or she will probably stress that the needs of the hearing-impaired child are the same as the needs of the normal-hearing child—love, guidance, consistent discipline, and so forth. Then the special problems can be discussed which seem to be caused, or are intensified, by the hearing impairment.

Group sessions are most successful when handled as round table discussions, ending in a talk by a counselor who summarizes and gives some general suggestions. Some parents like to put into a hat a number of their questions for general discussion.

The area of a child's social and emotional development, however, cannot just be dealt with in a group session. During the weekly therapy visits, the clinician can give invaluable support and guidance when the parent reports problems which have occurred each week at home. The clinician does not always have to play the part of passive listener. She may have to ask questions in order to elicit important information.

In the University of Denver program, a psychologist[1] was able to schedule an individual session with each mother approximately one hour every two weeks. Most of the mothers were seen about ten times. It had been explained that attendance was voluntary but desirable to learn about the child's behavior at home. In the first quarter, cooperation was good, the second showed fewer attendances. In the third quarter, not one of these mothers requested appointments but had impromptu meetings. These sessions served many purposes, and, in particular, a chance for the mother to talk about how difficult it was to have a hearing-impaired child, but not in so many words. The problems discussed included the following:

Toilet Training — This is not exceptional considering the age of children in a preschool program, but the mother's feeling of frustration in communication seemed greater.

Concerns About Disciplining Child — There is the feeling that it is unfair to punish a child who doesn't understand what is being said (if he can hear, then it's a sporting fight), and there are mixed feelings of knowing he needs discipline but feeling guilty when doing it. Parents have to be reminded that they use these terms when normal-hearing children do not yet understand them, but they will learn to understand because of the context in which they are spoken. Limited-hearing children will learn in the same way.

In particular, they feel that it is difficult to get subtle points or exact concepts across to young, hearing-impaired infants who are just developing language. Spoken language has a unique way of providing different shades of meaning, as for example, "You may not do this now, but *later.*" Parents feel that they encounter more temper tantrums (Murphy, 1979). Children also need to learn the consequences to expect when behavior is dangerous or unacceptable.

However, many discipline problems would not arise if parents knew that the key to raising any child is to show them how to behave, stand back and encourage them to try it, and then praise them for doing so. Too many parents spend all their energy berating their children for wrong doing but do not model the correct behavior.

Concern for Siblings, Grievances About Relatives, Etc. — There

---

[1]Dr. Esther Shapiro

is some connection with feelings of adequacy or inadequacy of the mother handling the child, feeling beset upon because of lack of cooperation; sibling jealousy, because attention to hearing-impaired child is greater, and so on. (There were many expressions of emotions regarding the discovery of the hearing loss. There was usually hostility toward the medical profession because of delay in diagnosing the hearing loss and referral for treatment. The mother expressed helplessness, anxiety, depression, and other problems.)

Concern for Progress of Child (especially in the area of expressive speech and elementary education).

Sleeplessness at Night — One of the problems frequently encountered by all parents when their children are two or three years old is a night time fear expressed in nightmares, restlessness, and refusal to go to bed alone. Some parents "dig their own graves" by permitting their children to stay up late, sleep in the parents' bed, or, vice versa, a parent stays in the child's room. But healthy children have to accept a quiet routine at a regular bedtime hour, and have to stay in their own beds accompanied by a favorite toy, blanket, and a night light. It is understandable that a hearing-impaired youngster fears the dark when he cannot hear or see the parents moving about the house. One solution is to let him wear one hearing aid at night, or to leave open the door and walk past it occasionally. In the case of a willful child, however, it may be necessary to lock the door.

In every case involving problems, it has been easy for the child to gain control because the parents have not dealt with their feelings of guilt and grief, and have not given clear-cut, consistent messages to define behavioral limits.

Difficulty in Group Participation — The solution is to cue into the conversation, especially when the topic changes, as for example, you can say, "We are talking about Mary's new puppy now." Then the hearing-impaired child is more likely to remain part of the group and not continually demand attention.

Sometimes taking turns at the dinner table with each child talking in a different order may help keep the hearing-impaired child involved. "Tonight _____ goes first," etc.

It is not always realized that this counseling must continue for a long time. The junior high school years are particularly difficult, not only for the hearing-impaired child, but also for the normal-hearing child. This is a time when the personality of the child begins to emerge and many

many parents will make the mistake of blaming everything that happens on the hearing loss. For example, one mother was very upset because she felt her daughter was not making friends in the normal-hearing junior high school. It was pointed out to her that the author's oldest son, who had normal hearing, had exactly the same experiences because both the children had similar personalities. They were more introverted and did not like to be part of a big group. It was also pointed out that at this age children become more selective about their friendships and it takes some time for them to find a truly congenial friend. In a large city school, children are grouped in different units for each subject and it takes time to become acquainted when one is moving around from group to group throughout the day. Some children need more companionship than others. Most important of all, the parents should not impose their own emotions on the child. Of course, there will be problems, but they are not necessarily *caused* by the hearing impairment. At this time the teenager may suddenly refuse to wear a hearing aid because he is becoming very aware of his appearance and feels that he will look different. It is especially important at this time to provide a special attachment to the telephone, or a TTD for the relay system, if this enables the hearing-impaired child to use the phone!

These are just a few of the problems which are discussed in parent groups.

It is most helpful to invite parents whose children are now in school to visit the group and discuss their own experiences. A long-term view for the new parent can only be taken vicariously.

Family and Community Life

Some of the discussions will center around the effect of a hearing loss upon each family member, the attitude of the neighbors, and other matters of importance. These have been well documented in a study by Gregory (1976) with English families.

Parents should be warned that they will encounter many stereotyped ideas. Unfortunately, they have to become aware that there will be great pressure placed upon them, usually with the best of intentions, to place their child in a deaf group. One mother described it thus: "I have had to put on blinders like a horse. I know my goal and right now I am just going to look in that direction only."

Luterman (1979) describes a number of excellent structured experiences for group participation, such as role playing, hypothetical families, and guided fantasies. For example, in role playing, two volunteers, a father and a mother *married to other spouses,* are encouraged to tell each other how they feel about having a hearing-impaired child, something which they find very difficult to do with their own spouses.

In hypothetical families, each parent in the group receives a short summary of a specific problem occurring in a family. A few details are given about the family members. The group discusses this problem and tries to find a solution. As they do so, they begin to reveal and gain insight into their own problems, which might be the behavior of the hearing-impaired child, the jealousy and behavior of a sibling, the impact on parents who do not agree about educational methodology, and so on.

New parents especially enjoy a session with parents of older children who describe their own experiences and answer questions. It is encouraging to hear that early problems were lived with and overcome. It is even more thrilling when young adults return to describe their life styles. New parents need hope above all else that their efforts will enable their child to lead an independent life.

It is very helpful to hold special rap sessions for the older siblings in a family. What is the impact of a hearing-impaired infant upon older, nonhandicapped children? Schwirian (1976) found that there was little effect in terms of responsibility placed upon them for child care or household chores until they become older. When siblings are encouraged to participate in the clinic sessions, they will frequently re-enact the session with the hearing-impaired child upon returning home, but a parent has to be cautious about directing the normal-hearing youngster to take responsibility. One mother described how she gathered her family together each week and said, "Our assignment for the week is to . . ."

Since siblings in general are less emotionally tied to each other than to their parents, they can protect each other and learn from each other (Murphy, 1979). For example, Susan's older sister insisted on inviting Susan to participate in all her play activities with neighborhood friends, and is still, although married, one of her sister's best friends. The sibling closest in age to the hearing-impaired child may experience more difficulties, however, because he may equate more *attention* to the hearing-impaired as more *love.*

One can also hold sessions for fathers only and for grandparents.

Parents have to be shown how to develop a positive attitude toward hearing losses within the community. One of the author's former patients, when a college student, wrote the following:

> Granted that the first handicap of deafness lies in communication, it has often seemed to me that a close second might be the attitude of hearing people toward it and that the former would be considerably lessened if we could do something to improve the latter. By turns I have been amused, annoyed, angry and frustrated by this attitude and its various manifestations. I have to remind myself that it is due to almost complete lack of understanding of the problems faced by those with a hearing loss and the narrowness and fear and insecurity bred of ignorance.

This student (whose mother was once told that "she might never learn to talk"—a very common occurrence unfortunately) has been so successful in changing the attitudes of those in her environment that one of her classmates described her in the following words:

> Mary has accepted the fact that she is hard of hearing and has proceeded to build her life around her capabilities, which, due to her determination, vary only slightly from those of a normal hearing person. In referring to her handicap Mary does not look for pity or sympathy, because she does not feel these things for herself. But most of all, she wants to be as everyone else, given a chance for the same opportunities and experiences that we all aspire to (Niemann, 1972).

Not all limited-hearing children will go to college, but all of them can be helped to "build a life around their capabilities."

Unfortunately, a great deal of newspaper publicity emphasizes the hearing *handicap* and tries to arouse *pity* within the community. On the contrary, we want to instill within the limited-hearing child the feeling that he does not have to be the *same* as a normal-hearing person (because he cannot be the same—he has a hearing defect) and that he can develop ego-strength on the basis of *who he is.* Therefore it is most important to instill a positive attitude within the normal-hearing community.

EDUCATION AND LEGAL IMPLICATIONS

For this topic, clinicians may invite local school representatives to describe the types of educational services available, and the regulations and policies which govern their programs. These are subject to change, but as described in Chapter 1, current federal laws, the IDEA and ADA, support the rights of hearing-impaired persons to take their place in the mainstream. However, the parents of children who have been educated in an Auditory-Verbal Program from an early age often have to fight for the type of educational placement they request.

Bonnie Tucker, a deaf lawyer, recounts in her book *The Feel of Silence* her experiences in advocating for a Native American boy whom the system wished to send to a residential school, four hundred miles from home. This was not an oral versus signing dispute, since the boy used "Total Communication" and could have received services in his local school, which under IDEA seemed to be his statutory right. Officials from the state school, however, insisted that the boy needed to be immersed in the Deaf culture until he was twenty-two years old. The judge was so entranced by the idea of Deaf culture that he ruled in favor of the state school. Tucker pointed out that she and many other hearing-impaired persons were successful in the mainstream, only to be told by the judge that she was an exception. So justice is not always served.

There have been other cases in which parents who requested an auditory-verbal or oral program were told that Total Communication includes auditory-verbal training. In order to help parents, the Alexander Graham Bell Association appointed Children's Advocates in various states.

In recent years, parents have been subjected to so much pressure to use sign language that the author advises them not to rush into enrollment in a special school because the majority of auditory-verbal children have the potential to compete in an educational program with normal-hearing peers. (See the outcome studies in Chapter 4.)

The advantages and problems of placement in a normal-hearing classroom must be discussed realistically. Although technological progress has made possible early detection and intervention, it has also resulted in acceleration and experimentation in the public schools which sometimes makes inclusion more difficult unless a cascade of services is available (Northcott, 1973). There is no single solution to the educational placement of a hearing-impaired child, but parents can be counseled not to set limits on their children (as special schools are apt to do), and to give them every opportunity to succeed in the least restrictive environment.

MAINSTREAMING IN AN
AUDITORY–VERBAL PROGRAM

The goal of an Auditory-Verbal Program is not first to segregate the child and then at some later date try to integrate him. From the first moment of early intervention, the Auditory-Verbal goal is to give each child the opportunity to become a fully participating citizen within the normal-hearing community to the degree permitted by his abilities and capacities, and with a consistent and continuous interaction within the home, community, school, and church; that is, in the mainstream of life (Bitter, 1973).

It is absolutely critical not to set limits upon a young child because of the degree of his hearing loss, but to take one step at a time, and to look at the whole child (Pollack and Ernst, 1973).

Reichenstein, in Israel (1978), concludes that with the four-point program, an early start, early binaural amplification, parental guidance and involvement, and integrated preschool education, it has become possible to make great changes in educational programming. He reports that the percentage of severely hearing-impaired children who go into integrated programs when they go to school is constantly growing, and that they have speech, language, and a learning potential way beyond what was dreamed of twenty or thirty years ago. Itano's studies in Colorado have proved this.

In an Auditory-Verbal Program, the author advises the following: if the hearing impairment was diagnosed at an early age, and if the child has received an auditory-verbal education with the full support of his parents, and is making progress as evaluated by language and achievement tests standardized on a normal population, he can be enrolled in a mainstreamed program. This means integration in a preschool or nursery school for normal-hearing children, kindergarten at six years of age, and so on, until it is proved beyond a doubt that the child cannot reach his potential without special education. We have often found that it is advisable for a child to repeat third grade in order to give him time to "catch up," vocabulary-wise.

Federal laws have mandated inclusion in the least restrictive environment, with parents participating with school personnel in drawing up an individualized educational plan (IEP) for each child. Amon (1995), in an excellent description of federal regulations, wrote:

> With an appropriate education, children with auditory disorders can learn, achieve, and grow commensurate with their chronological age, however this does

not often happen. The major obstacle to this occurring is the quest for a homogenous solution to the needs of a heterogenous set of students. Legislation alone neither ensures nor prohibits the provision of appropriate education. We as parents, consumers, service providers, and administrators must work in partnership to identify the needs of and goals for each child and design an IEP plan in response to these needs and goals, and to monitor growth constantly, changing our plans as needed.

SUMMARY

Information for parents in a parent-child program may include the following:

1. Hearing, hearing loss, amplification devices, genetics of hearing loss.
2. Care of the amplification devices.
3. Creation of a normal living, learning, and linguistic environment.
4. Normal child development and behavior management.
5. Normal speech and language development.
6. Problems in addition to hearing loss.
7. Alternative communication methods.
8. Relations to society.
9. Availability and utilization of community services (e.g., telephone relay service).
10. How to evaluate educational systems.
11. Legal rights.
12. Organizations which help the hearing-impaired.

RECOMMENDED READING

For books, pamphlets, and videotapes related to the topics listed above, the reader is referred to the catalogue published by the Alexander Graham Bell Association in Washington, D.C.

Other books for parents include:

Bertling, Tom: *A Child Sacrificed to the Deaf Culture.* Oregon, Kodiak Media, 1994.
Dreikus, Richard: *Children the Challenge.* New York, Hawthorn Books, 1964.
Gray, Daphne: *Yes, You Can, Heather!* Michigan, Zondervan, 1995.
Knox, Laura: *Parents Are People Too.* Nashville, Intersect.
Kushner, H.: *Bad Things Happen to Good People.* Schocken Books, 1981.
Stibbick, M., and Feibleman, P.: What parents ask of clinicians and counselors, in

Marlow, J. (Ed): *The Evaluation and Management of Communication Disorders in Infants.* New York, Thieme-Stratton, Vol. 2, No. 1, February 1982.

Tucker, Bonnie: *The Feel of Silence.* Philadelphia, Temple University Press, 1995.

Wright, D.: *Deafness.* New York, Stein and Day, 1969.

Chapter 14

MODIFICATION OF THE AUDITORY–VERBAL PROGRAM FOR THE HEARING–IMPAIRED WITH SEVERE LEARNING PROBLEMS

Thus far we have talked about a child with a hearing loss as one who can follow a normal development sequence with each simple skill providing the base for learning a more complex skill, which in turn becomes the base for an even more complex skill. Each step forward is the result of previous learning.

But every teacher has encountered children who do not progress in a normal, sequential manner, regardless of persistent and skillful teaching.

LEARNING DISABILITIES IN THE NORMAL–HEARING CHILD

Sensorimotor Integration

Normal learning presupposes not only the absence of brain damage or retardation, but that the child's senses are bringing back the correct information to his brain which will then organize, store, and recall that information for future learning, and plan an appropriate response to the environment.

Although the brain works in a "global" manner, it consists anatomically of two hemispheres, which have evolved in such a manner that one hemisphere is dominant for some functions. This lateralization and specialization of cerebral function enabled man to develop fine motor skills and speech. Thus, sensorimotor information from the peripheral organs is received in different areas of the brain, and integrated in a hierarchical sequence as the child matures.

The most important information or "feedback" comes from the following senses:

1. from the muscles, or the *kinesthetic* sense
2. from the skin, or the *tactile* sense

3. from the eyes, or the *visual* sense
4. from the ears, or the *auditory* sense
5. from the nose and taste mechanism, or the *olfactory* and *gustatory* sense
6. from the *vestibular* sense

In young children, we are dealing with a developing brain which is being programmed for a specific behavior pattern by each experience and within a normal time period. For example, a baby is usually born with a normal instinct to "root" for food, and to suck and swallow, but he has to learn how to chew and swallow food and drink from a cup. Many senses are involved in this learning: he feels the food, he tastes it, smells it, sees it, chews it, and swallows it. Thus, learning to eat involves the integration of many sensorimotor systems. Unfortunately, there are babies with poorly organized gustatory systems who suck and swallow poorly, and are not only poor eaters, but poor *speakers,* because the same muscles are used for speaking as for chewing and swallowing.

There are many other problems which indicate a disruption in the normal development of the neurologic system, and the causation is sometimes described as "brain dysfunction" or "brain difference."

In 1954, it was claimed that neurologic impairment occurs in 10 percent of full-term births. The rate among premature infants is higher. When screening studies were undertaken by the public schools, an amazing percentage of learning disabled children was found. Some of these may have been "slow blooming" or slow-maturing, rather than truly learning disabled, but this discovery necessitated a large, new group of remediation personnel in the public schools.

Cognitive Development and Sensorimotor Functioning

The connection between sensorimotor functioning and learning was described by two Europeans, Piaget and Montessori, who saw mental growth as an extension of physical growth, and in their view, the environment should provide nourishment or content for the growth of mental structures just as it does for the growth of physical organs. Some forms of environmental nourishment are more beneficial than others, and Montessori devised materials which had to be handled and organized sequentially.

Piaget (1973), who was more concerned with theory than practice, hypothesized that there are three stages in cognition, and he labeled the first one the sensorimotor stage during which an infant learns by moving around in, touching, and tasting his environment.

Piaget's formulation of early sensorimotor functioning as a foundation for *cognitive* development also implies that wherever important sensory deficits, motor deficits, or difficulties in integrating sensorimotor functioning exist, there will be some degree of interference with cognitive development for which a baby may not be able to compensate.

The Senses, Integration of Their Inputs and Their End Products

As shown in Table 14-I, when the inputs to the different senses are integrated normally, the end products show many strengths for learning and behavior, but if there is inefficient sensory processing, a number of problems result:

1. speech and language problems, as for example, dyslexia and dysarthria
2. postural muscle tone and coordination problems
3. behavior problems, as for example, hyperactivity, distractibility, and psychosocial problems.[1]

It will be readily understood that each child with learning disabilities is unique, with his own set of problems, depending upon which part or parts of the developing systems are affected.

1. Speech, Language, and Reading Problems

Dyslexia

One of the first group of learning disabled children to receive intensive study came to be known as *dyslexic:* a group of intelligent children who could see, hear, and speak normally yet were unable to coordinate this information and learn to read. Some of these children were found to have visual defects which could be corrected by glasses, others had normal acuity but poor depth perception, while others seemed to receive the information upside down and reversed. Visual exercises and special equipment were devised, as for example, "framing" a small area so that

---

[1]Currently called Attention Deficit Disorder (ADD).

TABLE 14-I

THE SENSES, INTEGRATION OF THEIR INPUTS, AND THEIR END PRODUCTS
By Jean Ayres

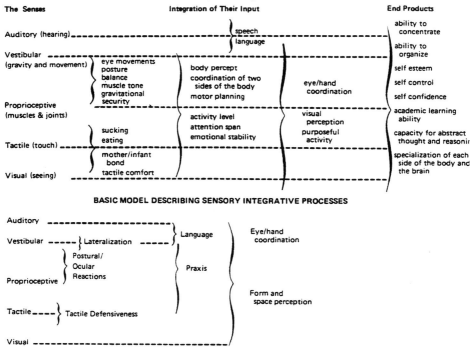

BASIC MODEL DESCRIBING SENSORY INTEGRATIVE PROCESSES

the child saw only one word at a time, or the sense of touch was substituted for vision and these children learned to read by tracing their fingers over sandpaper letters, and so on.

Visual dysfunction has received such prominent attention in the study of learning disabilities, as in Kephart's work (1960) that other equally important aspects of learning have been overlooked.

Language Learning Problems

Normal development of language depends on many processes which are closely interrelated, and a breakdown at any stage can result in a lack of normal communication, but it is always bewildering to parents who view their child as having normal hearing, vision, and no physical handicap. For example, B.B. came from a close and caring family unit, and was a well-behaved and friendly child who demonstrated adequate comprehension for a seven-year-old. Yet his ability to communicate grammatically was severely disturbed. He used sentence forms and pronunciation which were appropriate for a much younger child. Motor development was slow. Reading skills were poor because he showed visual memory and sequencing problems. The language of math confused him, and his writing showed many reversals. This is the kind of child who will count correctly 1, 2, 3, 4 . . . up to 13, and then reverse 14 to 41 and continue counting 42, 43, 44, etc. He may be able to count when numbers are in columns, but not when they are written across the page.

Apraxia. Sometimes the messages which are sent out to different parts of the body are abnormal because the information from each area of the brain is not coordinated or integrated normally. For example, a child is asked to move his tongue in a certain direction, or to speak a word which involves a number of movements of the tongue and lips, and he is unable to do this smoothly, not because his tongue is abnormally constructed but because the *motor-planning area* of his brain is dysfunctional; that is, the child has difficulty recalling, organizing, and sending a set of messages to the muscles involved in speaking. We usually refer to this problem as apraxia or dyspraxia.

Dysarthria. Sometimes the problem lies in the muscles themselves. A child with polio has suffered neurologic damage but the muscles have also atrophied and are incapable of performing a movement. In speech, we call this problem DYSARTHRIA. In more severe cases, all the sensorimotor associative aspects are involved: a child with cerebral palsy and a hearing loss receives poor information, has difficulty planning a response, and his muscles have difficulty carrying out the response.

2. Muscle Tone and Coordination Problems

Some of the most important functions of the vestibular system are associated with organizing many of our postural and equilibrium responses. Children with vestibular disorders often have poor co-contraction of muscles and poor protective extension of the arms and legs. They lack automatic adjustments of the trunk and legs which are normally made so that the arms do their job efficiently. Such deficits interfere with developing and maintaining a "body scheme" and cause postural insecurity. Other problems, such as poor coordination of both sides of the body and primitive reflexes are discussed in the next section about the work of the occupational therapists.

Ayres (1967) also mentions that some children with Learning Disabilities have a muscle twitch or chorea-like muscle contractions. Van Uden calls them "clumsy children." The author has seen similar tremors in the speech muscles of children who do not seem to be able to move jaw, tongue, and larynx in a smooth, coordinated manner.

3. Behavior Problems

The child with "brain dysfunction" is apt to give his parents and teachers more trouble than other children: he is fussy, overly sensitive, and cannot cope with everyday stress or new and unfamiliar situations. As a young child he is "all over the place." He may cry excessively or overreact through frustration.

Hyperactivity

One of the most obvious behavior problems stems from hyperactivity. The *hyperactive* child cannot keep still for more than a few seconds, it seems. He is up and down on his chair, constantly moving some part of his body, and often quite purposelessly. An excellent description of a hyperactive, learning disabled child is given in West's book (1968):

> You are energetic: a consummate understatement, which is like calling the cheetah not backward in moving forward. During one spell, you averaged only three hours sleep a night . . . People would never let their children play with you for reasons you never know about: you played exceedingly rough . . . It is clear that, more often than occasionally, something in your head doesn't work as it ought to.

The hearing-impaired child is not necessarily hyperactive because he seems physically very active. Before learning to use residual hearing, a youngster with a hearing loss has to check on his world visually, and often looks up or moves around. Before he develops speech, he uses his energy to explore his environment physically. However, if he is interested in an activity, such as an inlay puzzle, he sits and plays for a reasonable length of time.

Other Aspects of Learning Disabilities

Biochemistry

Although disordered sensorimotor integration seems to account for some aspects of learning disabilities, and enhancing it will make learning easier for those children whose problem lies in that domain, other parts of brain physiology, such as biochemistry, are recognized as equally important. Many learning disabled children are also treated by medication and special diets, especially when they are hyperactive, while others benefit from psychotherapy.

Emotional Aspect of Learning Disabilities

There are other professionals who look at the emotional aspects of the learning process and feel that disability may not be solely within the child but in the reinforcement contingencies in the environment. They view learning as an interweaving of affective and cognitive development, and state that if trust in an adult is not present, the child will lack self-control, will develop an aggressive or symbiotic psychosis, or will become distractible and hyperactive. Learning, that is, takes place only from a warm and nurturing person (Sapir, 1970). In addition to the parental reactions to having a defective child, other life situations could be associated with emotional problems, as for example, early hospitalization, death of a parent, severe marital problems, or child abuse.

THE ROLE OF PHYSICAL AND OCCUPATIONAL THERAPISTS

It was not until physical and occupational therapists became interested in the evaluation and treatment of learning disabilities that the high degree of coincidence between deficits in the perceptuomotor systems and sensorimotor problems in communication was realized. Since communication is a higher mental function founded upon biologic bases at various levels, it became imperative to ascertain that the neurobehavioral patterns were unfolding in an orderly manner. Higher brain functions will not develop normally if lower brain functions have not developed normally (Ayres, 1973).

Evaluation of Sensory Systems

Occupational therapists evaluate the following systems:

1. **The Olfactory System,** which is one system which seems to be less important to humans than to animals, nevertheless, learning-disabled children may be hyper-sensitive to perfumes, and other odors.

2. **The Tactile System,** which is probably more critical to human functioning than is generally recognized because it is a major source of information about the environment. Up to eight or nine years of age, the degree of integration of the tactile system is said to be a reasonably accurate index of sensory integration in general (Ayres, 1973).

3. **The Proprioceptive System,** which is also associated with the *kinesthetic system,* and which gives us information arising within our bodies, as from joints, ligaments, and receptors associated with bones. The kinesthetic sense is a more *conscious* awareness of joint position and movement, whereas proprioception is usually *unconscious* unless our attention is focused upon it. For example, we do not usually pay attention to the position of our tongue until we are directed to "stick it out."

4. **The Vestibular System,** which detects motion, and helps us to know whether sensory input is associated with body movement or is outside the body. The vestibular system has many interconnections with almost every other part of the brain, and the sensations it receives from gravity flowing through our nervous system helps to form a basic reference for all other sensory experiences. Man likes to stimulate his vestibular system: for example, babies like to be rocked. A child on a swing will move his body in response to the sensation of gravity and movement and this movement helps to reorganize those sensations.

5. **The Visual System,** which is of primary importance in form and space perception. Generally, it is used as a foreground sense, whereas hearing is multi-directional: we can hear, but cannot see, behind our backs.

Although the occupational therapist does not evaluate the sixth system, the auditory system (which evolved from the vestibular system), she does evaluate the other sensory systems when a child has a hearing impairment or is suspected of having an auditory perception problem.

Evaluation of Motor Mechanisms

Physical and occupational therapists evaluate a number of motor mechanisms which are the outcome of sensory deficits:

1. Postural and equilibrium responses.

2. Bilateral synchrony and orientation.
3. Oral-cephalic reflexes.

Postural and Equilibrium Responses

During the first year of life, we have reflexes which serve a purpose in the development of posture and equilibrium and then "fade out," as for example, the Moro's Reflex, a startle reflex which fades after sixteen weeks; the tonic neck reflex and the labyrinthine reflexes which are present up to the twelfth month; the Landau Reflex, a protective mechanism which appears around the fifth month and remains throughout one's life; and the Righting Reflex for turning over and getting into a sitting or crawling position.

If any of these reflexes do not develop normally, or do not fade out normally, subsequent learning is disrupted. For example, the author was examining a twelve-year-old with a severe articulation (speech) problem. She placed her finger on the outside of the girl's cheek and directed her to push it away with her tongue inside the cheek. Immediately the girl demonstrated a tonic neck reflex and her whole head turned as the tongue moved sideways, together with some movement of the arms. Years of speech therapy had been nonproductive because the basic underlying problem—noninhibition of a tonic neck reflex—had never been addressed. This girl was unable to move her tongue independently!

The importance of equilibrium responses to the vestibular system has already been discussed under Muscle Tone and Coordination.

Bilateral Synchrony and Orientation

The brain has two hemispheres which normally work together and then develop specialized functions. Thus, a baby begins to pat his hands together in the midline before he develops right- or left-handedness.

Deficits in this area cause failure to develop laterality or strong dexterity. There will be poor coordination of both sides of the body, poor inhibition of primitive postural reactions, poor left to right discrimination, and a poor body image. P.C., a child with these problems, could not catch a ball or walk on a balance beam, and he balked at building a tower of blocks or drawing a line across the blackboard without changing hands because he could not "cross the midline."

Oral Cephalic Reflexes

A neonate has a strong "rooting," biting, and sucking reflex which is later inhibited in favor of more sophisticated movements. If the primitive movements are present to varying degrees long after they are supposed to disappear, they interfere with voluntary control of fine motor movements and result in poorly articulated speech, as for example, closing the teeth instead of the lips, inability to bite the lower lip for *f* and *v* sounds, tongue thrusting, and inability to raise the tongue tip for *t, d,* and *l* sounds. Indeed, there are some children labeled motor apraxic who behave as if they have no "oral perception" at all: they do not receive feedback from the speech mechanism and cannot imitate or monitor their speech.

Types of Problems Encountered

A *combination* of some of the following behaviors should be warning signals to clinicians and parents, and indicate the need for multidisciplinary evaluation and remediation:

1. **Attention Deficits**
   These include: • fleeting eye contact
   - hyperactivity, with lack of awareness and control
   - impulsivity and distractability, showing an inability to screen out what is important and what is not
   - inappropriate emotional response
   - perseveration (inability to shift attention: the "needle gets stuck in the record")
   - inconsistent responses (as for example, responding better on some days than others)
   - chaotic, "driven" behavior

2. **Developmental Lags**
   These include: • primitive reflexes
   - balance problems (child staggers or falls frequently)
   - abnormal reactions to stimuli (child may cry uncontrollably or show tactile defensiveness; that is, he avoids touching or being touched)
   - defective sensorimotor adaptive responses to sensation (such as failure to cross the midline; failure to develop dominance, and left-right confusion)
   - slow maturation (these children seem much younger than their chronologic ages)

3. **Motor Problems**
   These include: • apraxia; that is, inability to form or recall motor patterns
   - spasticity or athetosis

- dysarthria; that is, poor coordination either of gross or fine motor movements and poor muscle tone
- denial of one side of the body (as for example, one hand is not used to assist the other)
- poor sense of rhythm and sequencing

4. **Language Learning Problems**

These include:
- failure to develop meaningful symbolic relationships, as for example, matching pictures to the wrong objects
- aphasia, or difficulty in understanding that a word represents a person or object
- poor memory and recall (a word seems to be erased shortly after it has been introduced; and it takes endless time before new words are a stable part of child's vocabulary, so new vocabulary has to be taught over and over).
- sequencing problems (particularly in arranging words into sentences)
- difficulty in transferring a meaning learned in one context to another context (Even a change of personnel in the room may "erase" or impede learning; so will a change of room.)

5. **Visual Problems**

These include:
- poor visual recognition
- poor visual memory
- ocular pursuit problems (for example, child cannot follow the pointed finger)
- figure-ground problems (an example of this would be a child who looks at a picture of a chest of drawers and sees only the circular knobs on the drawers and calls them "wheels" or "flowers")

REMEDIATION BY THE OCCUPATIONAL THERAPIST

Remediation by the occupational therapist does not teach specific skills: its activities are to enhance the brain's abilities to *learn* how to do these things; that is, to develop the capacity to perceive, remember, and motor plan. The therapist hopes to come close to altering the underlying neural dysfunction.

Unfortunately, without an occupational therapy program, energy for learning is diverted to adjusting to the sensorimotor deficits, or the child may select only one avenue for learning. The result is that only "splinter skills" are acquired as in the following case:

Case History

AB came to the Denver program at the age of 3.6 years. His mother had had rubella about the fourth week of pregnancy. He weighed less than five pounds at birth. His hearing loss was suspected at seven months. He had been fitted with a hearing aid at the age of two. One ear had an anomaly in the auricle, and was not fitted. He had been enrolled in a preschool group in another state where lipreading and visual skills were emphasized. His mother had followed a correspondence course and reinforced the group training in a most conscientious manner. She informed us that AB had been used in demonstrations as the best lipreader in the class, and that he could read and write a number of words, but he had never made any attempt to talk. He communicated by gestures and pointing. His audiogram was as follows (ISO Level):

Air Conduction	250 Hz	500 Hz	1000 Hz	2000 Hz	4000 Hz
Right Ear	80 dB	90 dB	105 dB	N. R.	N. R.
Left Ear	80 dB	90 dB	105 dB	N. R.	N. R.
Bone Conduction					
Right Ear	25 dB	50 dB	N. R.	N. R.	(vibration only)
Left Ear	25 dB	50 dB	N. R.	N. R.	(vibration only)

(One can obtain the same responses by putting the bone conduction unit on the child's knee.)

Unaided Voice Awareness:	95 dB
Aided Voice Awareness:	30 dB monaurally
	15 dB binaurally

The author observed that he was exceptionally small and immature for his age—his younger brother looked large in comparison—yet intelligence shone from his bright eyes. His motor development seemed unusual: he appeared to be unable to cope with steps, could not jump, and he put his arms in front of his face and closed his eyes when a ball was thrown (tactile defensiveness). He did not respond to environmental sounds and he did not vocalize.

He was visually obsessive—he jumped up and down from the chair many times, running to touch each object he saw in the room. Even with books, he turned the pages too rapidly. This hyperactive behavior persisted until he had learned to use his residual hearing.

He was referred to the occupational therapist when he was four years old for a perceptual motor evaluation, and the results were summarized as follows:

Several tests were not administered due to lack of communication. Several tests were unscorable because patient was unable to endure them. He resisted touch, hesitated and gestured to the therapist to go away. He was unable to tolerate the Southern California Kinesthetic and Tactile Perceptual test especially when his vision was occluded.

He is hypersensitive: tactile stimulation solicits immature reactions. He lacks body schema, lacks the unconscious awareness of his body position in relation to gravity which affects his balance. He lacks the integration of left to right due to his limited experiences with gross muscle activities.

His visual perception is highly developed. Many of his behavioral actions are due to strong visual stimulation.

He has some abnormal postural reflexes which affect his balance and increase his fear in performing the activities that involve postural adjustment.

A program was devised for tactile and kinesthetic training with emphasis placed on antigravity muscles, and also involving balance, postural adjustment and active physical participation with objects and people.

He responded well to listening activities, learning quickly to show his awareness of environmental sounds, and turning when his name was called at a distance of five to six feet. He especially liked to hold a block to his ear and build when he heard a noisemaker. He could detect all the noisemakers, except a small jingle bell, from any position in a large room. Within a short time he began to vocalize constantly, but his voice quality was typically "deaf." He tried hard to control his pitch and imitate a few phonemes. He experienced great difficulty at first in moving his tongue, and later in controlling its movements.

After six months he was integrating vision and audition and beginning to talk. His language development was intact. His left ear was fitted with an aid, and he enjoyed binaural hearing.

A neurologic workup was considered, but he made good progress with his new program which involved development of all kinds of perceptual-motor skills.

LEARNING DISABILITIES IN HEARING–IMPAIRED CHILDREN

We now recognize that many hearing-impaired children have the same learning disabilities as normal hearing children, and even a slight form of learning disability makes it much more difficult for the deaf than for the normal-hearing child. Unfortunately, peripheral hearing defect alone has usually been blamed for communication and educational deficits, and few teachers of the deaf have been taught to recognize and deal with the underlying neurologic impairment.

Textbooks are still written as if we were only teaching "deaf" or "hard of hearing" children. Rather, we are teaching a wide variety of children who happen to have varying degrees of hearing loss.

National Statistics

It is now known that at least 30 percent of hearing-impaired children have problems in addition to their hearing loss, and in some groups the number is as high or higher than 50 percent because more defective babies are surviving birth and diseases. The rubella epidemic of 1964–1965 left thousands of multiply handicapped babies (Schildroth, 1980).

The National Demographic Survey in 1976 showed the following statistics:

Total number of students: 49,427
Number with additional handicaps: 29,427

In the Acoupedic Program, during the same time period, twenty-eight children out of the total number of fifty-four had more than one handicapping condition.

The type of handicapping problems and the percentage found in a school for the deaf have been given in the following statistics from the 1976 survey:

Mental retardation	18%
Emotional/behavioral problems	17%
Visual problems	17%
Other	11%
Perceptual motor disorders	10%
Brain damage	8%
Cerebral palsy	7%
Heart disorder	6%
Orthopedic-disorder	4%
Epilepsy	2%

Etiology as Related to Learning Disorders in the Hearing-Impaired

Etiologically, there are four main groups of hearing-impaired children:

1. Genetic
2. Prenatal
3. Postnatal
4. Perinatal

However, the etiology is not always known, nor is the exact weight of every factor known.

Genetic

It is generally agreed that the majority of the genetic group usually show no other problems, especially in cases where Mendelian laws of inheritance count, and this may be the explanation for the achievement of deaf children of deaf parents. However, there can be different patterns within a family. At one time, the author taught two youngsters with the same parents who had hearing loss, visual problems, motor problems, and learning disabilities which were very severe in the older boy, and less severe, but still significant, in the younger girl. The etiology was Usher's syndrome. In another family, both the second and third girls, born several years apart, had language learning disabilities, with the older girl having a more severe hearing loss, dysphasia and special school placement, and the younger girl having less severe hearing loss, more subtle language problems and mainstreamed education. There was no other known family history of deafness but their father was dyslexic.

Prenatal

Among the prenatal causes of hearing loss which have been associated with learning disabilities are the RH negative factor, rubella, syphilis and toxoplasmosis. Sensorineural hearing loss is an important manifestation of viral infections in utero which can persist following delivery causing continuing damage to the Central Nervous System. Ernst (1974) studied twenty-three children in the Acoupedic Program who had all been born in 1964–1965, the period of a rubella epidemic which is known to have produced thousands of multiply handicapped children. Of the twenty-three studied, eighteen were of rubella etiology. Ernst found that only five of the twenty-three were "intact." The others had problems ranging from mental retardation, aphasia, deafness *and* blindness, to mild degrees of perceptuomotor dysfunctions.

Some of the problems associated with rubella have been labeled "auditory imperception," or the inability to process sound (Ames et al., 1970).

It is now suspected that the cytomegalic virus may be as devastating as rubella, and it can lead to developmental retardation and microcephaly.

Perinatal

The most significant perinatal problems occur as a result of actual brain damage caused by lack of oxygen or by trauma. These children may be labeled "cerebral-palsied." Other causes are an Apgar score of three or less, small weight for gestational age, and an abnormal hyperbilirubinemia. This type of child is often prone to disease and matures slowly.

Postnatal

The postnatal causes of hearing loss are those associated with childhood diseases and use of ototoxic drugs. Among the most significant are chronic otitis media, encephalitis, mumps, meningitis, with post meningitic cases being at higher risk for learning disabilities, because meningitis is a brain disease and the hearing loss is a secondary problem. The deafness and learning problems following bacterial meningitis may be apparent within several days of onset or may not occur for many months.

It has also been the author's experience that infants who have had heart surgery are also at risk for learning disabilities.

Environmental Factors

Regardless of the etiology of the hearing loss, it is the learning environment of a child which plays a most important role in overcoming a handicap. For example, Fiedler (1969) describes a hearing-impaired child with a typical problem who had no predictable framework to behave in, that is, the environment had ever-changing limits. These children need *more*, not less structure, and unfortunately, we usually find them in control of the family.

The author has seen many children with multiple problems complicated by lack of structure. E.L. presented with a history of open heart surgery soon after birth and the use of ototoxic drugs. Her mother was well educated but was on medication for epilepsy. This parent was often disorganized and withdrawn into her own activities during which time the children wandered away, unsupervised. When the situation became unbearable, a belt or the threat of a belt was used to "bring the children in line." The hearing-impaired child, whose loss was not profound, learned to imitate speech at an echolalic level and to use a few cliches, but she was a very slow learner. Her processing problem extended into picture recognition: she could not match pictures to objects without a long period of training. Unfortunately, no social worker assigned to the family experienced any real success in bringing some structure into the home environment, although the child was brought consistently to therapy.

Another case which caused much frustration among the clinicians was a rubella child who wore both glasses and hearing aids. The parents were very young, generally unhappy and unable to "cope." They moved five times within a year. Appointments, of course, were frequently "forgotten," glasses broken, hearing aids in poor shape, and so on. The child had a number of perceptuo-motor problems.

On the other hand, many of the learning-disabled children have come from "good" environments. One of these had meningitis at eight months and developed a profound hearing loss. His parents were supportive in every way, and the occupational therapist found few developmental lags. Nevertheless, at two years of age, it was obvious that he did not understand any natural gestures nor develop any signs of his own: behaviors which are atypical for a child who has only a hearing loss. In addition, he had dyspraxia, imitating few sounds without tactile clues. Eye contact for object, situation or person was momentary. Outwardly, he handled the everyday environment well, and did not seem to be frustrated by his lack of communication, which is also atypical.

By the time he was five years old, he was beginning to understand "labels" and to use visual cues, and he was referred to a total communication program where he became a visual-manual communicator. He did not become oral.

Some clinicians feel that it is more helpful to classify learning-disabled children on the basis of organic, developmental and emotional causation, recognizing that an emotional overlay may occur in all cases. The label "learning disability" usually implies intelligence within a normal range with *abnormal functioning* (Eisenson, 1972).

In summary, there does not seem to be strong evidence to support only one etiology of learning disorders in the hearing-impaired child: many factors have to be considered.

REMEDIATION FOR THE HEARING–IMPAIRED WITH SEVERE LANGUAGE LEARNING PROBLEMS

Symbolic Learning Problems

One of the outstanding characteristics of an "intact" child with a hearing loss is the normal "flow" of progress from one level to the next once a program is underway. But the "nonintact" or learning-disabled, hearing-impaired child demonstrates progress only during the early stages of learning to listen and respond to environmental and vocal sounds. Then it becomes apparent that he is failing to learn or retain any "labels," or names, even the names of "mama" and "dada." He may be unable to monitor his speech or recall speech patterns. Later, he has difficulty in learning syntax. Only a rigorous program of stimulus and reinforcement presentation—or operant conditioning—seems to work. In this approach, there is relative deemphasis on assumed processes within the child, and more emphasis on the specific task he needs to learn. Eventually, therapy does not always have to be systematic, because there is a danger in overemphasis on rote learning in that it may not actually represent *functioning* at that stage: forms may be taught and learned, but the child may have passed the substrate.

Operant Conditioning: A Case History

In the case of J.O., a bright-eyed, handsome, and profoundly deaf two-year-old, who had been fitted with amplification as soon as his loss was detected at eight months in another program, we were confronted by a child who was essentially "out of control." J.O. exhibited several classical behavioral characteristics of a child with learning disabilities: fleeting eye contact, distractability, impulsivity (in that he had to touch everything but did not really play with anything), and obsessive-compulsive behavior about the placement of objects which always had to be in a certain position and at a certain angle. (This is somewhat typical of a deaf child, but J.O. was *obsessed* by this.)

His relationships with people were inappropriate and he had no concept of communication. He also was not toilet trained for several years.

One of the most unusual behaviors was his development of a sequence of rituals to which he continually added other rituals, unless restrained. He would place an object in a certain manner, stand up, and position his chair. Then he would add "walk around the table" to this sequence, and so on.

The family history included other deaf relatives and a grandmother who was institutionalized for a mental disorder. Both parents were well educated and dedicated to helping their son.

During the first six months of treatment, J.O. was taught to use his residual hearing and began to respond to sounds in his environment, even to the telephone bell. He learned to play, and was enrolled in a preschool using Montessori equipment. He enjoyed this but group activities frequently aroused behavior which put him in a "time-out" chair.

Language or symbolic teaching required a highly structured, repetitive and nondistracting environment. The author faced the child across the table and used pictures rather than objects, as soon as J.O. could associate a picture with the appropriate object. He learned only when he had eye contact, but this was always so fleeting that we had to insist that he place both hands together on the table and look at the adult before any activity took place. He was taught to make an onomatopoeic sound for each picture, such as, *oooo* for a train, *wowow* for a dog, *mmmm* for an airplane, and so on, using only *one* sound and many different pictures of the same object in one lesson until he could do the following:

1. Pick up each picture when the author made the sound, from either auditory or visual cues.
2. Produce the correct sound himself when the adult held up, or pointed to, or turned over each picture (it was necessary to vary the routine for motivation and also to place a quickly edible reward upon each picture).

When three different pictures were correctly associated with sounds, the following routine was used:

1. The adult made the sounds representing each picture as she placed the picture and a reward on the table.
2. The adult made the sound and the child picked up the reward on the correct picture.
3. Pictures were then turned over and the child selected one and produced the correct sound by himself.
4. Later, the child had to recall and produce the correct sound as each picture was placed upon the table.

If we did not follow this repetitive and structured method, J.O. showed problems in motor planning, that is, remembering *how* to form the sounds; in recall, that is, remembering *which* sound; and perseveration, that is, difficulty in shifting from one sound to the next. Tactile cues (a sort of cued speech) were often necessary to help in recall.

After six months of twice weekly therapy and daily practice at home, these sounds were being used spontaneously together with a great deal of vocalization, greetings, and a marked improvement in eye contact and behavior. Real words were slowly added to the list and "onomatopoeic sounds" were dropped. Later he responded well to the McGinnis Method (as described in the next section).

J.O. was, in fact, a very intelligent child who was easily overstimulated. He was unable to organize mentally and recall all the information in his environment; thus, he always tried to control and organize it *physically.*

The occupational therapist felt that he was extremely bright and that he did not appear to have a sensori-integration deficit in his touch system. His gross and fine motor skills and also his visual-motor integration appeared to be above his chronologic age, but he had a need for vestibular stimulation.

In the Communicative Evaluation Chart, he performed above his age level in all tasks except speech and language, and in particular showed an excellent visual sequential memory. In speech and language, his progress was measurable from year to year.

His pure tone average remained virtually unchanged: 108 dB in the right ear and 105 dB in the left; however, his aided speech awareness threshold became 45 dB, or the level of a rather quiet voice. The configuration of his aided audiogram was that of a left corner loss, sloping from a response to 250 and 500 at 35 dB to an aided response of 75 dB at 2K, with no responses at 3K and 4K.

During the year between his third and fourth birthday, J.O. also received sessions of "play therapy" and his parents received counseling from the program family counselor for home management.

By school age, J.O. had learned "how to learn" and his parents chose placement in a private residential oral school.

Sequencing Problems

There is an increasing number of references to the fact that there is a central symbolic process underlying communication that is independent of any specific modality or channel of communication. One of the outstanding behaviors associated with learning disabilities is the difficulty in handling stimuli that *move in time,* or sequentially.

Sequencing problems show up, not in memory for pictures, colors, and so on, but for successively presented data, such as paper folding and block-tapping.

All communication systems move and are gone, whether lipreading, speaking, or signing, with the exception of the printed word. This remains stationary for as long as a disabled child needs to study it (visually or tactilely) and process it. Poizner et al. (1979) found that there is greater left hemispheric specialization for moving signs. Although visual information or signs are generally handled by the right hemisphere of the brain, and spoken language by the left hemisphere, the "global" form of language or any form of *processing* language, seems to be handled by the left.

The McGinnis Method

In 1968, McGinnis devised an Association Method for children with sequencing problems who seemed to be unable to process the spoken word. The most complete guidelines to using this method are given in DuBard (1974). It is a sensory-kinesthetic approach, designed to integrate all the sensorimotor information and to develop attention, retention, and recall. The McGinnis Method breaks up speech into simple elements and later combines them into syllables and words. In seven steps, the child has to feel, see, hear, write, and imitate each element and finally produce it from memory. For example, the child traces the letter *b* and learns to imitate the *b* sound. He learns to write this letter and produce its sound. Whenever he sees the letter *b,* he must recall its sound. He next learns to recognize and write the letters for a vowel such as *ee,* and say it. Later, he combines *b* and *ee* and must be able to recall and say the combination *bee* several times without looking at the written symbols.

Finally, the combination *bee* is associated with its meaning. Many other drills are used.

Emphasis is placed upon being able to reproduce the muscle movements correctly for a number of times because a dyspraxic child has great difficulty retaining and repeating a motor pattern; that is, daily routine actions do not develop into a skill. One postmeningitic child could not repeat *boo, boo, boo* three times; another changed "flower" to *fowl-lowl-low,* etc.

After approximately fifty nouns or words are learned in the McGinnis method, language learning proceeds in a more natural manner, but a great deal of sentence patterning is still required.

Case History

T.R., a profoundly deaf seven-year-old who had been aided and enrolled in a special preschool group since he was eighteen months of age, was brought to the Acoupedic Program because of failure to progress in Total Communication. He had never learned to speak, and indeed did not usually vocalize at all. His signing was limited to single words. He had always been a behavior problem in school and had been evaluated at a clinic for the developmentally disabled. The author began by fitting hearing aids that were more appropriate, and developed a basic auditory function following the sequence described in this book. She found that he was able to hear and imitate through his new aids most of the phonemes, including voiceless *p, t,* and *s. EE* and *K* were difficult because of a profound loss for the higher formants. He also learned the pragmatics of communication: good eye contact, greetings, such as *HI!*

to respond when called, and to call out himself. The McGinnis method was then initiated with two modifications: listening, not vision, was the first signal, and the i.t.a. symbols were used for those sounds which are reproduced by multiple spellings, as for example: the long sound *OH* can be written *o* as in go, *oa* as in boat, *oe* as in toe, *o-e* as in hole, *ough* as in dough, and so on. In i.t.a. only *o-e* is used, so that whenever T.R. saw *o-e* he could pronounce it. He transferred to regular spelling quite easily in school.

Although T.R. remains a "deaf" child who communicates manually, the benefits of this program have been far-reaching. He is no longer a behavior problem. His teacher reported that his attention span had improved to such an extent that he was the first child in his group to be mainstreamed for some subjects. He understood the phonics of the reading class, and later he joined a normal-hearing scout troop.

Cued Speech

Another method, which is becoming increasingly popular, was devised by Cornett (1967) for children who have difficulty processing language and learning to speak through hearing aids and/or lipreading. In this system, certain hand positions and configurations are used to distinguish between speech sounds which look alike on the lips, as for example, *p, b,* and *m.*

One disadvantage is that it adds yet another system for the child to process and detracts from the normal rhythm in speaking. If used with children who are not learning-disabled, it distracts attention from auditory cues, just as sign language does, because it requires constant visual attention (Clarke and Ling, 1976).

Nevertheless, it has helped some children develop spoken language (Nicholls, 1979; Nicholls and Ling, 1982).

Graphic Conversation and Fingerspelling

Van Uden (1981) studied ninety-five children between two-and-a-half and six years of age and found that 55 percent had no learning problems other than those caused by a hearing loss, and 45 percent had varying degrees of other problems. Therefore, he organized three separate departments in his school: group one was for the intact students, group two for the moderately dysphasic, and the third group, or smallest group, consisting of severe dyphasics who learned primarily through "graphic conversation," fingerspelling, and the use of a special typewriter. These children understood an "iconic" form of language, as for example, they could recognize a sign of rocking to represent a baby, or a throwing and catching motion to represent a ball, but they could not learn formal symbolic signs. In these cases, the performance IQ remained constant and within normal range, but the verbal IQ increased from age to age with special training. Van Uden found that too low an intelligence was rarely the cause of learning problems.

Sign Language

It is a common practice in the schools to refer hearing-impaired children to a sign language program if they fail to acquire adequate spoken and written language skills in an oral program, without considering the possibility that they have a central language processing dysfunction, which they will take into any program. Nor are their receptive sign language skills researched.

Dinner (1981), in her dissertation, *A Proposed Sign Language Battery for Use in Differential Diagnosis of Language/Learning Disabilities in Deaf Children,* pointed out that there are no standardized, diagnostic types of sign assessment tools. Dinner studied four groups of children, ages 7 through 11.5 years, who were assigned to groups on the basis of their total scores on the Pupil Rating Scales adapted for signing populations. Groups one and two exhibited behavioral characteristics of language/learning disabilities, ranging from mild to severe, whereas groups three and four did not. Dinner administered four receptive sign language tests individually in *Signing Exact English* (Gustafson, 1972). She found the presence of behavioral characteristics of L/L disabilities had a significant negative impact on receptive sign language performance, and that, generally, the greater the number and the more severe the behaviors, the poorer was the receptive sign language performance. The teachers of groups one and two complained of difficulties in comprehension of anything other than the simplest construction and of poor expressive skills.

Although sign language may be the best option for certain children who cannot learn adequately through an auditory-oral system, Dinner cautions clinicians, educators, and parents to be aware that the use of sign systems may be limited in its effectiveness in solving the problems of English language, comprehension, and production.

It is significant to note that the mean scores of subjects in Dinner's study who wore hearing aids were superior to the scores of the unaided subjects regardless of the group they were in, which supports the philosophy of this book; that is, the child who uses his residual hearing optimally will experience greater success in learning.

For pamphlets and for names and addresses of certified therapists, parents can write to:

The Center For the Study of
Sensory Integration and Dysfunction
78 N. Marengo Avenue
P.O. Box 1065
Pasadena, California 91102-1065

For in-depth study of Sensory-Integration, the author recommends:

Fisher, Anne; Murray, Elizabeth; and Bundy, Anita: *Sensory Integration, Theory and Practice.* F. A. Davis, Philadelphia, PA, 1991.

I do not expect my ideas to be adopted all at once. The human mind gets creased into a way of seeing things. Those who have envisaged nature according to a certain point of view during most of their career rise only with difficulty to new ideas. It is the passage of time, therefore, which must confirm or destroy what I have presented.

— Barber, quoting Levoisier (1962).

The following chapter tells what happened to many of the children mentioned in this book. In adulthood, some of them remained in the "hearing world," and did not relate to the "deaf world"; others had a foot, as it were, in both worlds, for they had a choice. But all of them could communicate independently.

Chapter 15

THIRTY YEARS LATER

MOLLY'S STORY

Molly was born with a sensorineural loss caused by rubella in the third month of pregnancy. She was fitted with binaural hearing aids at the age of one year. She began training one month later. She arrived at the clinic with the following audiological information:

	ISO Level via EEG Audiometry				
Air conduction	250	500	1000	2000	4000
Right Ear:	No response to right ear at that time.				
Left Ear:	50 dB	75 dB	90 dB	90 dB	82 dB
Bone conduction					
Right Ear:					
Left Ear:		NR	NR	NR	
SPEECH AWARENESS:		70 dB Unaided.			Turns to left.
		40 dB Aided.			

Molly was a very active child. She had walked alone at eleven months. She was the youngest of four children. After her first birthday she had several earaches and myringotomy was performed three times. Her voice quality was very loud and harsh. She did not respond when her name was called, but enjoyed loud noisemakers and music.

She attended the clinic for one-half hour, once a week. Her mother's diary describes her progress during the first year of training. It will be seen that this was a stormy year in some ways!

Molly's Diary

February: Chronological age—1.2 years; hearing age—2 months.

Today we tried putting a bonnet over the hearing aids and it worked! She wore them all morning and again after her nap. I did have a terrible time getting them in because she'd pull one out while I put the other in. We caught three new sounds today, very definite and repeated several times: mama, bab, and dada. She has never tried these before. She mumbles brightly all the time and we reiterate the sounds as often as possible. She seems to love the "make a noise, hand-to-ear" game.

* * *

We're so amazed to hear the change in her voice; it's much more human, her piercing scream has vanished, and in its place all of a sudden are all these lovely new consonants.

* * *

Bad luck this week. She has learned to pull the strap off her cap and we spent most of our time chasing her to replace the dangling ear molds.

* * *

She enjoyed our piano singing and nodded her head in time with the music.

* * *

I set up a schedule of morning and afternoon sessions to insure our getting down to business. A day can go so quickly with nothing accomplished. She is so wild and swift that it's hard to keep her attention for very long.

* * *

She seems so alert that I have difficulty remembering the importance of working hard. Altogether a very unproductive and somewhat discouraging week.

* * *

Molly's toleration of the aids seems to be about an hour and one-half. Then she tears them out. I think it's better to give her a break and then put them on later. I blew at Molly today and she blew back, with the same lip movement and sound. She didn't have her aids on.

* * *

I bought a hammer and peg set today and spent ten minutes with her completely alone and quiet. I could see what Mrs. Pollack meant by saying that I should constantly repeat single words like: in and out, hammer, etc. She responded beautifully for the whole time and then we said bye-bye and put it away.

We played the "knock-knock" game, and "calling her name" game with the other children at the front door. She enjoyed it.

* * *

She has an obsession with the piano. Plays with both hands and head swaying and babbles. She also loves to sit and peck at an old typewriter. She joined us in singing and clapped two blocks together like the other children were doing.

She also said *mama* loud and clear to me twice.

* * *

March:
(New ear molds made difficulty with feedback noise.)

* * *

(Very fussy with a cold.)

* * *

She is making a lot of clucking noises to herself. She only wears the aids half a day; however, when we did remove them she seemed to be looking around for them and constantly put her hand to her ear to feel for it. She loves to play the "eye and ear" game, and has said the words a few times.

* * *

Outside she heard a bird singing. I'm sure of it. She looked high above the house and waved. She cuddles her dolls and talks to them. Waves night-night spontaneously but hasn't said it. She starts murmuring the minute the earmolds go in and the sound is on.

* * *

April:

Molly had the right ear lanced. We didn't put the aid in and noticed a definite retrogression in her vocalizing: she went back to her old habits of screaming and screeching. Now she really likes wearing the aids and cries when we take them off. (No bonnet worn now.)

She points at everything and says *light* and *all gone.* One thing she hasn't improved much on is responding to her name.

* * *

Molly puts her hands to her ears a lot and indicates that she hears a noise. Once it was the coffee pot perking and she had trouble locating the source, so I unplugged the cord and said, *All gone.* She lit up and knew where the noise had been. She said *cook-cook* and pointed to the cupboard where the cookies are. This indicates to me that she has heard us use the name in this connection often enough to pick it up naturally like a normal hearing child would. She has learned to use "car" this same way, i.e. without exertion on our part to teach it. Her main love is lights. She has an obsession with them!

* * *

The pointing at things is something she really seems to enjoy. We now try to identify every object as simply as possible. For several reasons I did not get the aids on one day and several times she put her hands to her ears and said sorrowfully, *All gone.* She heard me say, *knock-knock* once, repeated the word quite well, jumped off the couch and marched to the door that we usually play the knocking game on.

She eats quite neatly now with a small fork and handles her own milk cup.

I called to my 4 1/2 year old who was sitting at the table and asked her to call Molly's name to see if she responded. When I called Lisa, Molly repeated it, and then when Lisa called Molly's name, she put her hand to her ear and strained to look round the corner to see who was calling.

* * *

May:

(quick summary) Chronological age—1.5 years; hearing age—5 months.

Says *good girl* quite often; *all gone* is favorite word. We hear her babbling *mama, baba, gaga* (not related to any object, though). When she points to something she always says *Da.*

She has improved greatly this month in heeding our instructions. Tongue clicking is a great joy to her. She has learned to do it and move her hands back and forth like a pendulum. We practiced *go* and *stop,* with Molly riding on our backs. The thing she learned was not the "go," but the bouncing and tongue clicking!

Down is something she understands, and says *da* for it. She loves the up and down game with blocks.

The candle still mystifies her.

* * *

We put something away and I said *bye-bye* without waving. A minute later I turned round and saw Molly wave and say *bye-bye* very clearly. She said *good girl* today and we think she says *baba* for bottle.

* * *

Molly has a bad temper. When she is angry with us she invariably pulls her earmolds out. It's a defensive trick.

* * *

Molly climbed in bed with us this morning and invented a game. She sat on her daddy's stomach, then lay back on his legs. She beat her breast, then pulled herself up. When she was sitting up again, she said, *Hi.* This was her own "knock-knock" game. We were impressed.

She definitely understands discipline now. She always wags her finger and says *Bad* very distinctly. This doesn't mean she avoids these "bads." But she imitates our tone and expression so vividly we almost always break out laughing.

* * *

She pushes a chair to the kitchen cupboard and looks for anything, matches, sugarbowl, cookies (her favorite word), . . . She needs constant supervision.

* * *

Molly seems not to experience pain as much as other children. She seldom cries when we spank her hand, seldom stops to cry when she bumps or falls down. She never stops moving or investigating. She is wild with curiosity. She learns so quickly we are amazed and thrilled with her progress.

> (Author's note: Imagine this child in a different program where she would have to sit and watch someone's face to lipread! In Acoupedics she is free to investigate and sounds are fed in naturally.)

She understands "Go get it" pretty well. One time we found her on the phone imitating conversation.

Turns around when called from about seven feet.

* * *

She sat at the family dinner table which she doesn't often do. We were discussing the new exercise in localization that the children could participate in. Lisa popped under the table and called Molly. Molly looked puzzled at each one of us and then she peeked under the table and saw Lisa. We all exploded with praise. Molly was elated.

The children have noise parades with her all the time and she joins in with gusto. A good marcher.

She offers her cup for more milk, her dish for more food, but she says *a-key* instead of milk. *Babbo* is bottle. We have a new dog which she loves and is very kind to. She doesn't say doggie but *dada*.

* * *

June:

Down and *up* she has clearly been saying. Also she can identify a cow (says *com*) and we have been looking at books and finding doggies, birdies, etc. She repeats beautifully *meow* and *tweet-tweet*.

She blew her father's birthday candle out, and blew at some candles in a picture. She responds almost 100 per cent of the time when we call her name, even out of the window when she is in the back yard.

* * *

She has her first book which she often reads to herself in a corner. She points to birds, cows, etc. and goes *tttt* for the clock.

(One eardrum burst. She went to the doctor and when he left the room she said *All gone,* and blew him a kiss.)

* * *

July:

Blows kisses a lot and says *good girl* and *bad girl.* Jumps off bottom stairs. Wants to hear *1-2-3-jump.*

Asks for things with real vigor but hasn't really attached separate sounds to different things. Mostly says, *ah-ah-ah* while pointing.

(Author's note: At this time, author was teaching an elderly stroke patient who used exactly the same form of communication.)

* * *

Responds very well to *no* and to her name.

When she goes swimming without aids on, we realize what a joy her aids are. She squeals loudly, and doesn't hear when we call her.

Says *birdy* and *ducky.* Clearly loves books. Says *more* sometimes when asking for more drink. Spends a lot of time talking to the dog.

* * *

Molly was playing ball with me in the living room and while her back was turned the ball rolled under the chair. I said, "Get the ball under the chair," and she went right for it.

Her first words, *Up* and *All Gone,* seem to have vanished. Actually she's had no new words in a week or so.

* * *

She repeated what the lambie and ducky said. She started to say *cup,* and *please* is another expression we are working on.

* * *

August 24: Chronological age—1.8 years; hearing age—8 months.

Molly has had many new experiences, and although her actual vocabulary has not increased measurably she shows many signs of new hearing awareness. She has also developed a fiery temper. We notice her hearing far-off noises: a model airplane being flown in the park across the street caught her attention although she could not see it. She made a waving motion with her hand as though she had caught the rhythm of it.

She has started a bit of incoherent conversation, no real words usually, but a human type voice with proper inflection and a great deal of facial expression to accompany her chatter.

* * *

She shows an understanding of sympathy. When one of the children is crying she often comforts them very tenderly. Her greatest virtue is her sense of humor. She is quite a clown and appreciates an audience.

* * *

September:

Molly definitely said "clock" and made her ticking noise with it. Today I locked the door so she had to stay outside and play. After a while she dragged a chair over to the back door and reached the doorbell which she proceeded to ring. We were amused.

I think I've detected a *thank you* a few times. We also think we've heard her say, *Bye Pop* twice.

* * *

Nothing but trouble! Ear molds chewed, and aids in the fishbowl. Active is too calm a word for Molly.

* * *

Two new words after her lesson with Mrs. Pollack: *home* and *more*. We are thrilled and repeat them all the time to her. The hiding game has been lots of fun. If I hear someone coming, I tell them quietly to stop around the corner and call Molly. She runs to look.

I think Molly repeated *Molly* today when Lisa was calling her. When I was sick in bed her daddy found her on the counter where she had mixed jello and Worcestershire sauce in a bowl, dumped a whole box of rice in it and crumbled a few graham crackers on top. Creative genius!

From mid-August to end of September we have spent $65.00 on ear molds. It used to take three of us to hold her down when they were made.

* * *

October:

I bought her a music box today. She wouldn't part with it. She wanted it back after her bath and kept handing it back to me because she could not hear it play. I helped her hold it close to her ear, but she was furious until we got the hearing aid back on, and she could hear it play again.

* * *

Molly put laundry away for me. I said, "Put this in Will's room," and she went tearing down the hall and stuffed them in Will's drawer. She got *Molly* right, but mixed up *Mommy* and *Tommy*.

* * *

She had heard several things without her aids which surprised me: a motorcycle and a dog barking. She imitated them. She likes to indicate any sound she hears, and sounds we take for granted, she likes to draw our attention to.

She loves to blow my recorder and pitch pipe, and to get out pan lids and clap together and march around.

She has learned *bang-bang* with a gun, and *grr* for tiger. *Birdy* has turned into *daddy* and it's hard to get the *b* back. *Doggy* is her best word now.

We have done a lot of *la-la* singing which she imitates beautifully. Working on different pitches has also been successful.

* * *

She has one sound *ma*, which seems to mean me, more, and milk. She uses *ba* to mean back, or put it back.

* * *

November: Chronological age — 1.11 years; hearing age — 11 months.

I had on my coat and was getting ready to leave. I told her she could not go this time and I expected a storm, but she calmly blew me a cheerful kiss.

* * *

She said *kitty cat* today. She carries a little book around with her with pictures of cats. Also she says a good *meow*. Lots of new words: *airplane, help me, find me,* and *book* —slightly blurred, but timely. Last night we worked on "apple" and she finally said *appee*. I've been saying *buzzing buzzing bee,* and tickling her. Now she's doing it to me. We learned snakes go *ssss* and wiggle on the ground. (She imitates *ssss*.)

* * *

December:

She is beginning to answer when you ask her a question—yes or no. She nods her head to agree. (Arm in a cast at this point.)

* * *

January:

Molly has made so much improvement in her behavior as well as her speech. New vocabulary: *please* (without the *l*), *turkey, monkey, fish* (*p* for the *f*), *button.*

She does puzzles well, and loves to string beads. She understands the concept of "just take one" or "two," but hasn't vocalized this.

* * *

February: Chronological age—2.2 years: hearing age—1.2 years.

She is starting to mimic our words and repeat them spontaneously. *Suddenly she has more words in her vocabulary than we can keep track of.*

Molly's first sentence: She came running into our room at 6:30 A.M. like a Keystone cop and put something back in my drawer. Then she went zooming back to join Lisa and Tommy and shouted: "Good girl, Molly, put back!" It woke us up with a shout of joy.

* * *

Thus, Molly, at age 2.2, after one year of therapy, had begun to catch up with an average normal hearing child. At age three, and again at age four, Molly's audiogram obtained by play audiometry was consistently as follows (ISO 1964 level):

Air Conduction	250	500	1000	2000	4000 Hz
Right Ear:	70 dB	95 dB	85 dB	75 dB	
Left Ear:	80 dB	90 dB	95 dB	85 dB	
Bone Conduction					
Right Ear:	30 dB	40 dB	50 dB	55 dB	65 dB

(The Bone Conduction responses may represent a conductive anomaly which could only be determined by middle ear surgery.)
Speech Reception Threshold: Unaided: 80–85 dB
Both Ears (aided): 35 dB

Molly's score on the Peabody test climbed slowly: 2.1 years when she was 3.6, and 2.7 years when she was 4 years of age. Using the Houston Language Test at 4.6 years, she scored primarily on four-year-level tasks, but her overall score of 43 placed her language development at five years. She was able to score on the six-year level for vocabulary and object counting.

Molly is a very intelligent child who was able to make rapid progress using the approach described in this book.

Postscript to Molly's Story (1984):

By six years of age, Molly's Peabody scores were two years above her chronologic age, an advantage she retained throughout her school days. A psychological evaluation at age 11-9 produced the following report:

> As measured on the Wechsler Intelligence Scale for Children (revised), Molly has a Verbal IQ of 136, a Performance IQ of 128. All her subtest scores are above average. She demonstrates an excellent facility and understanding of the nuances of language.
>
> As measured on the *Developmental Test of Motor Integration*, Molly is a year behind age level with some difficulty with spatial relationships which would affect her ability to perform rapidly on Math. Her Math skills are on age level but are not one of her strong areas. She demonstrates excellent artistic ability. Her language was easy to understand and only infrequently did she have to ask the examiner to repeat something that was said.

Molly was educated in private schools for the normal-hearing. She proved to have outstanding athletic ability and earned a great many accolades in her senior year, also "the respect and admiration of the entire soccer team," as her teacher wrote.

When in high school, Molly wrote the following:

> At this time my handicap gets little attention from me as it proves only to be a nuisance at times. It has made me what I am, and oh yes, I've stopped often to think of what I could have been, but I've found that this "nuisance" is really a blessing. I had a grand English teacher for three years in 7th grade where I came in with a poor reputation for not excelling in English, and I left in 9th grade from an Honors class with a straight A average. Last summer was a marvelous summer of adventure. I spent two months by myself in Europe, Germany and England. The trip was a step in my growing independence.

Molly went to Stanford University where she studied Human Biology and played varsity soccer. She graduated in 1987 and worked as a paste-up artist for a local newspaper for five years, gradually advancing to a senior designer position. She also freelanced as an illustrator and computer consultant helping different design companies in the Bay Area with their computer graphics needs.

Molly wrote the following:

In 1992, I decided it was time to go back to school, and in 1993 I started my first year in Boston University Law School. My ability to speak clearly and comfortably has been of immeasurable benefit to me. I believe that people have come away with new notions about hearing impairments after hearing or communicating with or even competing with me. My capacity to perform is never questioned. This is very important. A law professor early in my first year advised me that I should consider choosing another career when she heard that I had a hearing loss. She was sincere but didn't realize she really lit my fire! I believe that kind of thinking comes from a lack of exposure to any kind of handicap, with absolutely no understanding how versatile and tenacious these individuals will be.

I have performed in four moot trial competitions with the best oralist awards in two and the best brief in another . . . It has been an exciting three years. I am interested in developing greater trial advocacy but am interested in other areas of law . . . I am prepared for anything!

My early exposure to words has been a gift for life. I have a language. My poetry is my passion and words are my consolation. If this door had been closed to me, I would have been very bitter indeed . . . This is my life. I am happy to report that all is well.

Molly was recently married to a young man she met when she was a junior at Stanford.

* * *

JANICE'S STORY

Janice was identified in the newborn nursery. She never responded overtly to the test tones. She was tested by EEG audiometry with the following results (ISO level):

Air conduction	250	500	1000	2000 Hz
Right Ear:	50 dB	80 dB	N.R.	N.R.
Left Ear:	70 dB	80 dB	100?	N.R.
Speech Awareness:	70 dB unaided			
	40 dB aided			

She was fitted with one aid at the age of three months, and came to the clinic for training when she was seven months old. She attended once a week for half an hour.

She was very unresponsive to sound, and by ten months was walking, and hyperactive. She grew to be amazingly strong and, like Molly, was always getting into hazardous adventures. Her growth and development appeared normal to advanced.

At twelve months a second aid was purchased for the opposite ear.

Etiology is unknown, but her mother is RH- and Janice is RH-. The ophthalmologist reported coarsely granular pigmentation. She has one normal hearing sister, three years her senior, who has immature articulation for her age.

Janice's Diary

March: Chronological age—10 months; hearing age—7 months.

Janice is now responding to her name at close range. She also seems to respond from a distance when there are no distractions. Also she has developed an understanding of the word *No.* When she hears it she pulls back her hand and then teasingly pretends she is going to go ahead and get it. She seems to become increasingly happier and outgoing.

When we say *Up,* and hold her hands, she stands up; when I say *Down,* she will go into a stooping position. I have tried this repeatedly with her and she does this only when I say up and down. No new vocalizations, only *mamama.*

(Started to walk at this time.)

* * *

April:

When I say, "Where is the tree?" (or book or ball, and so on), Janice will look at the object and make a very excited sound.

(Author's Note: Two weeks later, she was pointing when they named objects; and pointing to objects she saw, for her parents to name. She began to like sounds as the mixer, the phone, the dog's collar jingling.)

* * *

May: Chronological age—1 year; hearing age—9 months.

She has developed many different vocalizations. She opened her mouth and exhaled a puff of wind and blew a match out! We have noticed a definite understanding starting lately. I can tell her to close a door, and she will. She understands "Look."

* * *

June:

When she misbehaves and you ask Janice if she wants a spanking, she shakes her head, NO.

* * *

Almost one year after starting training Janice's mother wrote:

She seems to have withdrawn back into a silent state. We haven't even heard the eight or nine new words she developed recently. We've come to the conclusion that she again has stopped to absorb the sights and sounds around her. We have noticed that she has started dancing when certain music is playing. (Music with a fast beat to it.)

(Author's Note: She was wearing a loaner aid for a few weeks, and seemed to hear less well.)

She was irritated by the loaner and was constantly pulling it out. When her own aid arrived, a look of pure joy and relief came over her face. She clapped her hands and jumped up and down. Since then, she has been getting her aids every morning, puts the harness over her head and comes to me so I can insert the molds and get ready for the day.

(Author's Note: The hearing aid industry needs to develop a sturdy aid just for small children. If only the manufacturers could see what the aids mean to a small child, and how critical time is lost when the aids are being repaired.)

* * *

November: Chronological age—1.6 years; hearing age—1.3 years.

This past week has brought many changes which have been exciting and amazing to us. The outstanding thing is that she is attempting to feed back words. It is her father's voice she attempts to mimic. She says, "mama, dada, hi." We think she is beginning to understand that when she yells it bothers us.

* * *

December:

She has continued to show an amazing understanding of the things that are said and done around her. She does not seem to be in the least frustrated because she is unable to express herself. Her vocalizations are starting to take on meaning. She makes certain sounds now that have a meaning to me. I'm sure in time these sounds will become refined into words.

* * *

February: Chronological age—1.9 years, hearing age—1.6 years.

Janice has very definitely shown us that she understands more than she says. You can now ask her if she wants you to help her, or get her something. This does not bring on a verbal response, but she will shake her head, NO.

Sunday brought another development. Janice had just gotten up. She had not yet put on her hearing aids. She had brought a book with pictures of cats out from the bedroom with her. She sat on the couch and was looking at pictures. Suddenly she pointed at one of the pictures and came out with a definite *meow* sound. It was a shock to us all!

(Author's note: We had used this many times and for many months, with a stuffed toy.)

Her listening and identification ability seem almost endless. She plays the discrimination game with noisemakers constantly. She derives great pleasure in showing how well she does this, to anyone who comes to our home. (Her range is between three and five feet.) She understands the meaning of "stop" and "go" in starting and stopping her toy tractor (a wind-up toy). She has become a pleasure for everyone to be around. People find it hard to believe she has a hearing loss. Her outgoingness and self-reliance are going to be great blessings to her.

(Author's Note: She also created panic: she was found up on a garage roof, and climbing a telephone pole.)

Her vocabulary hasn't been added to, nor has she used what she had developed up to this point. Working with her has become quite difficult. Her attention span seems shorter everyday. She spends most of her day with her sister and imitates her every move.) Perhaps she is learning to play imaginatively rather than with things?)

But two people have commented on the changes in her. One said that what she *does* say is very clear and that there is a noticeable straining on her part to talk.

* * *

This child progressed in spurts. At times she was hyperactive; at other times, very attentive. Her physical development was rapid. Her profound hearing loss would make speech development slow until she is old enough to help herself.

Janice's audiogram at 4.2 years, obtained by play audiometry, was as follows (I.S.O. 1964 level):

Air conduction	250	500	750	1000	1500	2000	4000
Right ear:		105	105	N.R.	N.R.	N.R.	N.R.
Left ear:		95	105	105	105	N.R.	N.R.
Speech Awareness:	95 dB						
Bone conduction							
Right Ear							
Left Ear		30	45	65 (vibration responses)			

Aided Speech Awareness: 55 dB

She was very definite about when she could hear and when she could not hear.

Such a severe loss makes integration of auditory and visual cues imperative, as soon as the auditory skills have been acquired.

This child continued to utilize her residual hearing by responding to voices and environmental sounds, and by vocalizing constantly for communication. But she did not remember words either visually or auditorily without an excessive amount of repetition and drill. Hyperactive and with poor eye contact until she was four years old, she suddenly began to settle down and help herself.

Her problems are representative of a number of children who appear to have great difficulty in the association area. If their hearing loss is profound, which slows down speech and language development, it is often difficult to diagnose their learning disability at an early age. If their loss is only moderate, difficulty in learning language can be diagnosed with confidence sooner.

* * *

Update on Janice:

In looking over Janice's medical records, we see that she ingested a large dose of aspirin at age three, requiring hospitalization. After this incident, Janice demonstrated a severe language learning disorder, which, however, could have been genetic since her father was dysgraphic and dyslexic, and a younger sister also had a severe hearing loss and moderate learning disabilities. Janice was evaluated at a Birth Defects clinic with essentially negative results, although it was noted that, as an infant, Janice used to swallow things such as scalding hot liquids which would be intolerable to other people, thus indicating a problem in proprioceptive or kinesthetic feedback. The occupational therapy report did show that dominance had not been established by age five, and that Janice had immature visual form and space perception, responding to details rather than wholes.

At age five, we changed to the McGinnis Method for Aphasic Children, but found that Janice had as much difficulty with a visual presentation as with oral. She had serious difficulties with motor planning (apraxia), recall and integration. At the Montessori preschool, the teacher reported "inability to remember" as a problem.

Janice received all her formal education in self-contained special education classrooms, oral and then total communication. She had many behavior problems. Sometimes she stayed with her father, sometimes with her mother. (Her parents were divorced.) As a teenager, she was transferred to the State Residential School for the Deaf.

At age eleven, a psychological evaluation showed a Verbal score of 49 and a Performance score of 114 on the WISC–R. At age 14-4, her Peabody vocabulary score was only 4-11, and her PIAT achievement scores were as follows:

Math	3.8 grade equivalent
Reading Recognition:	3.8 grade equivalent
Reading Comprehension:	4.4 grade equivalent
Spelling:	5.8 grade equivalent
General Information:	.3 grade equivalent
Total Score:	3.6 grade equivalent

School reports stated that Janice's strongest area was in gross motor skills and athletics; she beat the national record among the deaf for girl's discus throwing. She communicated orally and was very appreciative of that ability, but her mother feels that Janice never accepted her hearing loss, and since placement in the State School, developed a self impression that having a hearing loss means you are stupid.

From the State School, Janice went to a Community College to learn the traditional occupation of young deaf adults: Printing. She tired of this and tried a number of jobs, including driving passengers from outlying parking to their respective airlines. Eventually she went to the National Training Institute for the Deaf, but did not complete the course and returned home to resume printing.

Janice's younger sister, who also exhibited language learning disabilities, but to a lesser degree, attended parochial schools and is now a student at a local university. I recall that when she was three years old, she still did not understand that people had different names and called everyone by her own name. She has had many sessions of tutoring for reading, not in the mechanics, but in deriving the meaning of what she has read.

* * *

OTHER CASE HISTORIES

The following case histories demonstrate the uniqueness of every child who is labeled "deaf" and underscores the need for individual treatment.

K.K. (see Chapter 2) was conceived three months after a tubal pregnancy and was six weeks premature, weighing only 3 lbs. 11 oz. at birth. Her mother did have a virus but it was not thought to be rubella. During her first year, K. had many ear infections and cried a great deal. A hearing loss was suspected at nine months and she showed no response to Air Conduction testing. After medical treatment she was found to have a severe loss which improved in the left ear and deteriorated in the right ear (see Figure 2.1 in Chapter 2).

K.'s parents were very supportive of the program but had many personal problems and were divorced when K. was five. They each moved to a different state and K. alternated between them.

K.'s speech and language developed along normal lines, as shown in the following scores:

	May '77	*Dec. '78*	*Aug. '79*
Chronological Age:	3-2	4-9	6-0
Houston Language Test:			
(Part 2) Language Age:	3-0	4+	5-5
Peabody PVT:			5-11

In 1979, on the Boehm Basic Concept Forms B 1 and 2, K. scored 33 out of 50 correct, and on the TACL (Carrow Test of Auditory Comp.) her raw score of 87 was equivalent to a C.A. of 6-6. The Arizona Articulation test gave a score of 90.5, or within normal range, showing distortions on r, th, and sibilants.

K. also showed some visual perception problems and was slow to learn to read, but at age 9 she was reported by her school to be mainstreamed with little additional help and she loved to read.

K. visited the author in Colorado, where she is a freshman at a state university. She said that her elementary school years in New Mexico were difficult because the school population was divided into two "camps" —the Hispanics and the Caucasians. She disliked one boy in particular and was determined to "beat" him at skiing. Her teen years were spent in Steamboat Springs where there is a well-known ski school. K. became an international ski racer, but, she said regretfully, she did not make the Olympic team.

K. is enjoying university social life. She would like to be a writer living on the Aegean Sea, which she thinks sounds very romantic. K.'s speech is so natural that few people think she is deaf. K. said that she never told her teachers about her hearing loss, and only one of them noticed. This teacher told K.'s mother that K. should have her hearing tested! K.'s hearing in the most profoundly deaf ear was progressive and K. no longer wears a hearing aid in that ear. This appears to be a common occurrence in rubella cases.

* * *

S.R. was also a first born child whose hearing loss was not confirmed until he was almost three. (Late detection was the norm in his childhood.) His parents were both working as teachers and were able to help him a great deal, which was fortunate because there was no supportive help in his school at that time. He was a very aggressive, frustrated child when first seen. His speech and language developed slowly, and his PPVT scores remained several years behind his chronological age. He was always mainstreamed, but failed third grade. (He said his only good grades were in P.E. and handwriting.) He transferred to another school district, where he repeated third grade. He needed time to "catch up." In sixth grade, he was able to cope with a very large group in a team teaching situation, and by seventh grade was on the Honor Roll, and was elected president of the student council in a parochial school. He attended his neighborhood high school where he was very popular, won a number of awards, and was elected "Prom King." He won a football scholarship to Baylor University where he played as a linebacker in the Peach Bowl. He graduated with a degree in business administration. S. has held several different positions: with Pepsi-Cola, as an insurance agent, and as a financial analyst for ten years at Martin Marietta. S. is now working as an auditor and owns his own home. He is so enthusiastic about the Auditory-Verbal Program that he often speaks to parent and professional groups. He also served on the Board of the LISTEN Foundation. His audiograms have been stable for over twenty years and are as follows:

							P/T	Aided
Air Cond	250	500	1K	2K	4K	8K	Ave. SRT	Discrim.
Right Ear	60	80	95	100	90	NR	92 dB	
Left Ear	50	75	95	90	80	80	80 dB	
Binaural							48 dB	64%–60 dB

* * *

P.O. was adopted and the etiology of his profound sensorineural hearing loss is unknown. He received a heart catheterization for pulmonary stenosis in 1976 when he was 2 years, 3 months old. He was originally seen and fitted with two ear level aids in the UNIS–TAPS program in Minnesota, but the family moved to Colorado and enrolled him in Acoupedics at 22 months of age. The occupational therapist found that he had a slight limp and put all his weight on the right leg. He demonstrated some weakness (dysarthria) in the speech muscles and drooled excessively. He later showed faulty control of breathing, vocal pitch, and intensity.

P. suffered from a progressive loss, increasing from a pure tone average of 97 dB in the right ear and 100 dB in the left to 103 dB in the right and 118 dB in the left. His latest audiogram shows the following loss:

							P/T	Aided
Air Cond	250	500	1K	2K	4K	8K	SRT	Discrimination
Right Ear	95	100	115	95	85	NR	40 dB	64% at 65 dbHL

| Left Ear | 95 | 105 | 125 | 125 | 125 | NR 55 dB 33% at 80 dB |
| Aided Binaurial | 40 | 45 | 40 | 45 | | 45 64% at 65 dB |

P.'s speech and language developed along normal lines but slightly delayed:

	2/77	2/78	2/79	2/80	5/81
Chronological Age:	3-5	4-4	5-4	6-4	7-1
Houston Language Test (Part 2)	L.A.:	3-0	5-0	5-0	
PPVT:			3-10	3-11	5-6
Preschool Language Scale:		2-¼		4-8	
Draw A Man:		5-6			
Tacl:				4-½	4-3	5-7
Boehm Concepts:	⁵/₈1: Missed ¹³/₅0				

Goldman Fristoe Articulation and Ling Speech evaluation: distorts r, ng, z, j, th, and some l blends.
Speech Sample: Complex sentence level.
Metro. Readiness Test: at age 6-4.

A score of 57 places him in the 55th percentile. He is likely to succeed in first grade, but careful study should be made of his specific strengths and weaknesses and instructions planned accordingly.

P.O. attended a Montessori preschool through kindergarten, and was then mainstreamed in his neighborhood school where he received help. When P. was 8-4 years old, his family went to live in Australia. His parents wrote the following:

> In third grade, his reading is at grade-level. P. is in the top math group. He has an itinerant teacher twice weekly, a remedial reading teacher and speech therapist one hour a week. The school reports that there are no social problems: He has integrated well and he learns very willingly.

His parents felt that P. was "different" in some social situations from his normal-hearing friends, but overall they were very pleased with his progress.

By seventh grade, P.'s grades were age-appropriate and he had acquired an Australian accent. But children do not come with any guarantees. P. was hit by a car, thrown a considerable distance, and sustained a frontal lobe head injury. His parents say that the brain damage is far more devastating than his deafness. He is frequently "off base." P. tried returning to the United States, but stayed only a short time. He is now in a Center for Independent Living.

* * *

C.M., born in 1965, was legally deaf and blind, a rubella baby. Her parents came to the Acoupedic Program in February 1969, when C. was almost three. Although her visual defect had been diagnosed, she refused to wear her glasses. Her hearing had been tested at several centers both in and out of state, and the diagnoses had ranged from normal hearing, probably aphasic, to profound loss. Her parents complained that everyone had been interested in C.'s "case" but no one had given them a therapy program. At this time C. was obsessed by any source of light. She proceeded to "demolish" the author's office. However, in trying to work with C. on self-help skills and play activities, the author and the occupational therapist felt that C. was a bright child who could learn. Strict behavior management in therapy resulted in many temper tantrums and tears, but eventually C. wore both hearing aids and glasses. Her audiogram stabilized as follows:

Air Cond	250	500	1K	2K	4K	8K	P/T Aided Ave. SRT	Discrim
Right Ear	75	100	105	90	85	85	98 dB	84% at 60 db
Left Ear	70	95	85	85	75	70	88 dB	76% at 60 dB
Aided Binaural	10	20	35	30	20		30 dB	92% at 60 dB

As do many rubella children, C. had some continuing problems with one ear. Usually this is a form of tinnitus.

C. did not understand symbolic language until she was 5 years old, but her hearing age at that time was only 2. She attended the State School for the Deaf and Blind in her home town until she was in 4th grade, but as her teachers felt that she did not function like the deaf or the blind, she was partially mainstreamed. This was so successful that she has remained in the mainstream. The steady growth in her language and academic achievement is reflected in the following scores:

		1976	1977	1978	1979	
Chronological Age:		11	12	13	14-3	(in 7th grade)
PPVT		5-9			12-10	
PIAT:	Math (grade equiv.)	7.9	8.9	9.6	12.9	
	Reading Recognition	4.7	4.8	5.8	8.9	
	Reading Comprehension	3.2	3.1	4.4	5.5	
	Spelling	3.6	4.4	6.0	8.9	
	General Information	3.3	3.4	6.0	5.6	
	Total	3.6	6.3	6.0	7.7	

Between 1976 and 1978 we stressed a clinic and home program of listening for facts, drawing inferences, and vocabulary study in addition to conversational skills and articulation therapy. C.'s father took the responsibility to promote the growth of general information. C.'s parents also met with the family counselor.

A report from her parents when C. was in 10th grade shows that C.

had a CPG of 2.525, with grades of A's, B's and C's (A in Geometry). She became an accomplished pianist and took a modern dance class. For a long time she walked to and from school by herself, crossing busy streets. She went to visit a grandparent in California by herself and even changed planes.

C. graduated from high school and took some courses at a community college. When her father transferred to Texas, C. refused to accompany her parents. They placed her in a Center for Independent Living in a small college town. But C. felt that she did not fit into that group and found a small apartment where she occupied her time with her computer and keyboard. For a time she volunteered at the public library. She also loved to spend time talking on the telephone. Then she decided to return to her home town where she knew more people. Her mother arranged for an aide to clean the apartment and help C. with money matters. C.'s social skills are often lacking, because she has seen the world through a very limited visual field, and she really needs guidance, but she is determined to live independently. The social life of a deaf and blind person is unfortunately very restricted, but because C. uses her residual hearing and an excellent command of language, she has compensated by forming friendships on the computer network. C. also attended the Rochester Training Institute for the Deaf for a short time.

C. always referred to other deaf classmates as "those deaf children." When asked what she meant, she replied, "You know, the kids who can't talk."

* * *

Another example of severe multiple handicaps is L.R. whose older brother was also accepted in the Acoupedic Program until he could be enrolled in a school program for severely handicapped children. L.'s brother had nystagmus, physical handicaps (he could not walk), deafness, and mental retardation.

L. passed the neonatal screening but was followed as a high-risk baby.

At six months of age, she was aware of sounds and babbled in imitation but she did not localize. At nine months, she localized to the right speaker, even when sounds were emitted from the left speaker. Her parents were given a program for home stimulation training because L. had frequent ear infections. After medical treatment, L. showed a moderately severe hearing loss and a startle response to pure tones at 85 dB. She was fitted with hearing aids and enrolled in weekly therapy. Her speech and language developed along normal lines, but very slowly. Her spasticity increased, and it was found that she also had visual-motor problems and retardation, but of lesser degree than her brother. The etiology was determined to be Usher's syndrome, with the additional problems of spasticity.

The family moved to Kansas, where both children were enrolled in a program for the multicapped.

* * *

Ryan (see Chapter 3) was mainstreamed in his neighborhood schools using only the services of a speech pathologist. In elementary school he was a member of the "Brain Bowl." He conducted his Bar Mitzvah and part of the Saturday morning service in Hebrew and English. "There was not a dry eye in the Temple," said his mother. In high school, Ryan played football, served on the yearbook staff, writing some of the articles, and had an active social life. He was a member of the National Honor Society and of the "Blazer Buddies," an organization in which members helped young children with their schoolwork, and accompanied them in other activities. Ryan's buddy was a hearing-impaired boy whom he helped for three years and with whom he still corresponds. He told his mother, "Now I know how hard you have worked with me."

Ryan graduated in the top 8 percent of his class, with honors and two awards, one of which was the Principal's Award for the student who has overcome the most difficult situation.

Ryan is now a student at a large state university, majoring in architecture. He uses a note-taker. He works in the cafeteria to offset some of his board and accommodations. His mother says she has never seen him so happy, in spite of the fact that he is experiencing some difficulty because of the size of the classes, sometimes as many as 250 students. He has always used an FM unit in school. Guess what? The university wants him to learn sign language!

Ryan's parents were divorced before Ryan started school, but he and his younger brother spend some weekends with their father and his new wife. For example, they go skiing together. Ryan's mother has always worked in sales since the divorce. She says that she and Ryan are perfectionists and are a good combination.

Ryan appears on the A.G. Bell Pollack tape number 4, when he was almost four years old. He is still a charming and very bright young man.

The first audiologist to test Ryan told the family that Ryan would never learn to talk! Fortunately, they did not accept that verdict!

* * *

Dana G. (see photograph, Chapter 8) entered the Denver program at about one year of age. She had a severe hearing loss, etiology unknown because she had been adopted. It was a progressive loss and today it is profound. Dana was tested by our psychologist who said she was of average intelligence. However, she had a stimulating home environment and became an articulate young woman. Dana was mainstreamed in her neighborhood schools, attended a four-year state university, and graduated with a B.S. in Exercise Science. Dana enjoyed this work and enrolled in a technical college for a two-year program for physical therapy assistant. She graduated on the Dean's and President's lists. She is working for a company in Wisconsin.

A few years ago, Dana and her mother began a search for her birth mother, who was only seventeen when she gave up her baby for adoption. Dana has formed a friendship with her half-brothers and visits her birth mother.

Dana has always enjoyed athletics. She was once a junior golf champion, and she loves snorkeling, skiing, and so on.

* * *

When Laurie (see Chapter 10) was of school age, there was no program for the deaf-blind in Colorado. She was accepted at a well-known school in Massachusetts where she lived until her teen years. The author visited her and was told that her teachers were worried about some wasting of her muscles. This was diagnosed as muscular dystrophy. Eventually, Laurie returned home, which was now in a rural area of Colorado. She became too weak even to use her brailler. In the meantime, the author had retested Laurie's hearing and found that she had more residual hearing than was apparent. She was fitted with new behind-the-ear aids. At least, when Laurie was confined to a wheelchair during the last years of her life, she was able to communicate.

* * *

David (see Chapter 10) was a rubella baby with a severe to profound loss. His parents moved from another state to enroll David in the Acoupedic Program when he was two years old. He learned easily with a happy and humorous personality. However, he developed epilepsy which caused some learning difficulty. David wrote his own story:

> I am 32 years old and believe my life is evidence of what can be achieved through auditory-verbal training.
>
> I was placed in an integrated preschool when I was 4 years old, and mainstreamed from kindergarten through high school. Starting in first grade, after many requests by my persistent parents, the public schools agreed to provide an itinerant teacher to help me.
>
> I have always enjoyed soccer and played it until a few years ago. I earned a letter in high school.
>
> I met my wife, Lisa, in tenth grade, and we have just celebrated our tenth anniversary. I am the proud father of a daughter, who has just entered kindergarten, and a two-year-old son. Neither my wife nor my children are hearing-impaired.
>
> During junior and senior high school, I worked for the public schools in the school year and over the summer. After I graduated, I chose to go to work instead of college. I have been employed by a home improvement company for the last twelve years and recently was promoted to Receiving Department Manager where I am responsible for ordering and receiving goods for our store, in addition to supervising and training employees in my department. I also work part-time for United Parcel Service and was recently promoted to evening supervisor. We just bought another home and are excited about being part of a new community.
>
> Hearing aids are an integral part of me even when I am sleeping. I can't imagine what it would be like not to be able to talk with my wife, visit with my family, enjoy reading to my children, talking on the telephone, and working to support my family.

* * *

Luann (see Chapter 10), a child with a profound loss, entered the Acoupedic Program as a preschooler. She was a strong-willed little girl and, as the first child in the family, was spoiled by everyone, her mother admitted. Luann was mainstreamed with itinerant help in a small rural school. Her parents had applied to a well-known oral residential school, but after testing Luann, the application was declined. So, when Luann was in the sixth grade, she went to another residential oral school until ninth grade. The local educational system sent her to the "Lab School" associated with a state university. Her mother said that many of the children did not even wear hearing aids and left school, she felt, with few skills to cope with everyday life.[1] Luann attended a two-year community college for a while and then decided she wanted to learn cosmetology, which she did not enjoy either.

---

[1] This fact was discussed in an article, "Dialogue of the Deaf" by Lew Golan in the *Washington Post,* Weekly Edition, March 25 to 31, 1996.

When Luann's younger sister, T., was married, Luann set out to be married too. She married a young man she had known in Lab School. He has had two failed kidney transplants and is now on dialysis. His job opportunities were, in any case, very limited because he relied on signing. Both live on Social Security insurance. Their hobby is karate.

Mrs. T. reports regretfully that Luann was given many opportunities which she never took advantage of and never had any goals for herself. However, Luann is very independent and accomplishes anything she wants to do. She appears to be happy. Her sister, who is a teacher, says that Luann is so different from the hearing-impaired children she has taught. They either do not use their voices or have no inflections. They do not respond to their environment as Luann does. Luann communicates well with everyone.

* * *

Jay (see Chapter 3) attended N.T.I.D. in Rochester for several years. He traveled around the U.S. in a drama group and it was not until he was thirty-two years of age that he graduated with a degree in Engineering.

* * *

Jennifer (see Chapter 8) attended public school at first. Her mother remembers a special education teacher there saying that Acoupedics was making Jennifer into a little parrot! Jennifer then went to a parochial private school. During this time Jennifer suffered from a paralysis of one side of her face which was never satisfactorily diagnosed by the medical profession. Jennifer underwent several reconstructive surgeries with little success. Jennifer attended a university in Utah for two years and became a Mormon. She was sent on the required mission to the Deaf where she learned to sign. Jennifer married a Mormon who was severely hearing-impaired due to maternal rubella. Although he had much more residual hearing than Jennifer (who is very profoundly deaf), he was not taught to use this hearing and primarily depends on signing; therefore, Jennifer handles all the family affairs. Jennifer has worked as a laboratory technician but now is a homemaker with two children, one of whom is autistic. She is expecting their third child.

* * *

Debra (see Chapter 10) was adopted as a baby and her parents moved to Denver to enroll her in Acoupedics when she was about one year old. Debra only had residual hearing in the lower frequencies but made excellent progress. Today, she would have been recommended for a cochlear implant. When it was time for Debra to use sentences, the author observed that she had integration difficulties and recommended a sensorimotor evaluation, but Debra's pediatrician refused to give his referral, which was required at that time. Debra's mother also had a habit of talking without getting Debra's attention at a time when she needed to integrate vision with hearing.

Debra was placed in a number of educational settings from mainstreaming to special education. She then attended a private residential oral school, returning to a private parochial high school. She now attends Gallaudet where she is studying computers. Debra uses speech with hearing people and signing with the Deaf.

* * *

Bryce (see photo, Chapter 11) entered the Acoupedic Program after his first birthday. He had a profound loss. When he learned some nouns, he carried the pictures of them in a case and delighted in showing them to everyone he met. As he progressed, however, it became apparent that Bryce had learning disabilities. His elementary school years were passed in a school for children with LD. Seventh grade was spent in a private school for boys. Bryce transferred into his neighborhood high school with supportive services. He then attended a state college for five years where, he said, he had a "good time" and earned a degree in business.

As a Mormon, Bryce was required to go on a mission, which he did with some resistance, his father reported. He now works for a large office supply company where he is in charge of distribution and receiving. He rents an apartment in his married brother's house. The most outstanding characteristic of Bryce as an adult remains his outgoing personality . . . he loves to talk!

* * *

J.O. (Chapter 14) came back to his neighborhood schools until his junior year in high school, when he attended the state school for one year. He returned to his local high school because, he said, the state school was not challenging enough and he disliked the Deaf culture which did not encourage speaking.

The early indications that J. had difficulty processing auditory signals were correct. Today, J. has given up his hearing aids because, he says, he "hears, but it just sounds like a mumbo jumbo." He uses a combination of lip-reading and signing, but his best avenue of learning is reading. His father reports that J. "reads like a whizz." J. has always enjoyed drama. He has directed and acted in plays. His goal is to study writing and art. He would like to be a cartoonist.

J.'s parents divorced and his father has custody of his sons. J.'s father does not sign; they use spoken communication at home. At school, J. has an interpreter.

It is possible that if J. could have received a cochlear implant at an early age, he would have received much better auditory signals than he did with his aids, but the auditory processing problem would have remained. This case illustrates the importance of the regular evaluation of A–V Therapy and the modifications which must be made to meet the needs of certain children with hearing impairment and learning disabilities without sacrificing the goal of spoken communication.

* * *

J.S., the severely hearing-impaired triplet, was enrolled in the Acoupedic program at seventeen months of age. As he sat on the floor with his tongue hanging from his mouth, my first impression was that he was retarded. But after he was fitted with hearing aids, he stood up and slowly began to walk. Nevertheless, his progress was slow during the first year. His sisters always accompanied him into therapy and were great role models for conversation. They all loved the stories about the three bears and the three little pigs. One day, Jason ran ahead of the family, stretched his arms across my door and refused to let anyone enter. He had become very independent!

J. was mainstreamed throughout his school days with itinerant services, and graduated in the top tenth percentile. He enjoyed extracurricular activities, such as karate, helping a younger child with schoolwork (known as a blazer buddy), and soccer. He especially enjoyed being on the debate team. During his junior year, J. served as a resident counselor responsible for academic writing and public speaking at a summer camp. During his senior year, he went to Israel with his sisters for six weeks.

J. has recently graduated from Amherst with honors and is attending medical school in Boston. At one point, he was discussing speech therapy with another hearing-impaired student: "If my mother bugged me about my speech, I told her to back off" said the other young man. "My mother *never* backed off!" replied J. J.S. is an excellent example of an infant who would have failed an early test to predict whether he could succeed in an Auditory-Verbal program. This case points out the danger of a professional making program decisions for a family based on early tests.

APPENDIX A

NATIONAL/INTERNATIONAL SUPPORT PROGRAMS AND ORGANIZATIONS FOR PROFESSIONALS AND FAMILIES

Alexander Graham Bell Association for the Deaf
3417 Volta Place NW
Washington, DC 20007
(202) 337-5220 (V/TDD)

Alliance of Genetic Support Services
35 Wisconsin Circle, Suite 440
Chevy Chase, MD 20815-7015
(301) 652-5553
(800) 336-GENE

American Academy of Audiology (AAA)
1735 North Lynn Street, Suite 950
Alexandria, VA 22209-2022
(800) AAA-2336 (V/TDD)
(703) 524-1923 (V/TDD)

American Academy of Otolaryngology—Head and Neck Surgery (AAO–HNS)
1 Prince Street
Alexandria, VA 22314
(703) 836-4444 (V)
(703) 519-1585 (TDD)

American Academy of Rehabilitative Audiology (ARA)
P.O. Box 26532
Minneapolis, MN 55426
(612) 920-6098 (V)

American Hearing Research Foundation
55 East Washington Street
Suite 2022
Chicago, IL 60602
(312) 726-9670

American Speech-Language-Hearing Association (ASHA)
10801 Rockville Pike
Rockville, MD 20852
(800) 638-8255 (V/TDD)
(301) 897-5700 (V/TDD)

Auditory-Verbal International (AVI)
2121 Eisenhower Avenue, Suite 402
Alexandria, VA 22314
(703) 739-1049 (V)
(703) 739-0874 (TDD)

Beginnings for Parents of Hearing Impaired Children
1504 Western Boulevard
Raleigh, NC 27606
(800) 541-4327 (V/TDD)
(919) 834-9100 (V/TDD)

Captioned Films for the Deaf Modern Talking Picture Services, Inc.
5000 Park Street, North
St. Petersburg, FL 33709
(800) 237-6213 (V/TDD)

Cochlear Implant Club International (CICI)
Post Office Box 464
Buffalo, NY 14223-0464
(716) 838-4662 (V/TDD)

Cochlear Implant Hotline/Cochlear Implant Information Center
Cochlear Corporation
61 Inverness Drive East, Suite 200
Englewood, CO 80112
(800) 458-4999 (V/TDD)
(303) 790-9010

Dogs for the Deaf, Inc.
10175 Wheeler Road
Central Point, OR 97502
(503) 826-9220 (V/TDD)

John Tracy Clinic, Correspondence Course
806 West Adams Boulevard
Los Angeles, CA 90007
(213) 784-5481

National Center for Law and Deafness
Gallaudet University
800 Florida Avenue, NE
Washington, DC 20002-3695
(202) 651-5373 (V/TDD)

National Information Center for Children and Youth with Disabilities
Post Office Box 1492
Washington, DC 20013
(800) 695-0285 (V/TDD)
(202) 416-0300 (V/TDD)

National Information Center on Deafness
Gallaudet University
800 Florida Avenue, NE
Washington, DC 20002
(202) 651-5051 (V)
(202) 651-5052 (TDD)

National Institute on Deafness and
Other Communication Disorders—Clearinghouse
P.O. Box 37777
Washington, D.C. 20013-7777
(800) 241-1044 (V)
(800) 241-1055 (TDD)

Parent to Parent/House Ear Institute
2100 West Third Street
Los Angeles, CA 90057
(213) 483-4431 (V)
(213) 484-2642 (TDD)

Red Acre Farm Hearing Dog Center
109 Red Acre Road
Stow, MA 01775
(617) 897-8343 (V/TDD)
(617) 897-5370 (V)

Resource Point
Cochlear Corporation
61 Inverness Drive East, Suite 200
Englewood, CO 80112
(800) 523-5798

Self Help for Hard of Hearing People, Inc. (SHHH)
7910 Woodmount Avenue, Suite 1200
Bethesda, MD 20814
(301) 657-2248 (V)
(301) 657-2249 (TDD)

Sibling Information Network (Connecticut's University Affiliated Program)
991 Main Street East
Hartford, CT 06108
(203) 282-7050

SKI*HI Institute
Utah State University
Logan, UT 84322
(801) 752-4601

Tripod
2901 North Keystone Street
Burbank, CA 91504
(800) 352-8888 (V/TDD)
(818) 972-2080 (V/TDD)

APPENDIX B

PEDIATRIC CASE HISTORY FORM

(Reprinted with permission from the
Helen Beebe Speech and Hearing Center, Easton, Pennsylvania)

THE HELEN BEEBE SPEECH AND HEARING CENTER

Easton, Pennsylvania

Rec'd._____

APPLICATION FOR CLINICAL SERVICES

Please answer all questions as fully and accurately as possible. This information will assist the audiologist in planning for and conducting a more meaningful examination. The application must necessarily cover information which pertains to a number of different kinds of speech and hearing problems; therefore, some of the questions may not seem to relate to your problem. Do the best you can in answering all of the questions. If you have absolutely no idea of the answer, place a question mark (?) next to the number of the question. It would be better to indicate that you have no idea of the answer than to give an answer which could be misleading.

All information is for confidential use only.

PLEASE PRINT:

CASE HISTORY FORM — PEDIATRIC

Date: _____

Child's Name:_____ Birthdate: _____ Age: _____ Sex: _____

Mother's Name: _____ Father's Name: _____

Name of person completing this form or providing information: _____

Relationship to child: _____

Address: _____
          (street)   (city)   (state)   (zip code)

Home Phone: _____

Parent(s) work phone: Mother: _____ Father:_____

Referral source: _____

Physician's name:_____

Physician's address: _____

Reports   to: _____

_____

_____

2

State in your own words what it is about the child's speech and/or hearing which concerns you. Use an additional sheet if more space is needed.

_____

_____

_____

_____

Indicate below what specific services or information you would like the Helen Beebe Speech and Hearing Center to provide. We can best help you if you can indicate specifically the questions which you would like answered at the conclusion of the diagnostic evaluation.

_____

_____

_____

_____

Circle all statements below which seem best to describe the child's communicative behavior:

A. Acts as though there might be a hearing loss.
B. Has not yet started to talk.
C. Was late in starting to talk.
D. Is not developing speech as rapidly as expected.
E. Does not talk very much.
F. Not making speech sounds correctly which are expected for age.
G. People have trouble understanding the child.
H. Tries hard and seems to want to communicate.
I. Uses lots of gestures.
J. Has an unusual voice quality. (hoarse, harsh, whispery, etc.)
K. Speech too loud or too soft (underline which)
L. Pitch level is unusual (e.g., too high, too low).
M. Hesitates or repeats sounds and words excessively.
N. Does not seem to understand as well as expected.

_____

Age of onset hearing loss: _____Progression of hearing loss: _____

Severity of problem: severe _____ moderate _____ mild _____

Status of problem: constant _____ fluctuating _____

Number and duration of middle ear problems:

	Number	**Duration**	**How Treated**
Before Age 1	_____	_____	_____
2	_____	_____	_____
3	_____	_____	_____
4	_____	_____	_____
5	_____	_____	_____

3

MEDICAL HISTORY

If yes, describe (age, duration, severity, after effects):

Eye problems	Yes No	_____
High fever	Yes No	_____
Seizures	Yes No	_____
Serious accidents	Yes No	_____
Fainting spells	Yes No	_____
Surgery (operations)	Yes No	_____
Mouth breather	Yes No	_____
Frequent colds	Yes No	_____
Frequent sore throats	Yes No	_____
Frequent earaches	Yes No	_____

Has the child had any of the following illnesses or childhood diseases:

If yes, describe (age, duration, severity, after effects):

Measles	Yes No	_____
Chicken pox	Yes No	_____
Mumps	Yes No	_____
Whooping cough	Yes No	_____
Rheumatic fever	Yes No	_____
Scarlet fever	Yes No	_____
Influenza/meningitis	Yes No	_____
Pneumonia	Yes No	_____
Encephalitis	Yes No	_____
Epilepsy	Yes No	_____

Other illnesses or medical problems: _____

Diseases of eyes, ears, nose, or throat: _____

_____

Ear surgery: _____

Medications (describe type, quantity, frequency, duration, and for what problem) _____

_____

_____

Have the child's eyes been examined? By whom? When? Results: _____

_____

_____

HISTORY OF PREGNANCY

Health of mother during pregnancy: _____

Any illnesses or accidents: _____

Any history of miscarriages: _____

Previous pregnancy: _____

Medications taken: _____

Pregnancy length (in months): _____

4

BIRTH AND DELIVERY HISTORY

Duration of labor: _____ hours

Birth weight of child: _____ lbs. _____ozs.

Any difficulty at the time of birth: Yes _____ No _____

Was baby jaundiced: Yes _____ No _____

Need for transfusion: Yes _____ No _____ Anesthesia: Yes _____ No _____

Was baby placed in incubator: Yes _____ No _____

Caesarean section: Yes _____ No _____

Did baby come home from hospital at the same time as mother's discharge: Yes _____ No _____

DEVELOPMENTAL HISTORY

List ages for the following:

Age sat alone: _____ months

Age stood alone: _____ months

Age walked alone: _____ months

Age feeding self: _____ months

Age dressing self: _____ months

Bladder and bowel control/toilet trained: _____ months/years

Does the child have a hand preference: Right _____ Left _____

Child's physical development has been: Fast _____ Normal _____ Slow _____

Coordination: Good _____ Average _____ Clumsy _____

Would child separate easily from parent for therapy or testing: Yes _____ No _____

Chewing/feeding difficulty: Yes _____ No _____

SPEECH AND LANGUAGE HISTORY

Does child have a speech and/or language problem: Yes _____ No _____

Is child responsive to sounds or voice: Yes _____ No _____

When did child use his/her first word: _____ months   Examples:_____

When did child begin to use two or three words together: _____ months

Examples: _____

At what time were you first concerned about child's speech or hearing problem: _____

Can child be understood by parents: Yes _____ No _____

Can child be understood by other children: Yes _____ No _____

Can child be understood by strangers: Yes _____ No _____

Do you feel your child's speech or hearing problem is a handicap: Yes _____ No _____

What language is spoken in the home: _____

5

EDUCATIONAL HISTORY

Does the child attend school: Yes _____ No _____

Name of school: _____

    Grade: _____ Type of class: _____

    Teacher's name: _____

Does the child like school: Yes _____ No _____

Does he/she get along with school mates: Yes _____ No _____

Does he/she like his teacher: Yes _____ No _____

Is he/she a discipline problem: Yes _____ No _____

What are his/her difficult subjects: _____

_____

Attention span is: very short _____ average _____ longer than average _____

Does the child's peers understand his/her speech: very well _____ most of the time _____

    part of the time _____ not at all _____

Is the child's speech intelligible to other teachers and school personnel: Yes _____ No _____

What is the child's attitude toward his/her speech: unconcerned _____ embarrassed _____

    frustrated _____ enjoys attention _____

Special services: _____

                                                Name (if applicable)

Speech/language therapist   Yes _____ No _____   _____

Auditory/hearing therapist   Yes _____ No _____   _____

Interpreter   Yes _____ No _____   _____

SPECIAL EDUCATION INTERVENTION

Has the child ever been seen for a speech or hearing evaluation: Yes _____ No _____

If yes, please describe: _____

_____

Has the child ever been seen for speech and hearing therapy: Yes _____ No _____

If yes, please describe: _____

_____

Other special services provided to child: _____

_____

How often: _____ Date started: _____

Preferential seating: Yes _____ No _____

FAMILY HISTORY

Father's occupation: _____ Education: _____ Age: _____

Mother's occupation: _____ Education: _____ Age: _____

6

FAMILY HISTORY (continued)

Other children in family:	Name	Age	Sex	Present grade/placement
	_____	____	____	_____
	_____	____	____	_____
	_____	____	____	_____
	_____	____	____	_____

History of childhood hearing loss in family: Yes _____ No _____ Describe: _____

Do any other members of the family have hearing or speech/language problems: Yes _____ No _____
Describe: _____

Have there been any changes in the family group (such as death, divorce, frequent change of address, prolonged absence or illness of either parent, etc.)? Describe: _____

AMPLIFICATION

	Yes	No	Make and Model/Earmold
Wears hearing aid: Right Ear	_____	_____	_____
Left Ear	_____	_____	_____

Date first amplified: _____ Age of current hearing aids: _____

Hearing aid(s) fit by: _____

Hours of use per day/consistency of amplification: _____

Previous hearing aids: _____

Attitude towards aid(s): _____

MISCELLANEOUS

Tinnitus: Yes _____ No _____

Right _____ Left _____

Constant _____ Intermittent _____

Vertigo: Yes _____ No _____

Describe: _____

Noise exposure: Yes _____ No _____ Describe type, duration, etc.: _____

Thank you for your help. Your insights will enable us to do our best for you and your child.

BIBLIOGRAPHY

Adam, A., and Fortier, P.: Educating Children with Cochlear Implants: Tucker-Maxon Oral School. In Barnes, J., Franz, D., and Bruce, W. (Ed): *Pediatric Cochlear Implants: An Overview of Alternatives in Education and Rehabilitation,* Washington, D.C., A. G. Bell Assoc. for the Deaf, 1994.

American Speech-Language-Hearing Association. Definition of and competencies for aural rehabilitation. *ASHA, 26(5),* 37–41, 1984.

American Speech-Language-Hearing Association. Joint Committee on Infant Hearing Position Statement. *ASHA, 33(Supp. 5),* 3–6, 1991.

Ames, M., Plotkin, S., Winchester, R., and Atkins, T.: Central auditory imperception. *JAMA, 213(3):*419, July 1970.

Amon, Carol: Legislative impact on the education of children with auditory disorders. In *Roeser, Ross and Downs, M.P.: Auditory Disorders in School Children.* New York, Thieme, 1995.

Auditory-Verbal International: *Suggested protocol for audiological and hearing aid evaluation.* Easton, PA, 1991a.

Auditory-Verbal International: *Auditory-verbal position statement.* Easton, PA, 1991b.

Auditory-Verbal Position Statement: *Auricle.* Fall Vol. 3, 1991.

Ayres, J.: Remedial procedures based on neurobehavioral constructs. In *Proceedings of International Convocation on Children and Young Adults with Learning Disabilities.* Pittsburgh, Home for Crippled Children, 1967.

Ayres, J.: *Sensory integration and the child.* Los Angeles, Western Psychological Services, 1972.

Ayres, J.: *Sensory integration and learning disorders.* Los Angeles, Western Psychological Services, 1972.

Baldwin, A. L., and Frank, S. M.: In Courtney, C. (Ed.): *Language in early childhood.* Washington, D.C., Nat. Assoc. for Educ. of Young Children, 1972.

Balow, I. H., and Brill, R. G.: An evaluation of reading and academic achievement levels of 16 graduating classes of the California School for the Deaf, Riverside, CA. *Volta Review, 77:*255, 1975.

Barber, B., and Hirsch, J. W.: *The sociology of science.* New York, Free Press, 1962.

Barnes, J., and Franz, D.: La Voz de Ninos Oral School: Presbyterian Ear Institute's response to the educational needs of children with cochlear implants. In Barnes, J., Franz, D., and Bruce, W. (Eds.): *Pediatric cochlear implants: An overview of the alternatives in education and rehabilitation.* Washington, D.C., A. G. Bell Assoc., 1994.

Barr, B.: Pure tone audiometry for pre-school children. *Arch Otolaryng, 110(Supp.):*121, 1954.

Barr, B., and Wedenberg, E.: Prognosis of perceptive hearing loss in children with respect to genesis and use of hearing aid. *Arch Otolaryng* (Stockholm), *59(5):*462, 1965.

Bates, E., Bretherton, I., and Snyder, L.: *From first words to grammar: Individual differences and dissociable mechanisms.* Cambridge, MA, Cambridge Univ. Press, 1988.

Beebe, Helen: *A guide to help the severely-hard-of-hearing child.* New York, Basel, 1933.

Beebe, H., and Froeschels, E.: Testing the hearing of newborn infants. *Acta Otolaryng, 44:*710, 1946.

Beiter, A.: Evaluation and device programming in children. *Ear and Hearing, 12:*25S, 1991.

Bellugi, U.: The acquisition of negation. Cambridge, MA, Harvard Univ, Doctoral Dissertation, 1967.

Bench, J., and Bamford, J.: *Speech hearing tests and the spoken language of hearing-impaired children.* New York, Academic Press, 1979.

Bendet, R.: An investigation of the effects of auditory and visual input on selected language learning skills of hearing impaired students. Pittsburgh, PA, Univ of Pittsburgh, Doctoral Dissertation, 1977.

Bentzen, O.: Audiological treatment with binaural hearing aids. In Griffiths, C. (Ed.): *Proceedings of the international conference on auditory techniques.* Springfield, IL, Charles C Thomas, 1974.

Bentzen, O., and Jensen, J. H.: Early detection and treatment of deaf children: A European concept. In Mencher, G., and Gerber, S. (Eds.): *Early management of hearing loss.* New York, Grune and Stratton, 1981.

Berg, F.: *Educational audiology.* New York, Grune and Stratton, 1976.

Berg, F., and Fletcher, S.: *The hard of hearing child.* New York, Grune and Stratton, 1970.

Berko, Gleason R., and Fewell: *Play assessment scale.* Seattle, WA, University of Washington Press, 1984.

Bertling, Tom: *A child sacrificed to the deaf culture.* Oregon, Kodiak Media Group, 1984.

Bertram, B.: The importance of auditory-verbal education and the parents' participation after cochlear implantation of very young children. Paper presented at International Cochlear Implant, Speech and Hearing Symposium. Melbourne, 1994.

Binnie, C.: A comparative investigation of the visual perceptual ability of acoustically impaired and hearing children. Denver, CO, University of Denver, Doctoral Thesis, 1963.

Birch, Herbert G.: *Brain damage in children: The biological and social aspects.* Assoc. for the Aid of Crippled Children, 1964.

Bitter, G. (Ed.): *Parents in action: A handbook of experiences with their hearing-impaired children.* Washington, D.C., A. G. Bell Assoc., 1978.

Bitter, G., and Johnston, K.: *Systems O.N.E. Kit, Project Need.* Salt Lake City, UT, Univ of Utah Press.

Bitter, G., and Mears, E.: Facilitating integration of hearing impaired students into regular public schools. *Volta Review, 75(1):*13, Jan 1973.

Black, F., Bergstrom, L., Downs, M., and Hemenway, W.: *Congenital deafness.* Boulder, CO, Assoc. Univ. Press, 1971.

Bloom, L.: Comparison of language skills of two groups of hearing-impaired children: One trained in a visual oral approach and one trained in an aural/oral approach. Unpublished Masters Thesis. Mass., Emerson College, 1975.

Bloom, L.: *Language development: Form and function in emerging grammars.* Cambridge, MA, M.I.T. Press, 1970.

Bloom, L.: *One word at a time.* The Hague, Mouton, 1973.

Bloom, L.: *Structure and variation in child language.* Chicago, Soc. for Research in Child Dev., 1975.

Bloom, L., and Lahey, M.: *Language development and language disorders.* New York, Wiley, 1978.

Bluemel, C. S.: Double syllable words. *Speech and Hearing Dis, 24(3):*272, 1959.

Boehm, Ann E.: *Boehm test of basic concepts.* New York, The Psychological Corporation, 1967, 1970.

Boothroyd, A., Geers, A., and Moog, J.: Practical implications of cochlear implants in children. *Ear and Hearing, 12:*81s, 1991.

Bowlby, J.: The nature of the child's tie to his mother. *Int J Psychoanal, 39:*350, 1958.

Brackett, D., and Maxon, A.: Service delivery alternatives for the mainstreamed hearing-impaired child. *Language, Speech, Hearing Services in Schools, 17,* 115–125, 1986.

Brackmann, D.: Electric response audiometry in a clinical practice. *Laryngoscope,* Supp. No 5, *Vol LXXXVII,* No 5, Part 2, 1–33, May, 1977.

Brain, Sir R.: The neurology of language. *Speech Path Ther, 4(2):*47, 1961.

Brooks, D.: Otitis media in infancy. In Mencher, G., and Gerber, S. (Eds.): *Early management of hearing loss.* New York, Grune and Stratton, 1981.

Brown, R.: *A first language.* Cambridge, MA, Harvard Univ. Press, 1973.

Brown, R., and Bellugi, U.: Three processes in the child's acquisition of syntax. In Lenneberg, E. (Ed.): *New directions in the study of language.* Cambridge, MA, M.I.T. Press, 1964.

Bruner, J.: Cognitive consequences of early sensory deprivation. In Solomon, P. et al. (Eds.): *Sensory deprivation.* Cambridge, MA, Harvard Univ. Press, 1961.

Bullowa, M., Jones, L., and Bever, T.: The development from vocal to verbal behavior in children. In Bellugi, U., and Brown, R. (Eds.): *The acquisition of language. Soc. Research in Child Development, 29*(1), 1964.

Busenbark, L., and Jenison, V.: Assessing hearing aid function by listening check. *Volta Review, 88,* 263–268, 1986.

Calhoun, D.: *Comparisons and evaluations: Two methods of evaluation if evaluating play in children.* Fort Collins, CO, Colorado State University, 1987.

Castle, D.: *Telephone training for the deaf.* Washington, D.C., A. G. Bell Assoc., 1980.

Cazden, C.: *Child language and education.* New York, Holt, Rinehart & Winston, 1972.

Chomsky, N.: *Aspects of the theory of syntax.* Cambridge, MA, M.I.T. Press, 1965.

Chute, P.: Residual Hearing in Children. Paper presented at 100th NIH Consensus Development Conference: Cochlear Implants in Adults and Children. Washington, D.C., 1995.

Clark, J.: Counseling in a pediatric practice. *ASHA, 24:*521, 1982.

Clarke, R., and Ling, D.: The effects of using cued speech: A follow-up study. *Volta Review, 78:*23, 1976.

Clezy, G.: *Modification of the mother-child interchange in language, speech and hearing.* Baltimore, University Park Press, 1979.

Clinical Bulletin. Englewood, CO, Cochlear Corporation, 1990.

Clinical Bulletin. Englewood, CO, Cochlear Corporation, 1993.

Coggins, T., and Carpenter, R.: The communication intention inventory. *Applied Psycholinguistics, 2:*223–251, 1981.

Cohen, N.: The ethics of cochlear implants in young children. *Amer J Otol, 15:* 1, 1994.

Cohen, N., and Hoffman, R.: Complications of cochlear implant surgery in adults and children. *Ann. Otol. Rhinol. Laryngol., 100:*708, 1991.

Cole, Elizabeth: Promoting emerging speech in birth to three-year-old hearing impaired children. In Stoker, R., and Ling, D.: speech production in hearing-impaired children and youth. *Volta Review, 94*(4): Nov 1992.

Condon, W., and Sander, L.: Synchrony demonstrated between the movements of the neonate and adult speech. *Child Dev, 65:*456, 1974.

Conrad, K.: New problem of aphasia. *Brain, 77:*491, 1954.

Cornett, R. O.: Cued speech, *Amer. Ann. Deaf, 112:*3, 1967.

Council of Organizational Representatives (COR): Position Statement. Alexandria, VA, 1993.

Courtman-Davies, M.: *Your deaf child's speech and language.* London, Bodley Head, 1979.

Crickmay, M. C.: *Speech therapy and the bobath approach to cerebral palsy.* Springfield, IL, Charles C Thomas, 1966.

Crofts, J.: *A look at the future for a hearing impaired child of today.* Washington, D.C., A. G. Bell Assoc., Reprint No. 74C, 1974.

Crystal, D.: *Child language learning and linguistics: An overview for the teaching and therapeutic professions.* England, Edward Arnold, 1976.

Dahm, M.: Clinical experience in 17 children implanted at the age of 12 to 24 months. Paper presented at International Cochlear Implant, Speech and Hearing Symposium. Melbourne, 1994.

Dale, D. M. C.: *Applied Audiology.* Springfield, IL, Charles C Thomas, 1979.

Dale, D. M. C.: Units for deaf children. *Volta Review, 68(7):*496, 1966.

Davis, J.: Performance of young hearing-impaired children on a test of basic concepts. *J Speech Hearing Res, 17:*342, 1974.

Davis, J. M., Shephard, N. T., Steinmacher, P. G., and Gorga, M. P.: Characteristics of hearing impaired children in the public schools, Part 2. Psychoeducational data. *J Speech Hear Dis, 46,* 130–137, 1981.

Denes, Peter, and Pinson, E. N.: *The speech chain.* Baltimore, Williams & Wilkins, 1963.

Denver Ear Institute. Work in Progress, Englewood, CO, 1995.

Dicker, Leo: The rationale for total communication. Paper delivered at the Third

Annual Dinner Meeting for Principals and Teachers of the Deaf. Milwaukee, WI, Nov 1970.

Dinner, Berniece: A proposed sign language battery for use in differential diagnosis of language/learning disabilities in deaf children. Boulder, CO, Univ. of Colorado, Ph.D. Thesis, 1981.

Dix, S., and Hallpike, C.: The peepshow. *Brit Med J, 11:*719, 1947.

Doerfler, L., and McClure, G.: The measurement of hearing loss in adults by measurement of galvanic skin response. *J Speech Hear Dis, 19:*184, 1954.

Downs, M.: Baby auditory behavior index. In Northern, J., and Downs, M.: *Hearing in children.* Baltimore, Williams & Wilkins, 1974.

Downs, M.: The case for detection and intervention at birth. *Seminars in Hearing, 15:*2, May 1994.

Downs, M.: Universal newborn hearing screening—The Colorado story. *Int J Pediat Otol Rhino Laryngol,* 1995.

Dreikurs, R.: *Children: The challenge.* New York, Hawthorn, 1964.

DuBard, Etoile: *Teaching aphasics and other language deficient children.* Jackson, MS, Univ. Press of Mississippi, 1974.

Dunn, W.: The Sensori Motor Systems. A Framework for Assessment and Intervention. In Orelove, F. P., and Sobsey, D. (Eds.): *Educating children with multiple disabilities,* (2nd Ed.) In Press. Baltimore, Brookes.

Eilers, R. E., and Gavin, W. J.: Theories and techniques of infant speech perception research. In Reilly, A. (Ed.): *The communication game.* Racine, WI, Johnson and Johnson Co., Pediatrics Round Table Series:25, 1980.

Eilers, R., and Oller, D. K.: Infant vocalizations and early diagnosis of severe hearing loss. *J Pediatrics,* 199–203, 1994.

Eilers, R., Wilson, W., and Moore, J.: Developmental changes in speech discrimination in infants. *J Speech Hearing Res, 20:*766, 1977.

Eisenberg, Rita: *Auditory competence in early life.* Baltimore, University Park Press, 1976.

Eisenson, Jon: *Aphasia in children.* New York, Harper and Row, 1972.

Eissmann, S., Matkin, N., and Sabo, M.: Early identification of congenital sensorineural hearing impairment. *Hearing Journal, 40(9):*13–17, 1987.

Elliott, L., and Katz, D.: *Northwestern University—Children's perception of speech.* St. Louis, Auditec, 1980.

Erber, N.: *Auditory training.* Washington, D.C., A. G. Bell Assoc., 1982.

Erber, N.: Use of the auditory numbers test to evaluate speech perception abilities of hearing-impaired children. *J Speech Hearing Dis, 45(4):*527–532, 1980.

Erber, N.: Visual perception of speech by deaf children: Recent developments and continuing trends. *J Speech Hearing Dis, 39:*178, 1974.

Erber, N., and Alencewicz, C.: Audiologic evaluation of deaf children. *J Speech Hearing Dis, 41(2):*256–267, 1976.

Ernst, Marian: Report of the Porter Hospital study of hearing impaired children born during 1964–1965. In *International Conference on Auditory Techniques: Pasadena.* Springfield, IL, Charles C Thomas, 1974.

Estabrooks, W. (Ed.): *Auditory-verbal therapy.* Washington, D.C., A. G. Bell Assoc., 1994.

Estabrooks, W., and Birkenshaw-Fleming, L.: *Hear and listen! Talk and sing!* Toronto, Canada, Arisa, 1994.

Ewing, E. C.: Psychological variables in training young deaf children. *Volta Review,* 65–68, 1963.

Ewing, E. C.: In Hallowell Davis (Ed.): The young deaf child: Identification and management. *Acta Otolaryng, 206(Supp),* 1965.

Ewing, I., and Ewing, A.: *Opportunity and the deaf child.* London, Univ. of London Press, 1945.

Ewing, I., and Ewing, A.: *New opportunities for deaf children.* London, Univ. of London Press, 1961.

Fant, G.: *Auditory analysis and perception of speech.* New York, Academic Press, 1975.

Fant, G.: *International symposium on speech communication ability and profound deafness.* Washington, D.C., A. G. Bell Assoc., 1972.

Feigin, J., and Stelmachowicz, P. (Eds.): *Pediatric amplification: Proceedings of the 1991 national conference.* Omaha, NE: Boys Town National Research Hospital, 1991.

Ferguson, C., and Snow, C.: *Talking to children: Language input and acquisition.* Cambridge, Cambridge Univ Press, 1977.

Fiedler, M.: *Developmental studies of deaf children.* Washington, D.C., ASHA. Monographs, 13, Oct 1969.

Finitzo-Hieber, T., Matkin, N., Cherow-Skalka, E., and Gerling, I.: *Sound Effects Recognition Test (SERT).* St. Louis: Auditec, 1977.

Fisch, L.: The importance of auditory communication. *Arch Dis Child, 32:*230, 1957.

Fisher, A., Murray, E., and Bundy, A.: *Sensory integration, theory and practice.* Philadelphia, F.A. Davis, 1991.

Flexer, C.: *Facilitating hearing and listening in young children.* San Diego: Singular Publishing Group, 1994.

Fogerty, E.: *Speechcraft.* London, Dent and Sons, 1930.

Forner, L., and Hixon, T.: Respiratory kinematics in profoundly hearing impaired speakers. *JSHR, 20(2):*373, 1977.

Fowler, William: *Curriculum and assessment guides for infant and child care.* Boston, Allyn & Bacon, 1980.

Franz, D.: A team approach to pediatric cochlear implants, Paper presented at Auditory-Verbal International Conference. Cuyahoga Falls, OH, 1995.

Froeliger, V. (Ed.): *Today's hearing impaired child: Into the mainstream of education.* Washington, D.C., A. G. Bell Assoc., 1981.

Froeschels, E., and Jellinek, A.: *Practice of voice and speech therapy.* New York, Magnolia Exposition, 1941.

Fulton, R., Crnzycki, P., and Hull, W.: Hearing assessment with young children. *J Speech Hearing Dis, 40(3):*397, Aug 1975.

Furth, H.: *Deafness and learning: A psychological approach.* Belmont, CA, Wadsworth, 1973.

Gallagher, T., and Prutting, C. (Eds.): *Pragmatic assessment and intervention issues in language.* San Diego, College-Hill, 1983.

Gallaudet College: Language outline. Prepared by teachers at the Central Institute for the Deaf. *Amer Ann Deaf, 95:*353, 1950.

Gantenbein, A. R., and Noller, J.: Expressive inner language for the deaf through a descriptive grammar program. *Volta Review, 67(2):*136, 1975.

Gatty, J.: Teaching speech to hearing impaired children. In Stoker, R., and Ling, D.: Speech production in hearing impaired children. *Volta Review, 94(5),* 1992.

Geers, A., and Moog, J.: Effectiveness of cochlear implants and tactile aids for deaf children: The sensory aids study at Central Institute for the Deaf. *Volta Review, 96:*1–231, 1994.

Geers, A., and Moog, J.: Spoken language results: Vocabulary, syntax, and communication. *Volta Review, 96:*131, 1994.

Gilb, C.: Placement in an oral program: A due process procedure in California. *Volta Review, 81(3):*160, Apr 1979.

Goldberg, D., and Flexer, C.: Auditory verbal outcomes. *Volta Review 35:*363, 1995.

Goldberg, D., and Flexer, C.: Outcome survey of auditory-verbal graduates. *J Amer Acad Audiol, 189:*208, May 1993.

Goldfarb, William: The effects of psychological deprivation in infancy and subsequent stimulation. *Amer J Psychiat, 102:*18, 1945.

Goldstein, M.: *The acoustic method.* St. Louis, Laryngoscope Press, 1939.

Gray, D.: *Yes, you can, Heather!* Grand Rapids, MI, Zondervan, 1995.

Greene, M.: *Learning to talk.* New York, Harper, 1960.

Gregory, S.: *The deaf child and his family.* New York, Wiley & Sons, 1976.

Griffiths, C.: *Conquering childhood deafness.* New York, Exposition Press, 1967.

Griffiths, C., and Ebbin, J.: *Effectiveness of early detection and auditory stimulation on the speech and language of hearing-impaired children.* Contract No. HSM 110-69-431. Health Services Administration, Washington, D.C., 1978.

Grogan, M., Barker, E., Dettman, S., Blamey, P., and Shields, M.: Phonetic and phonological changes in the connected speech of children using a cochlear implant. Paper presented at International Cochlear Implant, Speech and Hearing Symposium. Melbourne, 1994.

Gustafson, G., Psetzinger, D., and Zawolkow, E.: *Signing exact english.* Roosmoor, CA, Modern Signs Press, 1972, 1973, 1975, 1980.

Haas, W., and Crowley, D.: Professional information dissemination to parents of preschool hearing-impaired children. *Volta Review, 84(1):*17–23, 1982.

Halle, Morris: The acquisition of language. *Child Dev,* Monograph No. 92, *29(1),* 1964.

Hamilton, P., and Owrid, H.: Comparison of hearing impairment and sociocultural disadvantage in relation to verbal retardation. *Brit J Audiology, 8:*27, 1974.

Hanners, B.: The role of audiologic management in the development of language by severely hearing impaired children. Presented at The Acad of Rehab Audiology, Detroit, 1973.

Hanners, B.: The audiologist as educator: The ultimate aide. In Nix, G. (Ed.): *Mainstream education for hearing impaired children and youth.* New York, Grune and Stratton, 1976.

Hardy, W., and Pauls, M. D.: Test situation of PGSR audiometry. *J Speech Hearing Dis, 17:*13, 1952.

Harford, E., and Musket, C.: Binaural hearing with one hearing aid. *J Speech Hearing Dis, 29:*133, 1964.

Harris, J. D.: *Some relations between vision and audition.* Springfield, IL, Charles C Thomas, 1950.

Harris, Susan: The hearing impaired advocate. *Judicature, 67(2):*95, Aug 1983.

Haskins, H.: A phonetically balanced test of speech discrimination for children. Unpublished master's thesis. (Cited by J. O'Neill and H. Oyer, in *Applied audiometry.* New York, Dodd, Mead & Co., 1966.)

Hayakawa, S. I.: *Language in thought and action.* New York, Harcourt-Brace, 1939.

Hernandez-Peon, R., Sherrer, H., and Jouvet, M.: Modification of electrical activity in cochlear nuclei during attention in unanesthetized cats. *Science, 123:*331, 1956.

Higgins, Paul: *Outdoors in a hearing world.* Beverly Hills, CA, Sage, 1980.

Hocken, S.: *Emma and I.* London, Sphere Books, 1977.

Horton, K.: Mainstreaming the primary-aged child. In Watrous, B., (Ed.): *Developing home training programs for hearing-impaired children.* New Mexico, Indian Health Service and Univ. of New Mexico, 1976.

Hubel, D. H., Henson, C. O., Rupert, A., and Galambos, R.: Attention units in the auditory cortex. *Science, 124:*279, 1959.

Huizing, H.: Deaf-mutism—Modern trends in treatment and prevention. *Advances in Oto-Rhino-Laryngology, 15:*74. Basel/New York, Karger, 1959.

Huizing, H., and Kruizinga, R. J. H.: *Whispered voice in audiology.* International Audiology Conference, 1962.

Hutchison, J.: Listening function: A diagrammatical analysis. *Auricle,* Summer Vol. 7, No 3, 1994.

Ivemey, G.: The written syntax of an English deaf child: An exploration in method. *British J Dis Communication, 11:*103, 1976.

Jacobsen, J., Seitz, M., Mencher, G., and Parrott, V.: Auditory brainstem response: A contribution to infant assessment and measurement. In Mencher, G., and Gerber, S. (Eds.): *Early management of hearing loss.* New York, Grune and Stratton, 1981.

Jensema, C. J., Karchmer, M. A., and Trybus, R. J.: *The rated speech intelligibility of hearing impaired children.* Washington, D.C., Office of Demographic Studies, Gallaudet College, 1975–1978.

Jensema, C. J., and Trybus, R.: *Communication patterns and educational achievement of hearing impaired students.* Washington, D.C., Office of Demographic Studies, Gallaudet College, Series T. No. 2, 1978.

Johnson, D.: The language continuum. In Sapir, S., and Nitzburg, A. (Eds.): *Children with learning problems.* New York, Bruner/Mazel, 1973.

Johnson, N., Bagi, P., Parbo, J., and Eberling, C.: Evoked acoustic emissions from the human ear. *Scand Audiol, 17:*27–34, 1988.

Johnston, C.: *I hear the day.* South Waterford, ME, Merriam-Eddy, 1977.

Kankkunen, A., and Liden, G.: Respiration audiometry. *Scand Audiol, 6:*81, 1977.

Kaplan, Louise: *One-ness and separateness.* New York, Simon and Schuster, Touchstone Press, 1978.

Karchmer, M., and Trybus, R.: *Who are the deaf children in mainstream programs?* Washington, D.C., Office of Demographic Studies, Gallaudet College, Series R. No. 4, Oct 1977.

Kearsley, R.: Neonatal response to auditory stimulation: A demonstration of orienting and defensive behavior. *Child Dev, 44:*582, 1973.

Keith, R.: An acoustic reflex technique of establishing hearing aid settings. *J Amer Audiolog Soc, 5:*71, 1979.

Kelsall, D.: The team approach to pediatric cochlear implants. Auditory-Verbal International Conference. Cuyahoga Falls, OH, 1995.

Kemp, D.: Stimulated acoustic emission from within the human auditory system. *J Acoust Soc Amer, 64:*1388–1391, 1978.

Kemp, D., Ryan, S., and Bray, P.: A guide to the effective use of otoacoustic emissions. *Ear and Hearing, 11:*93–105, 1990.

Kennedy, P., and Bruininks, R.: Social status of hearing-impaired children in the regular classroom. *Except Child, 40:*336, 1974.

Kennedy, P., Northcott, W., McCauley, R., and Williams, S.: Longitudinal sociometric and gross-sectional data on mainstreaming: Implications and preschool programming. *Volta Review, 78:*71, 1976.

Kenworthy, O. T.: Early identification: Principles and practices. In Alpiner, J., and McCarthy, P. (Eds.): *Rehabilitative audiology: Children and adults.* Baltimore: Williams & Wilkins, 53–71, 1993.

Kephart, N.: *The slow learner in the classroom.* Columbus, OH, Merritt Books, 1960.

Kessler, M.: Parent diary: A technique for sampling the expressive language of hearing-impaired children. *Volta Review, 85(2):*105, Feb–Mar, 1983.

Kirk, K., Osberger, M., Geers, A., and Moog, J.: Speech intelligibility of implanted children who use oral or total communication. Paper presented at International Cochlear Implant, Speech, and Hearing Symposium. Melbourne, 1994.

Killion, M.: Earmold plumbing for wide-band hearing aids. *J Acoustical Society of Amer, S62:*59, 1976.

Killion, M.: Earmold options for wide-band hearing aids. *J Speech Hearing Res, 46:*10–20, 1981.

Kirkman, R.: An experiment in early education for hearing-impaired children: Arkansas study. Summary report In Kirkman, R. (Ed.): *Peabody J of Educ, 51(3):*203, 1974.

Klima, E., and Bellugi, U.: Syntactic regularities in the speech of children. In Lyons, J., and Wales, R. (Eds.): *Psycholinguistic Papers.* Edinburgh, University Press, 183, 1966.

Knox, L.: *Parents are people.* Nashville, TN, Intersect Pub, 1978.

Knutson, J.: Psychological and social issues in cochlear implant use. Paper presented at 100th NIH Consensus Development Conference: Cochlear Implants in Adults and Children. Washington, D.C., 1995.

Korcybski, A.: The abstraction ladder. In Hayakawa, S.: *Language in thought and action.* New York, Harcourt, Brace, 1939.

Kothman, W.: Classroom auditory trainers. *Hearing Aid J,* Dec 1981.

Krech, D., and Crutchfield, R.: *Elements of psychology.* New York, Knopf, 1959.

Kushner, H.: *When bad things happen to good people.* New York, Schocken, 1981.

Laguna (Andrus de), Grace: *Speech: Its function and development.* Bloomington, IN, Indiana University Press, 1963.

Lane, H.: *The mask of benevolence disabling the deaf community.* New York, Alfred Knopf, 1992.

Leckie, D.: Creating a receptive climate in the mainstream program. In Northcott, W. (Ed.): *The hearing impaired child in a regular classroom.* Washington, D.C., A. G. Bell Assoc., 1973.

Lee, Laura: Developmental sentence types: A method for comparing normal and deviant syntactic development. *J Speech Hearing Dis, 31(4):*311, 1966.

Lenneberg, Eric: *Biologic foundations of language.* New York, Wiley, 1967.

Levine, E.: *The Psychology of Deafness.* New York, Columbia University Press, 1960.

Levitt, H., McGarr, N. S., and Geffner, D.: Development of language and communication skills in hearing-impaired children. *ASHA,* Monograph 26, 1987.

Lewis, M., and Freedler, R.: Mother infant dyad: The cradle of meaning. In Pliner, P., Kramer, L., and Alloway, T. (Eds.): *Communication and affect: Language and thought.* New York, Academic Press, 1973.

Libby, E. R.: Achieving a transparent, smooth, wide-band hearing aid response. *Hearing instruments, 32(10):*9–12, 1981.

Libby, R. (Ed.): *Binaural hearing and amplification.* Chicago, Zenetron, 1980.

Liberman, A., Delattre, P., and Cooper, F.: The role of selected stimulus variables in the perception of the unvoiced stop consonants. *Amer J Psychol, 65:*497, 1952.

Liberman, A., Cooper, F., Shankweiler, D., and Studdert-Kennedy, M.: Perception of the speech code. *Psych Rev, 74:*431, Nov 1967.

Liden, G., and Kankkunen, A.: Visual reinforcement audiometry. *Acta Otolaryngol, 67:*281–292, 1969.

Ling, A.: *Schedules of development in audition, speech language, communication for hearing impaired infants and their parents.* Washington, D.C., A. G. Bell Assoc., 1977.

Ling, D.: Early speech development. In Mencher, G., and Gerber, S. (Eds.): *Early management of hearing loss.* New York, Grune & Stratton, 1981.

Ling, D.: *Foundations of spoken language for hearing-impaired children.* Washington, D.C., A. G. Bell Assoc., 1989.

Ling, D.: *Speech and the hearing impaired child, theory and practice.* Washington, D.C., A. G. Bell Assoc., 1976, 1994.

Ling, D., Leckie, D., Pollack, D., Simser, J., and Smith, A.: Syllable reception by profoundly hearing-impaired children trained from infancy in auditory-oral programs. *Volta Review, 83:*451, 1981.

Ling, D., and Ling, A.: *Aural habilitation: The foundations of verbal learning in hearing-impaired children.* Washington, D.C., A. G. Bell Assoc., 1978.

Ling, D., and Ling, A.: Communication development in the first three years of life. *J Speech Hearing Res, 17:*146, 1974.

Ling, D., and Milne, M.: The development of speech in hearing-impaired children. In Bess, F., Freeman, B., and Sinclair, S. (Eds.): *Amplification in education.* Washington, D.C., A. G. Bell Assoc., 1981.

Lofchie, E.: Happiness is binaural hearing. *Audecibel,* Spring, 1970.

Los Angeles County Southwest School for the Hearing Impaired. *Auditory skills curriculum and test of auditory comprehension.* N. Hollywood, CA, Foreworks, 1979.

Luria, A.: *The working brain.* New York, Basic Books, 1973.

Luterman, D.: A comparison of language skills of hearing-impaired children trained in a visual/oral method and an auditory/oral method. *Amer Ann Deaf, 121:*389, 1976.

Luterman, D.: *Binaural hearing aids.* Paper read to National Conference on Parent-Infant Programs. Nashville, TN, Vanderbilt Univ., 1969.

Luterman, D.: *Counseling parents of hearing-impaired children.* Boston, Little, Brown and Co., 1979.

Lyons, Ruth K.: Integration of audition and visual spatial information in early infancy. *Soc Res in Child Develop,* April 1975.

Marlowe, Judith: Screening all newborns in a community hospital, *AJA, 22* Mar 1993.

Masters, L., and Marsh, G.: Middle ear pathology as a factor in learning disabilities. *J Learning Dis, 11:*54, 1978.

Markides, A.: Results of a four year experiment. In Libby, R. (Ed.): *Binaural hearing and amplification.* Chicago, Zenetron, 1980, Vol. II.

Markides, A.: The use of residual hearing in the education of hearing-impaired children: A historical perspective. In Cole, E., and Gregory, H. (Eds.): *Auditory learning. Volta, 88*(5), Sep 1986.

Martin, F.: *Introduction to audiology (4th ed.).* Englewood Cliffs, NJ, Prentice-Hall, 1991.

Mavilya, M., and Mignone, B.: *Educational strategies for the youngest hearing-impaired children.* New York, Lexington School for the Deaf, Educ Series Books 10, 1977.

Mawk, G., White, K., Mortensen, L., and Behrens, T.: The effectiveness of screening programs based on high-risk characteristics in early identification of hearing impairment. *Ear and Hearing, 12:*312–319, 1991.

Mead, Margaret: *Growing up in New Guinea.* New York, Morrow, 1930.

Meadow, Kathryn: *Deafness and child development.* Berkeley, CA, University of California Press, 1980.

Mencher, G.: *Early identification of hearing loss.* Basel, Karger, 1976.

Mencher, G., and Gerber, S. (Eds.): *Early management of hearing loss.* New York, Grune & Stratton, 1981.

Mendelson, M., and Haith, M.: *The relation between audition and vision in the human newborn.* Chicago, Monographs of the Society for Research in Child Development, No. 167, *41(4),* 1976.

Menyuk, Paula: *Sentences children use.* Cambridge, MA, M.I.T. Press, 1969.

Microsonic: *Custom earmold manual.* Cambridge, PA, 1994.

Mindel, E., and Vernon, McCay: *They grow in silence.* Silver Springs, MD, National Association of the Deaf, 1971.

Montgomery County MD Public Schools. *All about hearing aids.* Washington, D.C., A. G. Bell Assoc., 1975.

Moog, J., Biedenstein, J., and Davidson, L.: *Speech perception instructional curriculum and evaluation for children with cochlear implants and hearing aids.* St. Louis, MO, Central Institute for the Deaf, 1995.

Moog, J., and Geers, A.: *Early speech perception test.* St. Louis, MO, Central Institute for the Deaf, 1990.

Moog, J., and Geers, A.: Educational management of children with cochlear implants. *Amer Ann of the Deaf, 136:*69, 1991.

Moog, J., and Geers, A.: Effects of the nucleus cochlear implant on overall communicative competence in prelingually deaf children. Paper presented at International Cochlear Implant, Speech and Hearing Symposium. Melbourne, 1994.

Moog, J., and Geers, A.: Factors productive of literacy in the profoundly hearing impaired adolescence. *Volta Review 91:*59, 1989.

Moog, J., and Geers, A.: *Grammatical analysis of elicited language.* St. Louis, MO, Central Institute for the Deaf, 1980.

Morkovin, B.: *Through the barriers of deafness and isolation.* New York, Macmillan, 1960.

Morley, M.: *Development and disorders of speech in childhood.* London, Livingstone, 1957.

Moses, K., and Hecke-Wulatin, M.: The socio-emotional impact of infant deafness. In Mencher, G., and Gerber, S. (Eds.): *Early management of hearing loss.* New York, Grune & Stratton, 1981.

Moskowitz, Breyne: The acquisition of language. *Sci Amer, 239(5):*92, Nov 1978.

Mowrer, H.: *Learning theory and the symbolic process.* New York, Wiley, 1952.

Mulholland, A. (Ed.): *International symposium on deafness: Oral education today and tomorrow.* Washington, D.C., A. G. Bell Assoc., 1980.

Murphy, A. (Ed.): *The families of hearing-impaired children.* Washington, D.C., A. G. Bell Assoc., 1979.

Myklebust, H.: *Auditory disorders in children.* New York, Grune & Stratton, 1964.

Myklebust, H.: *The psychology of deafness.* New York, Grune & Stratton, 1950.

Myklebust, H.: *The psychology of deafness.* New York, Grune & Stratton, 1960.

Myklebust, H., and Brutten, M.: A study of the visual perception of deaf children. *Arch Otolaryng, 105(Supp.),* 1953.

MacDonald, B.: *Helping families grow: Specialized psychotherapy with hearing-impaired children and their families.* Denver, Listen Foundation, 1984.

McArthur Communicative Inventory: *Words and gestures.* San Diego, CA, Singular Pub., 1993.

McArthur, S.: *Raising your hearing-impaired child: A guide for parents.* Washington, D.C., A. G. Bell Assoc., 1982.

McClure, A.: Academic Achievement of mainstreamed hearing-impaired children with congenital rubella syndrome. *Volta Review, 79(6):*379, 1977.

McConnell, F.: The parent-teaching home: an early intervention program for hearing-impaired children. *Peabody J Educ, 51(3):*162, April 1974.

McConnell, F., and Liff, S.: The rationale for early identification and intervention. *Otolaryng Clinics of N. Amer, 8:*77, 1975.

McConnell, F., and Ward, P. H. (Eds.): *Deafness in childhood.* Nashville, TN, Vanderbilt University Press, 1967.

McGinnis, M.: *Aphasic children.* Washington, D.C., A. G. Bell Assoc., 1963.

McLaughlin, H.: Integration of deaf children with hearing society. From Ewing, A. W. G. (Ed.): *The modern educational treatment of deafness.* Manchester, Manchester University Press, 1960.

McNeill, D.: *The acquisition of language.* New York, Harper and Row, 1970.

National Institutes of Health: *NIH consensus statement—Early identification of hearing impairment in infants and young children, 11(1):* March 1-3, 1-24, 1993.

Negus, V. E.: Purposive inattention to olfactory stimulation. *Arch Otolaryng, 183(Supp.):* 99-102, 1963.

Newsom, E.: Visual and conceptual discrimination. *Speech Path Ther, 5(1):*3, 1962.

Nicholls, G.: Cued speech and the reception of spoken language. Montreal, McGill University Graduate Thesis, 1979.

Nicholas, J.: Sensory aid use and the development of communicative function. *Volta Review,* 96-181, 1994.

Nicholas, J., Geers, A., and Kozak, V.: Development of communicative functions in young hearing-impaired children. *Volta Review, 96:*113, 1994.

Nicholls, G., and Ling, D.: Cued speech and the reception of spoken language. *J Speech Hearing Res, 25:*262, June 1982.

Nickerson, R.: Characteristics of the speech of the deaf. *Volta Review, 342,* Sept. 1975.

Niemann, S.: Listen! An acoupedic program. *Volta Review, 74:*85, 1972.

Nix, G. (Ed.): *Mainstream education for hearing impaired children and youth.* New York, Grune & Stratton, 1976.

Nix, G.: The rights of hearing-impaired children. *Volta Review, 79(5),* Sept 1977.

Northcott, W.: *I hear that.* Washington, D.C., A. G. Bell Assoc., 1978.

Northcott, W.: *Reports on early childhood education program for hearing-impaired children, 0-6.* Minnesota State Dept of Education, St. Paul, MN, 1978.

Northcott, W., Nelson, J., and Fowler, S.: UNISTAPS: A family-oriented infant/pre-school program for hearing-impaired children and their parents. *Peabody J Educ, 51(3):*192, April 1974.

Northern, J., and Downs, M.: *Hearing in childhood* (3rd ed.). Baltimore, Williams & Wilkins, 1984.

Northern, J., and Hayes, D.: Universal screening for infant hearing impairment— Necessary, beneficial and justifiable. *Audiology Today, (6)* 5(2), 1994.

Northern, J., McChord, W. Jr., Fischer, E., and Evans, P.: *Hearing services in residential schools for the deaf.* Maico Audiological Library Series, XI(4), 1972.

O'Connor, Clarence: Children with impaired hearing. *Volta Review, 56(1):*437, 1952.

Osberger, M. J.: Audiological rehabilitation with cochlear implants and tactile aids. *ASHA, 32(4),* 38-43, 1990.

Osberger, M.: Cochlear implants: An update. Paper presented at A. G. Bell Assoc. for the Deaf Conference: A Sound Beginning. Denver, 1993.

Osberger, M.: Effect of Age at onset of deafness on cochlear implant performance. Paper presented at 100th NIH Consensus Development Conference: Cochlear Implants in Adults and Children. Washington, D.C., 1995.

Osberger, M. J., Maso, M., and Sam, L.: Speech intelligibility of children with cochlear implants, tactile aids, or hearing aids. *J Speech Hearing Res, 36:*186-203, 1993.

Osberger, M., Miyamoto, R., Zimmerman-Phillips, S., Kemink, J., Stroer, B., Firszt, J., and Novak, M.: Independent evaluation of the speech perception abilities of children with the nucleus 22-channel cochlear implant system. *Ear and Hearing, 12(4S):*66-80, 1991.

Osberger, M., Robbins, A., Todd, S., and Riley, A.: Speech intelligibility of children with cochlear implants. *Volta Review, 96:*169, 1994.

Owens, E., Kessler, D., Raggio, M., and Schubert, E.: Analysis and revision of the minimal auditory capabilities (MAC) battery. *Ear and Hearing, 6(6):*280–290, 1985.

Owens, E., Kessler, D., Telleen, C., and Schubert, E.: The minimal auditory capabilities (MAC) battery. *Ear and Hearing, 34(9):*32 and 34, 1981.

Pappas, D.: A study of the high-risk registry for sensorineural hearing impairment. *Arch Otolaryng Head Neck Surg, 91:*41–44, 1983.

Pappas, D.: *Diagnosis and treatment of hearing impairment in children: A clinical manual.* San Diego, College-Hill Press, 1985.

Pappas, D., and McDowell, C.: The sooner, the better: Identification and rehabilitation of the child with bilateral sensorineural hearing impairment. *J Med Assoc. State Alabama, 52:*34–37, 1983.

Paradise, J. L., and Bess, F.: Universal screening for infant hearing impairment: Not simple, not risk free, not necessarily beneficial nor justified. *J Peds, 93:* 332–334, 1994.

Parisier, S., and Chute, P.: Speech production changes in children using multichannel cochlear implants: Performance over time. Paper presented at International Cochlear Implant, Speech and Hearing Symposium. Melbourne, 1994.

Piaget, J.: *Play, dreams and imitation in childhood* (trans. by Gattegno and Hodgson). New York, Norton, 1945, 1962.

Piaget, J.: *The origins of intelligence in children.* New York, International University Press, 1952.

Piaget, J. L.: *The child and reality.* New York, Viking Press, 1973.

Plastner, G.: A factor analysis of variables related to academic performance of hearing-impaired children in regular classes. *Volta Review, 82(2):*71, 1980.

Poizner, H., Batterson, R., Lane, H.: Cerebral asymmetry for perceptions of Amer sign language: The effect of moving stimuli. *Brain and Language, 7(3):*351, 1979.

Pollack, D.: An Acoupedic Program. In Ling, D. (Ed.): *Early intervention for hearing-impaired children: Oral options.* San Diego, College Hill Press, 1984.

Pollack, D.: Binaural hearing aids in an acoupedic program. In Libby, R. (Ed.): *Binaural hearing and amplification.* Chicago, Zenetron, 1980, vol. II.

Pollack, D.: Denver's acoupedic program. *Peabody J Educ, 51(3):*180, 1974.

Pollack, D.: *Educational Audiology for the Limited Hearing Infant.* Springfield, IL, Charles C Thomas, 1970.

Pollack, D.: *Educational audiology for the limited-hearing infant and preschooler (2nd ed.).* Springfield, IL, Charles C Thomas, 1985.

Pollack, D.: *Preparation of severely hearing-impaired children, ages 0–6, for mainstreaming.* Washington, D.C., Office of Education, Personnel Preparation Grant, 1978.

Pollack, D.: *Teaching strategies for the development of auditory-verbal communication:* 5 one hour color videotapes. Washington, D.C., A. G. Bell Assoc., 1981.

Pollack, D.: The experiences of a congenitally deaf law student in a simulated courtroom competition. *A. G. Bell Assoc., Newsounds,* Oct 1982.

Pollack, D., and Ernst, M.: Don't set limits: Expectations for pre-school children. In

Northcott, W., (Ed.): *The hearing impaired child in a regular classroom.* Washington, D.C., A. G. Bell Assoc., 1973.

Poole, I.: *The genetic development of the articulation of consonant sounds.* LaVerne, Preston, 1934.

Probst, R., Coats, A., Martin, G., and Lounsbury-Martin, B.: Spontaneous click- and toneburst-evoked otoacoustic emissions from normal ears. *Hearing Res, 21:*261–275, 1986.

Pugh, B. L.: *Steps in language development for the deaf.* Washington, *Volta Review,* 1955.

Quigley, S.: Reading achievement and special reading materials. In Kretschmer, R. (Ed.): *Reading and the hearing-impaired individual. Volta Review, 84(5):*95, 1982.

Quigley, S.: *The influence of fingerspelling on the development of language communication and educational achievement in deaf children.* Urbana, IL, Institute for Research on Exceptional Children, 1969.

Quigley, S., and Kretschmer, R.: *The education of deaf children.* Baltimore, University Park Press, 1982.

Quigley, S., Wilbur, R., Montanelli, D., and Steinkamp, M.: *Syntactic structures in language of deaf children.* Urbana, IL, Institute for Research on Exceptional Children, 1976.

Rainer, J., Altshuler, K., and Kallman, F.: *Family and mental health problems in a deaf population.* Springfield, IL, Charles C Thomas, 1969.

Razran, G. H. S.: Conditioning and perception. *Psychol Rev, 72:*83, 1955.

Reich, C., Hambleton, D., and Houldon, B.: The integration of hearing-impaired children in regular classrooms. *Amer Ann Deaf, 132:*534, 1977.

Reichenstein, J.: Integrated kindergartens for severely hearing-impaired children. In *Proceedings of the International Conference on Pre-School Education of the Hearing Impaired Child, 1978 and After.* Tel Aviv, Israel, Micha Society for Deaf Children, 1978.

Riesen, A.: Studies of early sensory deprivation in animals. In Griffiths, C. (Ed.): *Proceedings of the International Conference on Auditory Techniques.* Springfield, IL, Charles C Thomas, 1974.

Ringler, N.: A longitudinal study of mother's language. In Waterson, N., and Snow, C.: *The development of communication.* New York, Wiley, 1978.

Rodda, M.: *The hearing-impaired school learner.* Springfield, IL, Charles C Thomas, 1970.

Rogers, D. (Ed.): *On being and becoming: Helping your child develop his/her potential. Birth to age six.* Vermont, New Creation Pub, 1981.

Ross, M.: Position statement on cochlear implants. *SHHH Journal.* Jan/Feb:32–33, 1994.

Ross, M., and Lerman, J.: *Word intelligibility by picture identification (WIPI).* Pittsburgh, Stanwix House, 1971.

Ross, M., and Randolph, K.: *The auditory perception of alphabet letters test (APAL).* St. Louis, Auditec, 1988.

Roth, R.: *The mother-child relationship evaluation.* Los Angeles, Western Psychological Services, 1961.

Ruben, R., and Rupin, I.: The plasticity of the development of the auditory system. *Ann. Otol. Rhinol. and Laryngol., 89:*303–311, 1980.

Rubin, M.: Hearing aids for infants. In Mencher, G., and Gerber, S. (Eds.): *Early management of hearing loss.* New York, Grune & Stratton, 1981.

Rush, M.: *The language of directions.* Washington, D.C., A. G. Bell Assoc., 1977.

Russell, R.: *Brain in memory and learning.* Oxford, Oxford University Press, 1969.

Sachs, O.: *Seeing voices.* New York, Harper, 1989.

Sanders, D.: *Aural rehabilitation.* Englewood Cliffs, NJ, Prentice-Hall, 1971.

Sapir, Selma G., and Nitzburg, Ann C. (Eds.): *Children with learning problems.* New York, Brunner-Mazel, 1973.

Schildroth, A.: Public residential schools for deaf students in the United States, 1970–1978. *Amer Ann Deaf,* April 1980.

Schlaegel, N., and Jelonek, S.: Selecting the right earmold for a high frequency fitting. *Hearing J, 44(3):*15–18, 1991.

Schlesinger, H., and Meadow, K.: *Sound and sign.* Berkeley, CA, University of California Press, 1972.

Schwirian, P.: Effects of the presence of hearing-impaired children in the family on behavioral patterns of older "normal" siblings. *Amer Ann Deaf, 121:*373, 1976.

Scollon, R.: *Conversations with a one year old.* Honolulu, HI, University Press of Hawaii, 1976.

Shah, C., Chandler, D., and Dale, R.: Delay in referral of children with impaired hearing. *Volta Review, 80(4):*206–214, 1978.

Shallop, J.: A team approach to pediatric cochlear implants. Paper presented at Auditory-Verbal International Conference. Cuyahoga Falls, OH, 1995.

Shannon, C., and Weaver, W.: *The mathematical theory of communication.* Urbana, IL, University of Illinois Press, 1962.

Shatz, M.: *The relationship between cognitive processes and the development of communication skills.* Nebraska Symposium on Motivation, University of Nebraska Press, 1977.

Silverman, Richard: The education of children with hearing impairments. *J Pediat, 62:*254, 1963.

Sitnick, V., Rushmer, N., and Arpan, R.: *Parent-infant communication.* Beaverton, OR, Dormac, 1977.

Smith, B.: Some observations concerning premeaningful vocalizations of hearing-impaired infants. *J Speech Hearing Dis, 47(4):*439, Nov 1982.

Smith, B., and Oller, K.: A comparative study of pre-meaningful vocalizations produced by normally developing and Down's Syndrome infants. *J Speech Hearing Dis, 46:*46, 1981.

Smith, C.: Residual hearing and speech production in deaf children. *J Speech Hearing Dis, 18(4):*795, 1975.

Sohmer, H., and Feinmesser, M.: Cochlear action potentials recorded from the ear canal in man. *Ann Otol, 76:*427, 1967.

Spitz, R.: *A Genetic field theory of ego formation.* New York, International Universities Press, 1959.

Staller, S., Beiter, A., and Brimacombe, J.: Use of the nucleus 22-channel cochlear implant system with children. *Volta Review, 96:*15, 1994.

Staller, S., Dowell, R., Beiter, A., and Brimcombe, J.: Perceptual Abilities of Children with the nucleus 22-channel implant. *Ear and Hearing, 12(2S):*345–475, 1991.

Star, R.: *We can!* (vols 1 and 2). Washington, D.C., A. G. Bell Assoc., 1980.

Stark, Rachel, (Ed.): *Sensory capabilities of hearing impaired children.* Baltimore, University Park Press, 1974.

Stengel, E.: A psychological study of echo reactions. *J Men Sc, 95*(55):5398, 1947.

Stibick, M., and Feibelman, P.: What parents ask of clinicians and counselors. In Marlowe, J. (Ed.): *The evaluation and management of communication disorders in infants.* New York, Thieme-Stratton, 3(1):88, 1982.

Stoker, R., and Ling, D.: Speech production in hearing impaired children and youth. *Volta Review, 94(4):* Nov 1992.

Stone, P.: Auditory learning in a school setting: Procedures and results. *Volta Review, 85(1):7*, 1983.

Stovall, D.: *Teaching speech to hearing impaired infants and children.* Springfield, IL, Charles C Thomas, 1982.

Streng, A.: *Syntax, speech and hearing.* New York, Grune & Stratton, 1972.

Streng, A., Kretschmer, R., and Kretschmer, L.: *Language, learning and deafness.* New York, Grune & Stratton, 1978.

Strong, C., Clark, T. C., Barringer, D. G., Walden, B. E., and Williams, S. A.: SKI–HI home-based programming for hearing-impaired children: demographics child identification and program effectiveness. *SKI–HI Institute.* Logan, UT, Utah State University, 1992.

Sullivan, Annie: *Letters and education,* a supplementary account to Helen Keller's *Story of my life.* New York, Doubleday, 1961.

Sutton-Smith, Brian and Shirley: *How to play with your children (and when not to).* New York, Hawthorn, 1974.

Suzuki, T., and Ogiba, Y.: Conditioned orientation audiometry. *Arch Otolaryng, 74:*192, 1961.

Teacher guide. Englewood, CO, Cochlear Corporation, 1994.

Tell, L., Feinmesser, M., and Levi, C.: Management and follow-up of early detected hearing impaired children. In Mencher, G., and Sanford, S. (Eds.): *Early management of hearing loss.* New York, Grune & Stratton, 1981.

Tobey, E., Geers, A., and Brenner, C.: Speech production results: Speech feature acquisition. *Volta Review, 96:*109, 1994.

Tobey, E., and Hasenstaab, M.: Effects of a nucleus multi-channel cochlear implant upon speech production in children. *Ear and Hearing, 12:*48S, 1991.

Tonokawa, L.: Results with cochlear implants in children: What have we learned? In Barnes, J., Franz, D., and Bruce, W. (Ed.): *Pediatric cochlear implants: An overview of alternatives in education and rehabilitation.* Washington, D.C., A. G. Bell Assoc., 1994.

Tough, J.: *Talking, thinking, growing.* New York, Schocken, 1974.

Trammell, J.: *Test of auditory comprehension.* Portland, OR, Foreworks, 1981.

Trehub, S., Bull, D., and Schneider, B.: Infant's detection of speech in noise. *J Speech and Hearing Res, 24(2):*202, 1981.

Tripp, S. Ervin: An overview of theories of grammatical development. In Slobin, D. (Ed.): *The ontogenesis of grammar.* New York, Academic Press, 1971.

Tsappis, A.: Can a hearing aid further impair hearing? *Audiology and Hearing Educ J,* *5(4):*17, 1979.

Tucker, Bonnie: *The feel of silence.* Philadelphia, Temple University Press, 1994.

Tyler, T.: Speech perception with the nucleus cochlear implant in children trained with the auditory/verbal approach. *Amer J Otology, 11(2):*99–107, 1990.

Urbantschitsch, V.: *Auditory training for deaf mutism and acquired deafness.* (New translation by Dr. R. Silverman) Washington, D.C., A. G. Bell Assoc., 1982.

Urbantschitsch, V.: In Goldsmith, T.: *The determination of the degree of interaction between auditory and visual sense thresholds.* New York, Fordham University, 1958.

Uzgiris, I., and Hunt, J.: *Assessment in infancy: Ordinal scales of psychological development.* Urbana, IL, University of Illinois Press, 1975.

Van Uden, A.: *A world of language for deaf children. Part 1.* Amsterdam, Swets and Zeitlinger, 1977.

Van Uden, A.: Early diagnosis of those multiple handicaps in prelingually profoundly deaf child which endanger an education according to the purely oral way. *J Brit Assn Teachers Deaf, 5(4):*112, 1981.

Vaughn, G., and Clark, R.: *Extraoral and intraoral stimulation technique for improvement of articulation skills.* Springfield, IL, Charles C Thomas, 1979.

Vaughn, P. (Ed.): *Learning to listen.* Washington, D.C., A. G. Bell Assoc., 1981.

Vigotsky, L.: *Thought and language.* Cambridge, MA, M.I.T. Press, 1962.

Vodehnal, S.: *They do belong.* Denver, Listen Foundation, 1981.

Waltzman, S., Cohen, N., and Shapiro, W.: Factors Affecting Postoperative Performance in Children with Cochlear Implants. Paper presented at International Cochlear Implant, Speech and Hearing Symposium. Melbourne, 1994.

Watrous, B. (Ed.): *Developing home training programs for hearing impaired children.* Indian Health Service and the University of New Mexico, 1976.

Watson, T. J.: The use of residual hearing. Part IV: Auditory Training. *Volta Review, 63:*487, 1961.

Weber, H., and Northern, J.: Selection of children's hearing aids. In Libby, R. (Ed.): *Binaural hearing and amplification.* Chicago, Zenetron, 1980, vol. II.

Webster, D. B., and Webster, M.: Neonatal sound deprivation affects brain stem auditory nuclei. *Arch Otolaryng, 103:*392, 1977.

Webster, D. B., and Webster, M.: Mouse brain stem auditory development. *Ann Otol. Rhinol. and Laryngol., 89(Supp. 68):*254–256, 1980.

Wedenberg, E.: Hearing measurements of infants. *Nord Psychiat Tidskr, 191(2):*106, 1955, 1961.

Wedenberg, E.: Prenatal tests. In Davis, H. (Ed.): The young deaf child: Identification and management. *Acta Otolaryng, 206(Suppl.):*28, 1965.

Wiener, Norbert: *The human use of human beings: Cybernetics and society.* New York, Doubleday, 1954.

Weir, R. H.: *Language in the crib.* The Hague, Mouton, 1962.

Wepman, Joseph: Aphasia: Language without thought or thought without language. *ASHA, 18(3),* March 1976.

West, Paul: *Words for a deaf daughter.* New York, Harper and Row, 1968, 1970.

Westby, Carol: Assessment of cognitive and language abilities through play. *Language, Speech and Hearing Services in the Schools, Vol. X, No. 3,* July 1980.

Wilson, J., and Moore, W.: Visual reinforcement audiometry with infants. In Gerber, S., and Mencher, G. (Eds.): *Early diagnosis of hearing loss.* New York, Grune & Stratton, 1977.

Woodruff, A.: *Basic concepts of teaching.* San Francisco, Chandler, 1961.

Wright, D.: *Deafness.* New York, Stein and Day, 1969.

Wyatt, Gertrude: *Patterns of therapy with stuttering children and their mothers.* U. S. Public Health Service. Small Grant M-2677-A, 1957.

Yamada, O., Ashikawa, H., Kodera, K., and Hitoshi, Y.: Frequency-selective auditory brain-stem response in newborns and infants. *Arch Otolaryng, 109:*79, 1983.

Yaremko, R., and Gibson, W.: Cochlear implants in deaf children who previously utilized hearing aids successfully or suffered a deteriorating loss. Paper presented at International Cochlear Implant, Speech and Hearing Symposium. Melbourne, 1994.

Yater, V.: *Mainstreaming of children with a hearing loss.* Springfield, IL, Charles C Thomas, 1977.

Yoshinaga-Itano, C.: Language assessment of infants and toddlers with significant hearing loss. *Seminars in Hearing, Vol. 15, No. 2,* May 1994.

Yoshinaga-Itano, C., and Apuzzo, M.: *Early identification and intervention.* Boulder, CO, University of Colorado, 1994.

Yoshinaga-Itano, C., Apuzzo, M., Coulter, D., and Stredler-Brown, A.: *The effect of early identification on development.* Boulder, CO, University of Colorado, 1995.

Yoshinaga-Itano, C., and Pollack, D.: *A description of children in the acoupedic method.* Englewood, CO, Listen Foundation, 1988.

Yoshinaga-Itano, C., and Pollack, D.: *A retrospective study of the acoupedic method.* Englewood, CO, Listen Foundation, 1988.

Yoshinaga-Itano, C., and Stredler-Brown, A.: Learning to communicate: Babies with hearing impairment make their needs known. *Volta Review, 95:*107–129A, 1992.

Yoshinaga-Itano, C., Stredler-Brown, A., and Yancosek, E.: From Phon to Phoneme: What can we understand from babies? *Volta Review, 94:*288–314, July 1992.

INDEX

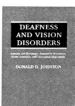
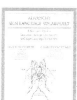

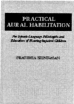

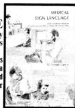